# Understanding
# Newborn Behavior &
# Early Relationships

# Understanding Newborn Behavior & Early Relationships

## The Newborn Behavioral Observations (NBO) System Handbook

by

J. Kevin Nugent, Ph.D.

Constance H. Keefer, M.D.

Susan Minear, M.D.

Lise C. Johnson, M.D.

Yvette Blanchard, Sc.D., PT

*with invited contributors*

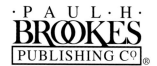

Baltimore • London • Sydney

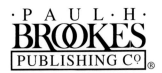

**Paul H. Brookes Publishing Co.**
Post Office Box 10624
Baltimore, Maryland 21285-0624

www.brookespublishing.com

Typeset by Maryland Composition, Inc., Glen Burnie, Maryland.
Manufactured in China by JADE PRODUCTIONS.

The vignettes in this book are based on real cases, but names and identifying
features have been changed to protect the privacy of the individuals.

Photographs © Matthew J. Lee. All photographs in this book and on the cover are used
by permission of the individuals pictured or their parents and/or guardians.

Eighth Printing , March 2017.

**Library of Congress Cataloging-in-Publication Data**
Understanding newborn behavior and early relationships : the newborn
behavioral observations (NBO) system handbook / by J. Kevin Nugent ...
[et al.].
    p.  cm.
  Includes bibliographical references and index.
  ISBN 978-1-55766-883-7 (alk. paper)
  1. Parent and infant—Handbooks, manuals, etc.   2. Infants—Family
relationships—Handbooks, manuals, etc.   3. Newborn infants—
Development—Testing.   4. Behavioral assessment of infants.   I. Nugent,
J. Kevin.

HQ755.84.U53 2007
306.874--dc22                                                      2007009391

British Library Cataloguing in Publication data are available from the British
Library.

# CONTENTS

# About the Authors

**J. Kevin Nugent, Ph.D.,** Professor, University of Massachusetts, Amherst, Massachusetts 01003; Director, The Brazelton Institute, Children's Hospital Boston; Lecturer, Harvard Medical School, Boston, Massachusetts 02215

Dr. Nugent is a developmental psychologist and Founder and Director of The Brazelton Institute at Children's Hospital Boston. He is co-author with Dr. Berry Brazelton of the Neonatal Behavioral Assessment Scale (NBAS) and has directed the NBAS training program since 1978. Dr. Nugent has conducted research on newborn behavior and parent–child relations in different cultural settings around the world and has published extensively on topics in infant and child development. In addition, he has written the manual *Using the NBAS with Infants and Parents* (March of Dimes Foundation, 1985) and is senior author of the series *The Cultural Context of Infancy* (Vols. 1 and 2; Ablex 1989, 1991). Dr. Nugent is editor of *Ab Initio,* the international journal for professionals working with infants and families.

**Constance H. Keefer, M.D.,** Faculty, The Brazelton Institute, Children's Hospital Boston; Assistant Professor, Harvard Medical School, Boston, Massachusetts 02215

Dr. Keefer, a board-certified pediatrician, has worked as a researcher and teacher in the field of infant–parent relations for 30 years. She has conducted research on newborns and young children in Kenya, has worked as a community physician, and was Director of the Newborn Nursery in the Brigham and Women's Hospital (BWH) in Boston, where she developed a curriculum in primary care neonatology for residents and the PEBE (the combined physical and behavioral neonatal examination) to help promote a more parent-centered approach to newborn care. Currently, Dr. Keefer is an attending pediatrician in the BWH Newborn Nursery and is also on the faculty of The Brazelton Touchpoints Center at Children's Hospital Boston, where she trains providers in aspects of early childhood development.

**Susan Minear, M.D.,** Director, Birth to Three Program, Boston Medical Center; Assistant Professor of Pediatrics, Boston University School of Medicine, Boston, Massachusetts 02118

Dr. Minear (formerly O'Brien) practices primary care pediatrics and is a board-certified behavioral and developmental pediatrician and a graduate fellow of the Zero to Three Leadership Development Initiative. From 1997 to 2005, Dr. Minear served as Medical Director of the Newborn Nursery at Boston Medical Center, where she worked to transform a traditional newborn nursery practice into a developmentally rich service for newborns and families. Dr. Minear incorporated the NBO into newborn care and into medical student and resident education. She implemented an infant massage program and was a cochairperson of the Baby Friendly task force through which Boston Medical Center achieved the World Health Organization's Baby Friendly status, a designation for hospital organizations that successfully follow the Ten Steps program to provide support for breast-feeding mothers.

**Lise C. Johnson, M.D.,** Director, Well Newborn Nurseries, Brigham and Women's Hospital; Instructor in Pediatrics, Harvard Medical School; Faculty, The Brazelton Institute, Children's Hospital Boston, Boston, Massachusetts 02215

Dr. Johnson is a board-certified pediatrician. Prior to focusing her clinical work and teaching on newborns, she worked for 10 years as a primary pediatrician in the greater Boston area. She integrates the NBO into her practice with newborns and their families and into her training of residents and medical students.

**Yvette Blanchard, Sc.D., PT,** Associate Professor of Physical Therapy, University of Hartford, West Hartford, Connecticut 06117; Faculty, The Brazelton Institute, Children's Hospital Boston, Boston, Massachusetts 02215

Dr. Blanchard teaches the pediatric curriculum of the physical therapy program at the University of Hartford and is a faculty member of The Brazelton Institute where she is the lead NBAS trainer and an NBO trainer. She is also an early intervention provider for the East Hartford Birth to Three Program in Connecticut. Dr. Blanchard has published more than 15 articles and 4 book chapters relating to the field of pediatric physical therapy and early intervention with high-risk infants.

# ABOUT THE CONTRIBUTORS

**Sarah A. Birss, M.D.,** Infant, Child, and Adult Psychiatrist; Faculty, Infant Parent Training Institute, Center for Early Relationship Support, Jewish Family and Children's Service of Greater Boston, Waltham, Massachusetts 02451

Dr. Birss has worked clinically with infants and parents for 20 years. She has trained in developmental pediatrics, adult and child psychiatry, and adult and child psychoanalysis. Dr. Birss is guest faculty at the Boston Psychoanalytic Society and Institute, and Clinical Instructor in Psychiatry at Harvard Medical School. She has an interest in assessment and treatment of early emotional disorders, and currently teaches infant observation and early emotional development. She has a private practice in infant, child, and adult psychiatry in Cambridge, Massachusetts.

**Kristie Brandt, RN, CNM, N.D.,** Director, Parent–Infant & Child Institute, Napa, California 94559

Dr. Brandt, a board-certified nurse–midwife and nurse practitioner, has a doctorate in nursing and more than 30 years of experience in both clinical practice and public health administration. Her research has focused on the parent–child relationship, factors influencing breast-feeding success, infant–parent mental health therapeutic services, and nurse home-visiting models. She has co-authored chapters and journal articles and produced assessment tools and protocols under state grants. Dr. Brandt created and conducted research on a Touchpoints Nurse Home Visiting pilot project in the Napa Valley. She also developed the Napa County Therapeutic Child Care Center and co-developed the Infant–Parent Mental Health Fellowship Program; both programs have received national awards of excellence. Brandt is a reviewer for *Pediatrics,* the journal of the American Academy of Pediatrics, and lectures and trains internationally with Dr. T. Berry Brazelton.

**Matthew J. Lee,** Staff Photographer, *The Boston Globe,* Boston, Massachusetts 02107

Matthew J. Lee studied at Santa Barbara City College and San Francisco State University and attended the last photo workshop taught in Yosemite National Park by Ansel Adams. After internships at the *Peninsula Times Tribune* and the *Philadelphia Daily News,* Mr. Lee received his first staff position at the *Charlotte Observer's* Union County North Carolina Bureau in 1987. In 1988 he began work at the *Oakland Tribune* and later accepted a staff position at the *Long Beach Press-Telegram.* In 1998 he joined the staff of the *Miami Herald* and stayed there for one year before leaving for *The Boston Globe*, where he has been a staff photographer since 1999. Mr. Lee received the 1990 Pulitzer Prize for News Photography, as part of the team that covered the Loma Prieta earthquake.

# FOREWORD

Parents are often hungry to understand and respond to their newborn infant and wish they had a definitive manual to tell them the best way to do this. The Newborn Behavioral Observations (NBO) system is designed to do just that: It enables clinicians to share behavioral observations of an infant's capacities and temperament with parents, and it offers clinicians an opportunity to enter into a partnership with parents in their desire to understand and respond to their newborn infant. Often, as a result of the confidence gained from using the NBO, parents become more interactive with their infant from the beginning.

Sharing their infant's behavior with a professional who has been trained to demonstrate the child's states of consciousness and to observe his capacity to respond appropriately in each state (e.g., sleeping, fussing, alert) can provide parents with a window into their newborn's temperament. An infant has the capacity to reach out to her new parents and has the competence to protect herself from being overloaded by the stimuli in the environment. An infant's reflex behaviors demonstrate motor capacities. His sensory responses at birth demonstrate an ability to be alert to his new world and to shut it off when he needs to sleep. By sharing and marking this individual behavior with parents early, clinicians can achieve several valuable goals:

- They can capture and focus the new parents' passionate response to their newborn.

- They can help parents understand the importance of different states of consciousness and how an infant's responses depend on her state.

- They can show parents how to promote their infant's optimal states for interaction and protection (e.g., sleep).

- They can observe the parents' responses to their infant during the NBO session and use those responses as a guide to understanding the parents' relationship with their new child. Parents' excitement in response to their infant's behavior suggests that a positive attachment will develop between them and their infant. If the parents are very concerned about their infant's behavior, this may be signaling the beginning of a stressful parent–infant relationship and will demand careful watching and guidance on the part of the clinician.

- They can become part of the parent–infant system from the beginning, advising parents about follow-up opportunities and home visits and planning early office visits to make up for shortened hospital stays.

The NBO can be seen as complementary to the Neonatal Behavioral Assessment Scale (NBAS). While the NBAS can be used as a diagnostic tool—as an assessment of neurological or dysgenetic defects—the NBO is designed to enable clinicians to share observations of the new infant with parents and to make an immediate connection with them. If there are questionable responses observed in the course of the NBO, the clinician should request a consultation and a full evaluation from a professional trained in the use of the NBAS.

Studies of newborn behavior from around the world have found that parents who have been given a demonstration of their infant's behavior become more confident as new parents. The evidence from hundreds of documented studies show that both infants and parents have profited on a wide range of variables, from increased self-confidence to greater father involvement. Hence, our goal for the NBO is to make such a shared observation between parents and clinician more universal by providing a demonstration of the infant's individuality. The following vignette demonstrates how practitioners can use the NBO in clinical practice:

*

After eight years of waiting, the Stones finally had their first child. Because the pregnancy was uneventful, they expected the infant to be perfect. Still, like most pregnant couples, in the back of their minds they worried that the delivery could result in an imperfect, damaged child. Mrs. Stone's labor started on time, but it went on and on. When the infant finally arrived, both mother and father were exhausted. It was a boy and they named him Jon. Jon cried right away—a high-pitched squeal that delighted everyone except his anxious father, who wondered: "Is that cry normal?" Jon soon quieted down and started breathing, choking up his mucous. His initial Apgar score was 8 out of 10, and at 10 minutes, he had an excellent 9 out of 10 score.

Everyone rushed to reassure the Stones that Jon was indeed a "perfect infant"—quiet and exhausted but breathing easily with good color. When the parents had a few minutes with their son, they examined him in minute detail. They could see that he had a soft bruise on the top of his skull and one eye was swollen and the other bruised. But the delivery crew had been reassuring, and he showed none of the abnormal features that they'd read about and feared. Besides, they hadn't had a chance to express their fears or ask any questions.

When Jon was 8 hours old, a nurse in the nursery who was trained to demonstrate an infant's behavior using the NBO went to see Jon's parents. The NBO is used to answer parents' questions and help allay their fears by focusing on the infant's strengths and individuality. The nurse prepared to perform the NBO on Jon and to share her observations of Jon's behavior with his parents. She sat down with both parents to review the notes in her chart about the pregnancy and the long labor. "Do you have any questions about your infant? That long labor and his misshaped head must worry you." The father replied, "It seemed like the labor took forever, but after he finally came and the crew in the delivery room read us off the Apgar, we were reassured." The nurse replied, "If you have any questions as we observe him, I hope you'll share them with me."

As Jon lay on his back, wrapped in a blanket, breathing deeply and noisily, the nurse used a flashlight to shine light in his closed eyes. Jon startled, throwing out his arms and moved around in his wrappings. With each repeated flash, he moved less and less, finally suppressing his responses. His breathing deepened, as he went into a deep sleep. "He has done what we call habituation," commented the nurse. "He responded to the first few lights, so you can see that he has the capacity to shut out disturbing stimuli, to protect himself from becoming overloaded in a busy, noisy world." Then the nurse shook a rattle near his head, and again he startled, even letting out a little cry. As the nurse repeated the rattle, he shut down again. "He's done it!" The parents looked at each other as if for reassurance. The nurse pointed out to them that Jon had come from a sleep state to a responsive state, but then was able to quiet himself and go back into a sleep state again. His brain was able to manage state changes and keep him from being overwhelmed. The mother, who had been gripping the bedside, began to relax.

As Jon was uncovered, he began to cry—long extended wails. His parents were startled and reached out for him. But when the nurse leaned over and spoke softly into his ear, Jon stopped crying to listen and let out a few more wails, becoming more active as he did. He cried and startled again. The startle led to another cry. The nurse grasped each arm to inhibit the startles that followed each wail. As she contained his arms, and the startles subsided, she talked quietly to him. He not only quieted, but he also stopped moving. His face became alert and he cocked open the less swollen eye. "He's listening to her," his mother whispered to her husband with awe.

When the nurse picked him up gently to rock him, Jon's eyes came half open. "He's moved from his fussy state to an alert one," she said. "What a responsive boy!" As she spoke to him, his face became alert. His whole body was quiet as he followed her talking face back and forth and up and down. His parents were excitedly watching all of this responsive behavior, their faces glowing. "He's all right!" said his mother.

The nurse held the infant up in the air in front of her, one hand under his head, the other hand under his buttocks. She pointed out to the parents how easy it was to handle him this way. They hungrily imitated her posture with their arms out. They were learning all they could. She then asked the mother to speak to the infant, first on one side and then on the other. The infant turned to his mother's voice right away. His mother almost wept as she leaned in to kiss and stroke him. "You know me already," she said. When Jon turned to his father's voice, the father took the infant from the nurse and said, "You know *me*. You and I are already buddies." By this time, the mother was weeping with joy and relief. Her husband had his arm around her. "We can't thank you enough. We didn't dare think about it, but we had so many questions after that long labor."

After this shared observation, the parents were not only euphoric, they also were ready to ask a few questions. "What is the mark on the back of his head?" "When will both of his eyes open?" "When can I expect my breast milk?" "Can you help me get him on my breast to suck?" The NBO, which took less than 10 minutes to perform, had been an intervention for the infant's future. The parents now felt that they were ready to parent their newborn.

✳

My dream is that all neonatal centers will train professionals in the use of the NBO to help them share observations of newborn infants with their parents. However, when professionals find unusual or deviant behavior in the neonate, they should also be able to turn to a trained NBAS observer to conduct the NBAS. I would like every center to have the NBO for relationship building and the NBAS for a more detailed diagnostic assessment of neonatal behavior. As a relationship-based approach, the NBO constitutes an important step toward family-oriented medicine. When a clinician shares the infant's behavior with parents, parents feel that they have been respected and valued. Parents, in turn, are likely to develop a warm trusting relationship with a professional who gives them such a valuable start toward understanding their newborn infant.

*T. Berry Brazelton, M.D.*
*Founder and Chief Emeritus,*
*Child Development Unit, Children's Hospital Boston*
*Professor Emeritus, Harvard Medical School*

# ACKNOWLEDGMENTS

Firstly, we would like to acknowledge our indebtedness to T. Berry Brazelton, whose teaching and supportive mentoring inspired the development of the Newborn Behavioral Observations (NBO) system. Over the years, Dr. Brazelton has informed our understanding and appreciation of newborn behavior and has shaped our clinical stance toward parents and families. His pioneering work with the Neonatal Behavioral Assessment Scale (NBAS) on the nature of individual differences in newborn behavior and his positive approach to working with parents influenced both the content and clinical approach of the NBO. We have attempted to preserve in the NBO his philosophy and his overall respect for infants and their parents.

We would like to thank Cynthia O'Hare, RN, M.P.H., for her unique contribution to the development of the NBO when it was known as the Clinical Neonatal Behavioral Assessment Scale. She played an indispensable role as a faculty member in shaping the direction of the NBO training program. NBAS Master Trainer Jean Cole's clinical work with the NBAS provided many ideas for the development of the NBO, and we would also like to acknowledge the contributions to the development of the NBO in the initial stages of Dr. Zachary Boukydis, the Erikson Institute, Chicago, and Dr. Sherry Muret-Wagstaff, Children's Hospital Boston. We would like to thank Joao Gomes-Pedro and his colleagues in Portugal, who modified the NBAS for clinical use; Tiffany Field, who developed the Mothers Assessment of the Behavior of the Infant; Ida Cardone and Linda Gilkerson, who developed the Family Administered Neonatal Activities; and Rebecca Kang, Kathryn Barnard, John Worobey, Donna Karl, and Joylene Pearson, all of whom made original adaptations to the NBAS in their clinical work. We also would like to thank Jennifer Gillette of The Brazelton Institute for her contribution to the training curriculum as an NBO faculty member.

We would like to thank the NBAS trainers from around the world. Tomitaro Akiyama, Nadia Bruschweiler-Stern, Drina Candilis-Huisman, Alain Caron, Carme Costas-Moragas, Adrienne Davidson, Marie-Paul Durieux, Guy Frankard, Claire De Vriendt-Goldman, Joao Carlos Gomes-Pedro, Marie Fabre-Grenet, Dan Griffith, Joanna Hawthorne, James Helm, Beth Higley, Elise Holloway, Betty Hutchon, Chisato Kawasaki, Nittaya Kotchabhakdi, Cecilia Matson, Hannah Munck, Shohei Ohgi, Roberto Paludetto, Thembi Ranuga, Gherardo Rapisardi, Marie Reilly, Jose and Jane Saraiva, Karin Stjernqvist, Byounghi Park-Synn, Toshiya Tsurusaki, Beulah Warren, Inga Warren, Judi Withers, and Dieter Wolke are among those whose ideas influenced the development of the NBO. We offer a special word of thanks to Jay Killough, Julio Gonzalez, Judith Wides, and Marie Curtin-McKenna, whose feedback contributed to the NBO's evolution in the context of the University of Massachusetts study on the effects of the NBO as a form of intervention.

Dr. Heidelise Als's work and personal commitment to infants and families has influenced our ideas about infants and about the nature of clinical work with infants, especially those at high risk. Daniel Stern's work has played a major role in our thinking about the transition to parenthood, while the work of John Kennell and Marshall and Phyllis Klaus has influenced our approach to our work with parents. We also thank Ed Tronick, Chief, Child Development Unit, Children's Hospital Boston, for his ideas and support over the years, and Marjorie Beeghly, Karen Olson, Katherine Weinberg, and all of our colleagues at the Child Development Unit, as well as John Hornstein, Maureen O'Brien, Jayne Singer, Ann Stadtler, and our many colleagues at Touchpoints. We would also like to acknowledge the contributions of Amy Alberts, Simona Bujoreanu, Kate Buttenweiser, Kate Campbell, John Cloherty, Dorith Wieczorek-Deering, Catherine Donohue, Heidi Feldman, the late Emily Fenichel, Esther Gerendas, Sheila Greene, Mary Grimanis, Ann Halstead, Desmond Hourihane; Jackie Kelleher and members of Doulas of North America; Arnold Kerzner, Nancy Kloczko, Barry Lester, Martha Levine, Susan McQuiston, Lynn Murray, Carmen Norona, Joan Pernice, Maggie Redshaw; Jack Shonkoff; the Smith-Richardson Fellows; Jan Tedder, John F. Travers, Marge Wilson, Peter H. Wolff, and Barry Zuckerman; and the many practitioners whose clinical work with the NBAS and the NBO have influenced our thinking. We thank Bonnie Petrauskas and Kathleen Tara of the Johnson and Johnson Pediatric Institute for their ideas, the nurses and doctors at the Connors Center for Women and Newborns at the Brigham and Women's Hospital Boston, the nurses and staff at the Boston Medical Center, and all of those who have been using the NBO in their practices for their feedback and support.

We would like to thank our colleagues, Drs. Marvin Wang, Mary Allare, Leslie Kerzner, and Beth McManus, who made important contributions to the development of the NBO in their roles as faculty members for the NBO training program. We offer a special word of thanks to our administrative associates Patricia Lambkin, Gillian Blake, and Kimberly Rose and to Dr. Joseph Nugent for his critical reading of parts of the manuscript, and we acknowledge the role of the late Kate Neff, who added so much richness to our lives and whose ideas contributed so much to our efforts to meet the needs of children and families over the years.

We would especially like to thank Dr. Judith Palfrey, Chief, General Pediatrics at Children's Hospital Boston, for her support and encouragement of our work at the Brazelton Institute.

We also want to acknowledge the support of The Brazelton Foundation; the Commonwealth Fund; Eileen and Jack Connors Jr.; Hill, Holliday, Boston; A.L. Mailman Family Foundation; Ronald McDonald House Charities; and the Noonan Family Foundation for their support. Thanks also to the March of Dimes, and, in particular, Dr. Scott Berns, Dr. Jennifer L. Howse, and Liza Cooper, who facilitated the use of the NBO in the different sites across North America in the March of Dimes NICU Family Support program.

Finally, we would like to thank our own families—our spouses, mothers, fathers, daughters and sons, grandparents, aunts, uncles, nephews, and nieces. Our professional involvement with the growth and nurturance of newborns and their parents draws its strength and spirit from our personal experiences within own families and communities.

*To Una, Aoife, and David Declan—le mo bhuíochas, mo ghrá go deo (JKN)*

*To the memory of my parents, Fleming and Sybil Riva Keefer (CHK)*

*To all of my patients, who have taught me so much, and to my husband
Paul for his untiring love and support (SM)*

*To Bergljot and Howard, to Hiram, and to Kjartan, Abraham, and Lilly (LCJ)*

*To my parents, Lucien and Rita Blanchard, for all your love and support (YB)*

# INTRODUCTION

The birth of a child provides clinicians with a remarkable opportunity to support parents at a time when they may feel anxious, alone, and vulnerable. The transition to parenthood can be especially difficult for single or adolescent parents, parents who are isolated or poor, parents of premature or disabled infants, parents who suffer from postpartum depression or have a history of mental illness, or, indeed, for any parents who feel unprepared for their new role as mothers or fathers. We developed the Newborn Behavioral Observations (NBO) system as a means of supporting parents during this critical life transition.

The NBO was designed to help practitioners sensitize parents to their child's competencies and uniqueness and thus contribute to the development of a positive parent–infant relationship from the very beginning. The NBO consists of 18 neurobehavioral observations that describe the newborn's capacities and behavioral adaptation from birth to the third month of life. While it describes the infant's capacities, the NBO provides parents with individualized information about their infant's behavior, so that they can appreciate his or her unique competencies and vulnerabilities and thereby understand and respond in a way that meets their child's developmental needs. The 18 NBO items include observations of the infant's

- Capacity to habituate to external light and sound stimuli (sleep protection)

- Quality of motor tone and activity level

- Capacity for self-regulation (including crying and consolability or soothability)

- Response to stress (indices of the infant's physiological stability and threshold for stimulation)

- Visual, auditory, and social-interactive capacities (degree of alertness and response to both human and non-human stimuli)

Although the NBO attempts to reveal the full richness of the newborn's behavioral repertoire, the clinical focus is on the infant's individuality—that is, on the aspects of behavior that make him or her unique. In other words, the NBO provides the infant with a "voice," a "signature." It gives the child an opportunity to let the caregiver know who he or she is, what his or her preferences and vulnerabilities might be, and in which areas he or she may need support. The NBO was designed to enable the infant to reveal his or her own profile of behavior and temperament or behavioral style and thus diminish the possibility of premature labeling based on a priori medical or social background data. By providing this behavioral profile of the infant's strengths and challenges, the NBO can provide clinicians with the kind of individu-alized guidance that can help parents meet their child's needs. This, in turn, will help the parents develop the kind of confidence they need to support their infant's development and enjoy the experience of being the parent of a newborn. In sum, the NBO is an individualized, infant-focused, family-centered system of learning and communicating. Although the infant's behavior is at the heart of the observation ses-sion, the NBO is designed to foster a positive relationship between par-ents and their infants and to promote communication between clini-cians and parents.

For clinicians who work with children and families, the newborn period and the first months of life may well be the *teachable moment par excellence* because it is a major transition period in the life of the child, in the lives of the parents, and indeed in the life of the whole family. A wide range of research studies underscores the need for strengthening parents' knowledge, confidence, and practical skills in caring for their children, especially during the transition to parenthood and during the months after discharge from the hospital. The NBO can be used to pro-vide parents with vital knowledge and resources to meet their infant's needs and thus bridge the gap between parental expectations and pro-fessional competence.

National surveys of attitudes of parents toward the health care system report that what mothers and fathers want from their health care clinicians today is more information and support on child behav-ior and development (Young-Taffe, Davis, Schoen, & Parker, 1998). Fortunately, as Blumberg and colleagues (2003) pointed out in their in-troduction to the National Survey of Early Childhood Health, because of their regular contact with infants and parents, health care profes-sionals and educators (e.g., doctors and nurses, infancy specialists, physical and occupational therapists, child life specialists and social workers, psychologists and psychiatrists, doulas, early intervention specialists, infancy specialists, parent educators, and home visitors) are uniquely positioned to give parents the kind of support they need to meet their child's needs. However, there is some evidence to suggest that while health care professionals conscientiously counsel parents about topics such as safety and nutrition, they are much less likely to offer guidance on developmental or behavioral topics (Bethell, Peck, Abrams, Halfon, Sareen, & Collins, 2002; Bethell, Peck, & Schor, 2001). Moreover, many clinicians are often overwhelmed by heavy workloads and shrinking resources, which may prevent them from providing a more relationship-based form of care to parents and their young chil-dren. We realized, therefore, that we needed to create a tool that was developmentally robust, conceptually and clinically rich, and at the same time flexible and easily integrated into everyday practice—whether in a newborn physical examination, as an integral part of a home visit, as part of a lactation consultation, as a "stand alone" ses-sion with parents at discharge from the NICU, or as part of a clinic or follow-up early-intervention home visit. This handbook rests on the as-sumption that because the NBO is flexible and easy to use, it can be an

important resource for health care professionals to enable them to provide the kind of information and emotional support today's parents
need during the transition to parenthood.

To study the usefulness of the NBO for practitioners, 222 pediatric
professionals from 10 settings around the United States, representing
inner-city, suburban, and small-city sites, were trained in using the NBO.
Program evaluation revealed that 98% of the practitioners reported that
the NBO was excellent or good in helping parents learn about their newborns, 91% maintained that parents became more confident in their parenting as a result of the NBO, and 99% maintained that the NBO en-
hanced their relationship with parents. In a follow-up study, there was a
significant difference in how clinicians interacted with the families as a
result of adopting the NBO. They reported that parents learned new information about their infants (p<.01) and became better observers of
their infant's behavior (p<.001), and that they, the clinicians, felt more
"connected to" or "tuned in" to parents' needs when they used the NBO
(p<.05) (Philliber, 2001). Similarly, in a 9-month follow-up, McQuiston,
Kloczko, Johnson, O'Brien, & Nugent (2006) found that teaching pediatric residents to use the NBO in both nursery and outpatient settings resulted in positive changes in the residents' assessments of newborn behavior and their interactions with parents of newborns (p<.001). In a
study of the efficacy of the NBO as a nursing intervention, Sanders &
Buckner (2006) reported that the NBO was a feasible and cost-effective
intervention for nurses and was effective in enhancing mother–infant engagement in first-time mothers.

Although conceived as a flexible and easy-to-use teaching tool, the
NBO was created to foster a more inclusive relational approach to the
examination and care of the infant and his or her family. The NBO em-
bodies, therefore, a personalized relationship-based approach to clinical work with new parents, transforming the classic model of clinician-
led patient care into a collaborative model of family-centered care
(Brazelton & Cramer, 1990; Harrison, 1993; Inui, 1996; Stewart, Brown,
Weston, McWhinney, McWilliam, & Freeman, 1995). The Pew Health
Professions Commission and the Fetzer Task Force for Advancing
Psychosocial Health Education emphasized that the best way for pediatric professionals to communicate information to parents is by including them as partners in the decision-making process (Tresolini & the
Pew-Fetzer Task Force, 1994). By valuing the parents' attempts to reach
out and understand their child, the clinician using the NBO provides
parents with a more nurturing and supportive context. This positive,
nurturing, nonjudgmental experience becomes gradually internalized
and incorporated into the parents' own internal representation of
themselves as mothers and fathers.

This handbook is written for professionals who work directly with
new parents and their infants and for faculty, clinical supervisors, and
mentors who are responsible for preparing students or trainees for
work with parents and young infants. Because the NBO is based on the
assumption that parents who understand their child's behavior and
development will be more confident in their ability to meet their child's

needs, the handbook provides clinicians with information on newborn behavior and development and on parent development. The first part of the handbook (Chapters 1 and 2) describes the NBO and provides the theoretical and clinical principles that guide its use. The second part (Chapter 3) is the NBO manual for the administration and recording of the behavioral observations. The manual provides interpretative material, including implications for caregiving and guidelines for anticipatory guidance. In the third part (Chapters 4 to 8), the focus is on the relationship-building aspects of the NBO and how it can be applied to different clinical settings—from hospital to clinic to home—and how it can be used in a culturally appropriate way.

It is our hope that the NBO itself and the material in this handbook will provide clinicians with a deeper appreciation and understanding of newborn behavior and early relationships, and thus enable them to provide parents with the kind of information and support they need during this critical life transition and to assist them in making the kinds of informed choices that best serve their infant's needs and foster their own sense of competence.

## REFERENCES

Bethell, C., Peck, C., Abrams, M., Halfon, N., Sareen, H., & Collins, K.S. (2002). *Partnering with parents to promote the healthy development of young children enrolled in Medicaid: Results from a survey assessing the quality of preventive and developmental services for young children enrolled in Medicaid in three states.* New York: The Commonwealth Fund.

Bethell, C., Peck, C., & Schor, E. (2001). Assessing health system provision of well-child care: The Promoting Healthy Development Survey. *Pediatrics, 107*(5), 1084–1094.

Blumberg, S.J., Olson, L., Frankel, M., Osborn, L., Becker, C.J., Srinath, K.P., et al. (2003). Design and operation of the National Survey of Children with Special Health Care Needs. *Vital Health Statistics 1, 41,* 1–136.

Brazelton, T.B., & Cramer, B.G. (1990). *The earliest relationship.* Reading, MA: Addison Wesley Longman.

Harrison, H. (1993). The principles of family-centered neonatal care. *Pediatrics, 92*(5), 643–650.

Inui, T.S. (1996). What are the sciences of relationship-centered primary care? *The Journal of Family Practice, 42*(2), 171–177.

McQuiston, S., Kloczko, N., Johnson, L., O'Brien, S., & Nugent, J.K. (2006, Summer). Training pediatric residents in the Newborn Behavioral Observations (NBO) system: A follow-up study. *Ab Initio,* www.brazelton-institute.com/abinitio2006summer/art0.html

Philliber Research Associates. (2001, March). *The Clinical Neonatal Behavioral Assessment Scale (CLNBAS): Training outcomes.* New York: Accord.

Sanders, L.W., & Buckner, E.B. (2006). The Newborn Behavioral Observations (NBO) system as a nursing intervention to enhance engagement in first-time mothers: Feasibility and desirability. *Pediatric Nursing, 32*(5), 455–459.

Stewart, M.A., Brown, J.B., Weston, W.W., McWhinney, I.R., McWilliam, C.L., & Freeman, T.R. (1995). *Patient-centered medicine: Transforming the clinical method.* Thousand Oaks, CA: Sage Publications.

Tresolini, C.P., & the Pew-Fetzer Task Force (1994). *Health professions education and relationship-centered care.* San Francisco: Pew-Health Professions Commission.

Young-Taffe, K., Davis, K., Schoen, C., & Parker, S. (1998). Listening to parents: A national survey of parents with young children. *Archives of Pediatrics and Adolescent Medicine, 152,* 254–262.

# 1

# AN INTRODUCTION TO THE NEWBORN BEHAVIORAL OBSERVATIONS SYSTEM

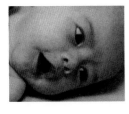 This chapter is divided into three sections. The first section describes the history, content, and uses of the Newborn Behavioral Observations (NBO) system; the second section presents the underlying theoretical assumptions of the NBO; and the third section presents a series of clinical principles that govern the use of the NBO.

## BACKGROUND OF THE NEWBORN BEHAVIORAL OBSERVATIONS SYSTEM

This section describes the history, content, and uses of the Newborn Behavioral Observations (NBO) system.

### History

The development of the NBO is based on more than 30 years of research and clinical practice with the Neonatal Behavioral Assessment Scale (NBAS) and was shaped by the authors' clinical work in a variety of environments working with infants and families. It also was inspired by the formative influence of T. Berry

Brazelton, whose teaching and mentoring have shaped the authors' understanding and appreciation of newborn behavior on the one hand and molded their clinical stance toward parents and families on the other hand. His pioneering work with the NBAS on the nature of individual differences in newborn behavior and his respectful, nonjudgmental clinical stance toward parents in his clinical teaching influenced both the content and the clinical approach of the NBO.

In terms of helping both scientists and practitioners understand the newborn infant, it is widely recognized that the single most important advance in the study and the assessment of the newborn infant was the development and publication of the NBAS by Dr. Brazelton and his colleagues in 1973 (Brazelton, 1973, 1984; Brazelton & Nugent, 1995). For much of the 20th century, it had been assumed that the newborn infant was a *blank slate*—a reflex organism that operates at a brain stem level. However, a new body of research on newborn capabilities in the 1960s and 1970s and the introduction of the concept of *newborn behavioral state* by Wolff (1966) led to a greater appreciation of the human newborn as a responsive organism capable of organized behavior, which, in turn, contributed to the development of a new generation of neonatal scales. Because it yields a comprehensive description of newborn competencies on the one hand and identifies individual differences in newborn behavior on the other hand, the NBAS can be said to have begun where other scales left off.

Extensive research has shown that the NBAS is sensitive to a wide range of perinatal variables, such as the effects of intrauterine growth restriction; the prenatal ingestion of cocaine, alcohol, caffeine, and tobacco; or the effects of prematurity. The NBAS remains the most comprehensive assessment of newborn behavior available; as such, it can be said to have played a major role in expanding the understanding of the phenomenology of newborn behavior.

Although the NBAS has been used primarily as a research instrument, it also has been used as a clinical or educational tool to attune parents to their infant's capabilities (Nugent, 1985; Nugent & Brazelton, 1989, 2000). The scale has been adapted or modified to render it more effective as a teaching tool for parents. A number of scales were developed for use in clinical environments, as a form of parent education or intervention. Field et al. (1978) developed the Mother's Assessment of the Behavior of the Infant to involve mothers actively in the assessment of their child. By incorporating behavioral items and concepts from the NBAS into the routine physical pediatric examination, Keefer (1995) developed the combined physical and behavioral neonatal examination to help promote a more parent-centered approach to pediatric care. Gomes-Pedro et al. (1995), in their efforts to sensitize parents to the behavior of their newborns, effectively tested a shortened version of the NBAS for use as the newborn pediatric discharge examination. Cardone and Gilkerson (1990) also used the concepts of the NBAS to develop the Family Administered Neonatal Activities.

With the growing recognition of the importance of the newborn period as a unique opportunity for preventive intervention with families, Nugent (1985) developed a manual for clinicians, providing guidelines on how to use the NBAS as a teaching tool in clinical environments. The approach itself and the manual can be said to be the precursor to or the first iteration of the NBO and the training material described in this handbook. A series of studies, summarized by Brazelton and Nugent (1995) and Nugent and Brazelton (1989, 2000), showed that demonstrating the newborn infant's behavioral capacities to parents can serve as a mechanism for helping parents learn about their new infant, thereby strengthening the relationship between parent and child and supporting the family adjustment. Specifically, a number of studies consistently have reported positive effects of exposure to the NBAS on variables such as maternal confidence and self-esteem, paternal attitudes toward and involvement in caregiving, parent–infant interaction, and developmental outcome. Parker, Zahr, Cole, and Brecht (1992), for example, invited mothers to participate actively in the behavioral assessment of the infant in the neonatal intensive care unit environment, and Rauh, Achenbach, Nurcombe, Howell, and Teti (1988) used the NBAS serially in the neonatal intensive care unit as a teaching tool with mothers of low birth weight infants. Studies by Anderson and Sawin (1983), Beeghly et al. (1995), Gomes-Pedro et al. (1995), Hawthorne-Amick (1989), Myers (1982), Rauh et al. (1988), Widmayer and Field (1981), and Worobey and Belsky (1982) and the meta-analysis by Das Eiden and Reifman (1996) all reported positive effects of the NBAS on various developmental and parenting outcomes. The results from these controlled studies encouraged us to develop the Newborn Behavioral Observations system as a tool clinicians could use to support parents and strengthen their relationship with their infant.

## Content and Uses of the NBO

The NBO system, initially known as the Clinical Neonatal Behavioral Assessment Scale, comes from this tradition and grew from the authors' desire to provide clinicians with a scale that retained the conceptual richness of the NBAS but shifted the focus from assessment and diagnosis to observation and relationship building. The underlying concepts of newborn behavior, therefore, are complemented by theoretical principles that describe the transition to parenthood and the nature of the parent–infant relationship and by clinical principles that describe the nature of relationship building in clinical practice. Moreover, the NBO was designed to be flexible and easy to use so that it could be integrated easily into the care of newborn families, whether in hospital, clinic, or home environments.

The NBO was created to sensitize parents to their infant's competencies, with a view to helping them understand their infant's behavior and thereby promote positive interactions between parents and their new infant and contribute to the development of a positive parent–infant relationship. It is conceived of as an interactive system, one in which parents play an active role in both the observations of their infant's behavior and the identification of appropriate caregiving strategies. Therefore, although the theoretical principles that guide the use of the NBO and the accompanying training program include many of the conceptual themes that informed the NBAS, they also are informed by theoretical and clinical principles from the fields of child development, behavioral pediatrics, nursing, developmental and clinical psychology, physical and occupational therapy, early intervention, and infant mental health.

The NBO is made up of 18 behavioral observations. These items were selected to operationalize the theoretical framework on which the NBO was based. They draw on the understanding of the richness of the newborn's behavioral repertoire, on the appreciation of the wide range of variability in newborn behavior, on the understanding of the developmental agenda of the human newborn across the first months of life, and on the understanding of the developmental challenges that parents face in these early months. The items that are included in the NBO also incorporate the understanding of the ontogeny of the parent–infant relationship in the transition to parenthood and the influence of the infant on the parent–child relationship. The NBO items include observations of the infant in sleep, awake, and crying states and the degree to which the states are integrated or organized. The individual behaviors were selected to represent the developmental tasks that newborns face across the first months of life and were designed to capture the process by which the autonomic, motor, organization of state, and responsivity (AMOR) domains become integrated. The autonomic domain is represented by observations of the infant's response to stress, such as the amount of color change, startles, or tremulousness. Observations of motor tone in the arms and legs, activity level, the crawl response, and sucking and rooting reflexes represent the motor domain. The infant's state regulation, or the organization of state domain, is captured by observations of the infant's capacity for habituation or sleep protection, the amount of crying, and the ease with which he or she can be consoled or his or her capacity for self-consoling and the nature of transitions between states. Finally, the infant's response to visual and auditory stimulation, including social interaction, represents the attentional-interactive domain, or the responsivity domain.

The NBO may take between 5 and 10 minutes to administer if all of the 18 behaviors can be observed, but its length and, indeed, its focus will be shaped not only by the infant's behavior and the needs of the parents but also by the nature and the clinical goals of each particular session. For that reason, it may take 5 minutes or 1 hour, depending on the goals of the clinician, the needs of the family, and the nature of the relationship between the clinician and the family. The NBO is appropriate for use from birth to the third month of life and can be used in a range of clinical environments, including in-hospital, outpatient, and in-home environments.

Administration of the NBO must be flexible, and the administration sequence is always driven by the infant's state. Therefore, if the infant is sleeping at the beginning of the session, then the NBO begins with the administration and discussion of the habituation items. If, however, the infant is crying, then the session begins with the soothability item, as befits the infant's state. In general, the administration is shaped by a number of factors, including the robustness or frailty of the infant, the focus or concerns of the parents, and the goals and the purpose of the NBO session itself. Most important, the parents' participation is central to the administration of the NBO. Their own previous observations of their infant's behavior, such as crying or soothing experiences, and their interpretation of these behaviors all inform and shape the direction of the session. Parents can be invited to administer parts of the NBO, such as eliciting the infant's response to the parents' voices or soothability, as a way of drawing parents further into the center of the interaction. The following are the NBO items:

Introduction and observation of infant state with parents

1. Habituation to light (flashlight)
2. Habituation to sound (rattle)

Uncover and undress (optional)

3. Muscle tone: legs and arms
4. Rooting
5. Sucking
6. Hand grasp
7. Shoulder and neck tone (pull-to-sit)
8. Crawling response
9. Response to face and voice
10. Visual response (to face)
11. Orientation to voice
12. Orientation to sound (rattle)
13. Visual tracking (red ball)
14. Crying
15. Soothability
16. State regulation
17. Response to stress (color changes, tremors, and startles)
18. Activity level

Although these 18 observations make up the full set of NBO observations, it should be pointed out that some of them are summary observations, such as crying, state regulation, response to stress (color change, startles, and tremors), and activity level.

In sum, the NBO can be described as an individualized, infant-focused, family-centered observational system that is designed for use by practitioners to elicit and describe the infant's competencies and individuality, with the explicit goal of strengthening the relationship between the parent and the child and promoting the development of a supportive relationship between the clinician and the family.

## UNDERLYING THEORETICAL ASSUMPTIONS

The theoretical assumptions underlying the NBO, which will be expanded and elaborated on throughout this volume, provide the clinician with a framework within which to understand newborn and infant behavior and development, on the one hand, and parent and family development, on the other, so that he or she can use the NBO in a way that is individualized, theoretically robust, and developmentally sound. Here, we will summarize some of the key theoretical principles on which the NBO is based.

### The Competent Infant

The NBO is based on the assumption that newborns come into the world with a wide array of mental skills and predispositions and a set of abilities that are uniquely suited to the critical needs of early life. Recent research has yielded an extensive taxonomy of newborn and infant behavior. The newborn infant not only can see but also has clear-cut visual preferences, as Fantz (1961) pointed out many years ago. Fantz reported that infants preferred to look at visual patterns that they had never seen before in contrast to patterns that they had seen. This has been confirmed by a number of more recent studies demonstrating that newborns can focus and visually track stimuli (Dannemiller & Freedland, 1991; Laplante, Orr, Neville, Vorkapich, & Sasso, 1996; Slater, Morison, Town, & Rose, 1985). Newborns have certain scanning preferences and are sensitive to eye gaze from the beginning. Not only can newborns track visually, but they also prefer the mother's face and can even discriminate their mother's face from that of a stranger (Pascalis, de Schonen, Morton, Deruelle, & Fabre-Grenet, 1995).

It therefore is clear that biology has programmed the human newborn to be a prosocial organism that actively seeks contact with the social and physical world, and the biological competencies at birth guarantee that the infant is able to interact with the physical and social environment. Newborns not only can distinguish between contrasting physical patterns but also are able to explore the internal features of the face and to gather cues about the partner's emotions (Blass & Camp, 2003; Trevarthen, 1993). Newborn infants seem to prefer the human face over all other stimuli, and are sensitive to eye gaze from the beginning. Farroni, Massaccesi, Pividori, and Johnson (2004), for example, showed that newborns looked significantly more at a face with direct gaze than at a face with averted gaze. The infant's gaze behavior not only regulates his or her internal physiological state but also signals his or her readiness to engage in communication. The infant's visual system, therefore, serves to elicit a dyadic form of interchange, which helps a parent recognize that the infant indeed is a fully responsive human being—a person with an individual personality.

In terms of sensitivity to the interpersonal context of their new world, there is evidence that infants are able to discriminate between different affective facial expressions (e.g., happy, sad, surprised) and even are capable of imitating these expressions (Field, Woodson, Greenberg, & Cohen, 1982). Indeed, newborns can imitate both in the visual and auditory modalities, which include not only mouth, tongue, and other facial movements but also eye blinking and sequential finger movements (Meltzoff & Moore, 1999). An equally important finding for the clinician who uses the NBO is the discovery by Als in her work with the Assessment of Preterm Infant Behavior and the current authors' work with the NBAS that gaze aversion suggests the need to withdraw from an overly demanding situation or the need to recover from the excitement of the interaction (Als, 1982, 1986; Brazelton et al., 1974; Brazelton & Nugent, 1995). The NBO is based on the assumption, therefore, that the main task or challenge that the newborn faces is to organize and integrate the new world of sights, sounds, faces, and voices in a way that is both understandable and predictable. In other words, the newborn seems to come into the world with a set of social capabilities that enable him or her to read and decipher the emotional expressions of the caregiver as well as to interact with the caregiver, playing a vital role in the development of the parent–infant bond (Klaus, Kennell, & Klaus, 1995).

The newborn also can hear and locate sounds (Muir & Field, 1979) and seems to prefer higher pitched voices or, more specifically, the mother's voice (Clarkson & Clifton, 1995; deCasper & Fifer, 1980; deCasper & Spence, 1991; Ecklund-Flores & Turkewitz, 1996; Fifer, 1993; Fifer & Moon, 1994; Moon, Cooper, & Fifer 1993; Morrongiello, Fenwick, Hillier, & Chance, 2004; Querleu, Renard, Boutteville, & Crepin, 1989; Spence & Freeman, 1996). Indeed, newborns can detect the overall patterns of rhythm and pitch that differentiate one person's voice from another's and can discriminate between languages (Nazzi, Floccia, & Bertoncini, 1998). There even is evidence to suggest that newborns can discriminate between two vowels (Moon et al., 1993) and between unfamiliar whispered voices (Spence & Freeman, 1996). Newborns can remember speech sounds (Swain, Zelazo, & Clifton, 1993) and specific musical sounds (Hepper, 1991). Newborns also seem to be able to detect the sounds of *any* language and can make fine-grained distinctions between many speech sounds (e.g., "ba" and "ga," "ma" and "na") and show a greater sensitivity to low-frequency sounds as compared with adults, who show maximum sensitivity to high frequencies (Aldridge, Stillman, & Bower, 2001). It is their adaptive value that renders these remarkable capacities so important to the newborn because, taken together, they serve one of the major developmental functions of the infancy period, namely, the promotion of mother–infant attachment.

Although infants have very specific visual and auditory capabilities, it is evident that they are competent in all five sensory modalities. Review of the evidence for the other newborn senses reveals that the newborn already has a sophisticated sense of smell and can distinguish the smell of the mother from that of a stranger. Taste, too, is well developed, and infants not only prefer sweet solutions over salty or bitter-tasting solutions but also prefer some types of sweet tastes over others. Newborn infants also are sensitive to touch. Touch is a fundamental means of interaction between parents and infants, and a substantial body of research demonstrates the positive effects of gentle stroking on the infant's behavioral development and on the parent–infant relationship itself (Field et al., 1986; Scafidi, Field, & Schanberg, 1993).

Infants are born with an array of reflexes and motor behaviors such as rooting, sucking, crawling, and muscle tone, all of which are included in the NBO. Although most newborn reflexes disappear during the first 6 months of life as a result of the increase in voluntary control over behavior as the cerebral cortex develops, many of the newborn reflexes such as rooting and sucking have clear-cut adaptive value for the neonate and serious implications for caregiving. The rooting reflex, which propels the infant to search for the mother's nipple, is displayed when the infant is hungry or when the cheek area is lightly stroked (Rochat & Hespos, 1997). Moreover, although the sucking reflex is involuntary, there is evidence to show that infants do have control over their sucking and can adjust their sucking pressure in response to the flow of the milk from the nipple (Craig & Lee, 1999). Indeed, research has demonstrated that newborns can learn to adjust their level of sucking to produce interesting sights or sounds. For example, newborns suck faster to be able to see visual designs or hear music and human voices (Floccia, Christophe, & Bertoncini, 1997). As Als pointed out, from a bioevolutionary perspective, newborn infants can be said to be perfectly designed to elicit from their new environment all the support they need for their survival and successful adaptation (Als, 1986).

That newborns can see and hear, have a refined sense of smell and touch, can shut out specific environmental noise, and have a number of highly adaptive reflexes is an impressive range of behavioral capabilities. As impressive as these competencies are, though, they can only hint at the very complexity of the newborn's overall behavioral organization. How these remarkable competencies are activated and integrated by the infant to respond to and make sense of his or her new world is one of the core questions that the NBO poses. It is the infant's capacity for organization—the degree to which he or she organizes these behaviors and the attempts to self-regulate—that are the focus of the NBO. For that reason, it should be pointed out that it is not the aim of the NBO to demonstrate, *show off,* or highlight discrete capacities, such as the infant's ability to turn to the sound of a rattle or track a red ball. The focus, rather, is on the overall quality of self-regulation and organization. The NBO yields a comprehensive profile of the newborn in terms of the level of behavioral organization and areas of disorganization or areas in which the infant needs environmental support. The NBO is used to help parents understand the integrative capacities of the newborn, how the newborn infant can produce organized response to his environment, and how much and which kind of support the newborn needs to reach this level of organization. Although describing the newborn's competencies is validating for parents, identifying the areas in which the infant needs environmental support, and arriving at the kinds of facilitation or scaffolding that the infant may need, make for a more balanced behavioral profile.

## Behavioral States

The first and perhaps the most obvious example of the newborn's capacity for organized behavior is the existence of predictable behavioral states. The concept of behavioral state is central to understanding the newborn and is, perhaps, the single most important concept that has contributed to current understanding of the newborn. Behavioral states can be defined as recurrent ensembles of behavior that have similar characteristics (Brazelton, 1973; Prechtl & Beintema, 1964; Wolff, 1959). These behaviors tend to co-occur and can be observed and identified reliably. There are six behavioral states:

1.  Deep sleep (non-REM sleep): regular breathing, eyes closed, no spontaneous movement, no rapid eye movement; startles may appear

2.  Light sleep (REM sleep): eyes closed, irregular respirations, more modulated motor activity; rapid eye movements are present

3.  Drowsy or semi-alert: eyes may be open or closed; activity levels are variable

4.  Quiet alert: alert with bright look; minimal motor activity

5.  Active alert: eyes open; considerable motor activity; fussing may or may not be present

6.  Crying

These behavioral states demonstrate that the newborn is not at the mercy of his or her environment and that the behavior of the newborn has an inherent organizational structure. Moreover, the NBO can demonstrate that the newborn infant has predictable, even unique, behavioral patterns. This has led to the understanding that *state* is a critical matrix on which to assess all reactions, sensory as well as motor, in the newborn (Brazelton, 1973). In addition, state is a powerful concept that helps parents to understand their infant's behavior, the appropriateness of their handling techniques, and the quality of the stimulation that they can provide to meet the needs of their infant. This discovery led to the important clinical principle that the newborn's behavioral states inevitably influence the quality of the newborn infant's responses. The concept of *behavioral states* provides the clinician and the parents with a frame, or a lens, to enable them to organize their own observations about the infant and to learn to read the infant's behavioral cues.

The body of research described previously has yielded an impressive catalogue of newborn competencies that have transformed scientific understanding of the human newborn. This understanding also has enabled a new generation of clinicians to help parents recognize that their newborn infants can see and hear and are capable of organized responses and thus to support the development of the relationship between the parent and the infant from the beginning (Klaus et al., 1995; Nugent & Brazelton, 2000). Understanding the newborn's more complex organizational capacities and the ability to describe and recognize the developmental agenda and adaptive challenges for both term and preterm infants during the first months of life is critical in informing the clinical approach to working with parents. In this way, clinicians can provide developmentally appropriate information and individualized guidance to parents during this important life transition.

## The Newborn Period and the Development of Self-Regulation

The first 3 months of life can be called a period of rapid developmental transition, as the infant's behavior and physiology shift from intrauterine to extrauterine regulation. The developmental agenda now centers on the regulation of the infant's states (Brazelton, 1992; Emde & Robinson, 1979; Mirmiran & Lunshof, 1996; Sander, Stechler, Burns, & Lee, 1979). This period is characterized by changes that are pervasive and enduring and involves major reorientations in person–environment relations (Emde & Robinson, 1979, 1987). There also is evidence that this is a special period of developmental change and reorganization in the patterns of infant attention and emotion (Lavelli & Fogel, 2005). Although there is a wide range of variability, simple attention during the first month seems to dominate face-to-face interactions, whereas during the second month, infants show a wide range of facial expressions and emotional responses, from interest to concentration to astonishment and pleasure. From the fourth through the sixth week of life, the earlier simple gaze now is accompanied by more active positive emotional expressions, by expressions of effortful concentration, and by smiling and often motor excitement. By the third month, the duration of smiles and cooing increases as smiles become more open and cooing more playful. This more active pattern of attention is accompanied by excited attention during face-to-face interactions. Clearly, the infant's response to the parent's face is emotional, so gaze/attention is not merely neutral or cognitive.

The scope of the NBO extends across this period and is designed to describe the infant's adaptation and development, specifically the capacity for self-regulation during that period. The task of self-regulation must be negotiated successfully before the infant can maintain prolonged moments of mutual gaze with his or her caregiver and develop the capacity for shared mutual engagement that constitutes the major task of the next stage of development (Adamson, 1996; Brazelton, Koslowski, & Main, 1974; Stern, 1995; Tronick, 2003).

It has been hypothesized that the newborn infant faces a series of hierarchically organized developmental challenges as he attempts to adapt to his new, extrauterine world, both the inanimate and the animate. Although these challenges or substages may not develop in an absolute sequence (and may be contemporaneous), there is an assumption of a hierarchical progression, such that each precedes the next. This includes the infant's capacity first to regulate his physiological or autonomic system, and then his motor behavior, his state behavior, and finally his affective interactive behavior, which develop in a stage-like epigenetic progression during the first months of life. From this developmental perspective, the NBO, when used serially during the first 3 months of life, enables the clinician to systematically study behavioral changes over time by describing the process of hierarchical integration of the different domains or systems of behavior.

The first and basic developmental task for the newborn is to organize his autonomic or physiological behavior. This involves dealing with stress related to homeostatic adjustments of the central nervous system. It involves the tasks of stabilizing breathing, reducing the number of startles and tremors, and being able to maintain temperature control. In the NBO, this is monitored by observation of the infant's startles, tremors, lability of skin color, and regularity of respiratory patterns.

When this homeostatic adjustment has been achieved, the newborn can move on to the second task: regulating or controlling motor behavior. This means gaining control over and inhibiting random motor movements, developing well-modulated muscle tone, and reducing excessive motor activity. The NBO facilitates observation of tone in the arms and legs; activity levels; and reflexes such as rooting and sucking, hand grasp, and crawl.

The third developmental task of this period is state regulation or organization of state. This is the ability to modulate behavioral states and includes the ability to develop robust and predictable sleep and wake states and what could be called sleep protection, or the ability to screen out negative stimuli while asleep. State control means that the infant is able to deal with stress, either through self-regulation strategies such as hand-to-mouth maneuvers or through communication with the caregiver by crying and thus being consoled with the caregiver's help. The NBO facilitates observation of the infant's capacity to habituate to light and noise stimuli while asleep and recording of the infant's state organization. Also observed are the amount of crying and the infant's capacity for soothability as indicators of his level of self-regulation.

The final developmental task for the newborn is the regulation of attentional-interactive, or social, behavior. This involves the capacity to maintain prolonged alert periods, the ability to attend to visual and auditory stimuli within his range, and the ability to seek out and engage in social interaction with the caregiver. During the NBO, the infant's responses to the human face and voice as well as to inanimate visual and auditory stimuli are observed.

In summary, the NBO can reveal where along this hierarchical continuum the individual infant falls, in which domain he or she needs support, and the kind of support that he or she may need. Nevertheless, this developmental agenda and the infant's capacity to protect sleep and develop predictable sleep–wake states, cope with stress, and respond to his or her environment can be achieved only with the support of the caregiver. The NBO is designed, therefore, to help the clinician and the caregiver identify where the infant needs support and how they can provide this support. Management of crying, feeding, and sleep, for example, are some of the most overwhelming concerns of parents in these early months (Anders, Halpern, & Hua, 1992; Barr, 1990; Brazelton, 1962; Papousek, 1998; Wolke, Gray, & Meyer, 1994), so the NBO can be used as a tool to provide parents guidance on the most appropriate ways to manage sleep, feeding, and crying behavior in a way that is responsive to the individual infant's needs (these are discussed in greater detail throughout the book).

## Synapse Formation in the Newborn Period

There is growing evidence to suggest that the newborn period and the first months constitute a major stage in the infant's adaptation to his or her new environment and marks an important transition period in the infant's behavioral development (Barr, 1998; Dobbing, 1990; Lavelli & Fogel, 2005; Rochat, 1998), but it also involves a major transformation in many neural functions (Als et al., 2004; Hopkins, 1998; Huppi et al., 1998; Rakic, 1995). New research on brain development indicates that whereas the infant's nervous system will mature in a programmed sequence as higher brain areas progressively take control of the newborn's mental life, the newborn infant's brain at birth is fully developed to ensure that the infant can survive. Although synapse formation begins in the cortex as early as 7 weeks' gestation, it continues through gestation and the newborn period and into the second year of life and beyond. This is defined as a sensitive period, a period of rapid brain development, a period when the brain seems to act like a sponge, taking in new information quickly and easily. However, it also is known that although genes program the sequence of neural development in infants, it is the quality of the infant's unique caregiving environment that shapes this development. Genes control the timing of myelination, whereas environmental factors, such as the kind of stimulation to which the infant is exposed, will affect positively or adversely the thickness of the wrapping around the individual axons.

What is important for the clinician to realize, therefore, is that all of the essential refinements of brain wiring—dendritic growth, synapse selection, and even myelination—are influenced by a child's early experiences (Huttenlocher, 2002). Everything the infant sees, touches, hears, feels, tastes, and thinks translates into electrical activity in just a subset of synapses, tipping the balance for long-term survival. Synapses that rarely are activated, whether because of the absence of appropriate parent–infant interaction, crying that never is relieved, smiles that never are reciprocated, or expressions that never are exchanged, will wither and die (Eliot, 1999). Once a given brain region has passed the refinement stage, its critical period has ended, and the opportunity to rewire it has been significantly limited. Therefore, the critical period for basic sensory abilities, such as vision and hearing, end much earlier than those for more complex skills such as language and emotion whose neural circuits prune their synapses and myelinate their axons during most of childhood. This critical period of brain development presents a window of opportunity during which experience will play a key role in shaping a child's mental skills.

## The Newborn Period as Formative in the Transition to Parenthood

From the parents' perspective, these first months can be considered a normative crisis, a period that is characterized by rapid change as they attempt to establish a relationship with their new infant (Cowan & Cowan, 1995, 2000; Klaus et al., 1995; Winnicott, 1975) and search for the *goodness of fit* between themselves and their infant (Thomas & Chess, 1977). In the case of mothers, Stern (1995) referred to this unique but normal psychological condition as the *motherhood constellation,* a condition or stage that every mother experiences. With the birth of an infant, a mother passes into a new and unique psychic organization, which will determine "a new set of action tendencies, sensibilities, fantasies, fears and wishes" (Stern, 1995, p. 171). Although the clinician who administers the NBO draws on the infant's behavior as the key informant in this intervention, he or she also must be aware of the challenges that parents are facing at this time if he or she is to enter into an empathic relationship and develop a therapeutic alliance with the parents.

This normative stage in the transition to parenthood therefore has its own protoclinical challenges, the resolution of which will have an impact on the ontogeny of the parent–child relationship, a stage that potentially is conducive to change in the parent's own life development. Winnicott (1975) has suggested that this is a period during which a mother has a heightened sensitivity to her infant, which he calls "primary maternal preoccupation," and that this sensitization is a necessary state to enable the new mother to "feel herself into her infant's place, and so meet the infant's needs." The core challenge for the new mother therefore is to engage her infant in such a way that "fosters the baby's development in a way that is authentic to her" (Stern, 1995, p. 173). This involves her ability to nurture and care for her infant, to help her infant to grow and thrive physically, to become attached, and to provide a secure environment for her infant. Fathers also face many of the same psychological challenges in their own transition to parenthood, as Birss points out in Chapter 2. Although there is a wide range of cultural variation in the role that fathers and other caregivers play in this early stage, it should be pointed out that in most societies, both partners have a unique role to play in the socialization process of the young infant (Nugent, Yogman, Lester, & Hoffmann, 1988; Parke & Buriel, 1998). Because it is family-centered, the NBO offers the clinician a unique opportunity to enter into a supportive partnership with parents at a time when they may feel vulnerable and in need of support.

## The Development of the Parent–Child Relationship in the Newborn Period and the First Months of Life

These early months also constitute a major transition stage in the development of the parent–infant relationship (Beckwith, 2000; Beckwith, Cohen, & Hamilton, 1999; Brazelton, 1992; Cowan & Cowan, 2000; Emde & Robinson, 1979; Greenspan, 1992; Konner, 1998; Sander et al., 1979; Stern, 1995; Trevarthen, 1979; Trevarthen, Kokkinaki, & Fiamenghi, 1999; Tronick, 2003). At this stage, the earliest patterns of interaction are taking shape, as infant and parent are in a heightened state of readiness to exchange their first communication signals in their efforts to achieve a mutually satisfying level of affective mutual regulation—what Stern (1985) referred to as *affective attunement.* During the first months of life, the infant develops the capacity for shared attentiveness (Adamson, 1996), so both parents and infant have already embarked on and are actively engaged in an interactive regulative system (Sander et al., 1979).

It is during this time that parents' perceptions of the infant begin to consolidate (Brazelton, 1982; Bruschweiler-Stern, 1997; Cramer, 1987; Stern, 1995; Zeanah et al., 1997). Although parents begin to develop perceptions of their infants during pregnancy by translating fetal movement patterns in behavioral terms such as, "She's very active," or, "He is so good," or, "She is very angry with me," it is only in the newborn period that they can test these attributions in the light of the child's observable patterns of behavior. The NBO can help parents develop realistic perceptions of their infants and help them to modify their prenatal perceptions in response to their infant's objectively observed behavior patterns. Cramer (1987) maintained that parents' perceptions of infant behavior play a crucial role in determining the unfolding of the parent–infant relationship.

Many parents may tend to have unrealistic perceptions of their newborns, although Freedman (1980), Hinde (1976), and Kaye (1982) argued that a certain amount of *adultomorphism,* or overestimation of the infant's capacities (e.g., "She has a mind of her own," "He understands everything I say") can be adaptive in that it motivates parents in their attempts to communicate with their infants with the expectation of engaging in reciprocal interaction. Conversely, negative attributions such as, "He doesn't seem to like me," or, "Every time I look at her, she looks away," present important clinical information to the clinician and may suggest that the parent–infant dyad could be at risk for future interactive disturbances.

Stern's (1995), Cramer's (1987), and Bruschweiler-Stern's (1997) work clearly indicated that the task of influencing parents' perceptions of their infant is complex because the meanings that parents attribute to their infant's behavior may have their origin in the parents' personal history and unconscious. Although the resolution of such distorted perceptions may be prolonged and painstaking, the NBO intervention can begin to contribute to the resolution of such perceptions by enabling parents to observe their infants' own unique behavioral makeup and the infants' own interaction capacities, thereby helping to prevent the development of noncontingent interaction patterns. (Chapter 2 presents a more comprehensive treatment of the meaning attribution process in parent–infant relations.) Fraiberg et al. (1980) illustrated this in her work on "ghosts in the nursery," in which she demonstrated how conflicts from earlier relationships may intrude on and interfere with the parents' current relationship with their infant. For example, a child may become a replacement for a deceased or lost object such that the parent is reacting to an imaginary child and not to the real infant before him or her. According to Fraiberg, parents often repeat with their infants their own childhood traumas "in terrible and exacting detail" (1980, p. 165). The result of such distorted perceptions may lead to what Stern (1985) referred to as *parental misattunements*, and it is proposed here that the NBO can be used to prevent this from happening.

The NBO is designed, therefore, to help the clinician and the caregiver, together, to identify where the infant needs support and how they can provide this support. Management of crying and sleep, for example, are two of the most overwhelming concerns of parents in these early months (Anders et al., 1992; Barr, 1990; Brazelton, 1962; Wolke et al., 1994). The NBO can be used as a tool to provide guidance to parents on the most appropriate ways to manage sleep and crying behavior in a way that is responsive to the individual infant's needs and enhances the parent quality of parent–infant interaction. From an interventionist point of view, it has become clear that this transition period provides the clinician with a remarkable opportunity to play a supportive role in promoting the infant's self-regulation on the one hand and facilitating the mutual affective regulation process between the parent and the infant on the other hand. Moreover, the quality of the clinician's relationship with parents is crucial because it is intended to have a transforming effect on the parents' relationship with their child.

## A Major Transition in Family Functioning

The early months are unique in that this period constitutes a critical transition point in the evolution of the family as a system (Cowan & Cowan, 2000; Minuchin,

1985; Stern, 1995). The entry of an infant into an already functioning system inevitably changes the dynamics of family functioning because the period after birth involves a vital redefinition of roles (Belsky, 1985; Cowan & Cowan, 2000; Minuchin, 1985). Indeed, it can be added that these profound life changes also are ecological transitions, as Garbarino (1992), Bronfenbrenner (2002), and Lerner, Rothbaum, Boulos, and Castellino (2002) pointed out, in that the birth of a child will irrevocably influence the family system and the wider circle of systems, including the family and the community, which potentially will influence the course of the new infant's future development.

The task of the family system is to accommodate the new member while maintaining a viable relationship among its elements and with its environment. The task of the clinician, then, is to help the family to maintain stability within its system and at the same time enable it to be flexible enough to adapt to and accommodate a new element into an already existing, integrated system. After birth, all family members—mothers, fathers, siblings, and grandparents—have to adjust to the presence of the new family member and to renegotiate their relationships and roles (Nugent, 1991). The NBO can facilitate this major developmental process by helping parents to understand the differential effects of the infant on the family and how the infant's behavioral makeup may influence family roles and functioning. (See Als and Lawhon, 2004; Barnard, Morisset, and Speiker, 1993; Beal, 1986; Candilis-Huisman, 1997; Fabre-Grenet, 1997; Murray, 1994; Murray and Cooper, 1997; and Myers, 1982, for studies emphasizing the importance of helping parents understand the impact of the infant on family relationships.)

What is unique about the NBO approach as a form of intervention or parent support is that the infant—the infant's behavior—is at the center of the encounter with parents; it is through the infant that clinicians hope to motivate and support parents in their efforts to understand and respond to their infants. It is *infant focused* because it yields a profile of the infant's behavioral repertoire or temperament and describes the behavioral adaptation of the infant from birth to the third month of life. It also is characterized as *family centered* not only because it is always conducted in the presence of parents and family members but also because it is designed to engage the parents and sensitize them to their infant's communication cues to enhance the quality of parent–infant interaction and family functioning. To provide support that is individualized to the infant and the family, one of the primary goals of the NBO is to help the parents understand their infant's behavior to identify the kind of support and stimulation that the infant needs for his or her optimal development. Specifically, the NBO provides information on the infant's sleep behavior; feeding and motor behavior; threshold for stimulation, crying, and soothability; and social interactive behavior. The ultimate goal of the NBO, however, is to promote relationship building to help parents understand and respond to their newborn infant and at the same time to help the clinician develop a partnership with the parents around the infant's behavior.

## CLINICAL PRINCIPLES THAT GUIDE THE USE OF THE NBO

This chapter has presented data to suggest that the newborn period and the first 3 months undoubtedly are an important period of development, but in terms of the implications for clinicians, there also is the possibility that the first months of life may be *the intervention touchpoint* or *the teachable moment* par excellence, across the life span. A teachable moment is a point in the child's or the family's development when providing the kind of developmental information and emotional support that parents need may have long-lasting effects on the parent–infant relationship and on developmental outcome. Following is a series of clinical principles that are designed to guide the clinician in the appropriate use of the NBO.

### First Clinical Principle: The NBO Is a Relationship-Building System

The NBO is, in essence, a relationship-building instrument that can be used to sensitize parents to the capacities and the individuality of their newborn infant and to foster the relationship between parents and infants. Not conceptualized as an assessment, per se, or as a simple demonstration of the infant's capacities, the NBO aims to capture the infant's uniqueness or individuality with the goal of fostering the bond between parent and infant. It provides parents with an understanding of their infant's behavior, on the basis of the shared observations of the NBO. It creates a profile of the infant's behavioral repertoire and thereby enables the clinician to provide important information to parents about their infant and identify the kind of support and stimulation that the infant needs for his or her optimal development. Each behavior is described in terms of what it reveals about the infant's temperament or personality and its potential for guiding parents on how to respond to their infant.

The NBO assumes, then, that the newborn infant is a competent, social organism who is predisposed to interact with his or her caregiver from the beginning. It documents the newborn's contribution to the parent–infant system, so it can be described as an observation of the infant in a dynamic interactional environment, not as a simple observation of the infant in isolation. It was never conceptualized as a series of discrete stimulus–response presentations but rather as an interactive observation in which the clinician plays a major role in facilitating the organizational skills of the infant. In this way, the clinician–infant transactions during the NBO simulate the parent–infant relationship and provide a window into the infant's contribution to the emerging parent–infant relationship. This process is described in more detail in Chapter 4.

Providing parents with information on their child's development and offering caregiving guidance should be presented in the context of a relational model of family-centered care if it is to have a significant effect on child growth and development. Karl, Beal, and Rissmiller (1995), Becker, Palfrey and Wise (1998), and

Green and Palfrey (2000), for example, demonstrated that a close relationship between the family and the primary care clinician helped to improve the pattern of health care utilization by families who lived in disadvantaged areas. The hope, then, is that this positive, nurturing, nonjudgmental relational experience becomes gradually internalized and incorporated into the parents' own internal representation of themselves as parents and of their child. For parents who are feeling alone and vulnerable, the opportunity to develop a relationship with a clinician who is supportive and caring can be the first step in enhancing parents' sense of worth. This in turn is an important condition in helping parents become more positively invested in their child.

The NBO in the neonatal period, however, is thought to provide only one glimpse into the continuum of the infant's adjustment to labor, delivery, and a new environment. Repeated NBO observation sessions can best demonstrate the infant's coping capacities and capacities for using his or her own inner organization as he or she begins to integrate and profit developmentally from the environmental stimulation. Serial observations in either clinic or home settings would reflect better the interaction between the infant's inborn characteristics and the environmental influences during the first weeks of life. Moreover, this shared experience allows for the relationship between parents and clinicians to develop so that the clinician–parent relationship can become a reliable safe base for the new parents.

## Second Clinical Principle: The NBO Is Infant Focused

At the heart of the NBO is the infant's behavior. The NBO provides the infant with a *voice*, with an opportunity to reveal his or her own profile of behavior and temperament or behavioral style and thereby prevent the possibility of premature labeling on the basis of a priori medical or social background data. However, an assumption underlying the NBO approach is that the infant's temperament or behavioral profile is a co-construction of the parent, the clinician, and the infant. The infant's behavior never is objective information in the sense that it stands on its own and is self-explanatory. Although it may be interpreted by the clinician, the clinician must be aware then of the mother's psychic processes and should recognize that her representations of herself and her infant will shape her understanding of the infant's behavior during the session, as Bruschweiler-Stern (1997) and Birss (in Chapter 2) pointed out.

What is unique about the NBO approach, therefore, is that the infant—the infant's behavior—is at the center of this shared observation, and it is through the infant that clinicians hope to motivate and support parents in their efforts to respond to their infants. The NBO reveals the power of the infant to elicit from his caregiving environment the nurturing and caregiving that he needs for his successful adaptation. The infant therefore becomes the catalyst in intervention environments by providing a powerful motive for positive change in the parents. The infant represents parents' hopes and deepest longings: "He stands for the renewal of the self; his birth can be experienced as a psychological rebirth for his parents" (Fraiberg et al., 1980, p. 54). All parents want the best for their child, so when the clinician shares this goal, the infant becomes the bond that unites the clinician and the parents in fulfilling their hopes for their infant. In this way, the positive adaptive tendencies that are inherent in the parent–infant relationship can be mobilized in the service of the infant's development.

The NBO reveals that the newborn is capable of communicating his needs, so the course of infant development depends to a great extent on the ability of the caregiver to read and respond to these communicative cues. The infant emerges both as being socialized and a socializer at the same time. It is a bidirectional process wherein the infant regulates, modulates, and refines the caregiver's behavior in the service of his or her own adaptation, and the caregiver in turn provides the scaffolding to help promote the infant's successful adaptation (Sander et al., 1979; Vygotsky, 1987). Several studies have examined the contribution of newborn behavior to parent–infant interactions and future developmental outcome (e.g., Crockenberg, 1981; Lester, 1984a; Linn & Horowitz, 1984; Murray & Cooper, 1997; Van den Boom, 1991, 1994, 1995; Waters, Vaughn, & Egeland, 1980).

In the context of the NBO, the infant becomes the key informant, and the clinician accepts whatever level of information or participation parents offer, at the pace at which they offer it. The NBO approach underscores the importance of respecting parents' defenses by neither directly eliciting clinical material nor predetermining the nature and the extent of parents' involvement at this time of transition in their lives. By following this approach, parents' degree of involvement and participation in the intervention tend to increase during the course of the interventions during the first months of life (Nugent, Hoffman, Barrett, Censullo, & Brazelton, 1987). By the third month, the parents and the clinician will have come to know the infant more as an individual because they have observed the infant's development during that period. By that time, the clinician in turn hopes to have laid the foundation for an enduring, supportive relationship with the family that will continue to grow as the neonate moves into infancy.

## Third Clinical Principle: The NBO Is an Individualized Development-Based System

Whereas the NBO can be carried out in many ways and may take different forms depending on the clinical environment, it is the capacity of this set of observations to bring out the individuality or the temperament of each infant that may constitute its effectiveness as a form of intervention. It is the individualized nature of the NBO that renders it responsive to the particular needs of individual infants and families. For this reason, it has been suggested that through the NBO session, although parents learn new information about their newborn's capacities, what is more important is the ability of the NBO to reveal the infant's unique traits or style of adaptation or temperament. This new knowledge in turn better enables parents to understand and respond to their infant as a unique individual and to learn the infant's communication cues.

The newborn's temperament emerges out of his or her engagement with these developmental challenges and his or her emotional response to the new environment. Demonstrating and identifying the child's behavioral style or temperament affects both the way parents feel about themselves and the way they function as parents (Carey, 1999; Carey & McDevitt, 1995). Carey and McDevitt pointed out that the newborn period is an optimal time to help parents understand their infant's cues. This can be done through the kind of shared behavioral observation with parents that the NBO offers.

The NBO does not describe what infants can do or even how they do it in generic terms. When clinicians introduce the NBO to parents, they do not say, "Did you know that infants can see and can even track a red ball?" or "Did you know that infants recognize their mother's voice?" Rather, they can say, "Let's see how your infant responds to what we present to her." The goal of the NBO is to personalize the infant for the parents by describing the infant in terms of the kinds of characteristics that make him or her unique. By focusing on the *how* of the infant's responses—the process rather than the product—the focus is shifted from what he or she does or does not do to what makes this infant unique. In this way, the infant's behavioral profile on the NBO becomes his or her behavioral signature.

By eliciting, describing, and interpreting the newborn's behavior, the clinician has an opportunity to participate with parents in identifying the kinds of demands that the infant will make on his or her environment and the kinds of caregiving techniques that best can promote the infant's organization and development. The NBO thus offers the clinician and the parent a forum to observe the infant's level of functioning during the first months and together arrive at a behavioral profile that captures the infant's individuality and temperament. Although the immediate goal of the NBO may be to help reveal to parents the infant's unique adaptive and coping capacities, the long-term clinical goal is to influence the infant–parent relationship positively by developing a supportive therapeutic alliance with the family at what could be called *the* formative moment in the development of the family system. The NBO thus is seen as the first stage in the development of a supportive relationship between the clinician and the parents that should continue beyond the newborn period.

## Fourth Clinical Principle: The NBO Is a Family-Centered System

With the birth of an infant, the family becomes an open system. This means that the pediatric clinician has a unique opportunity to enter into and become an integral part of the family support system. In high-risk environments, this entry point can provide the clinician with a unique opportunity to support the family and thereby counterbalance the risk that is present within the microsystem itself

(Garbarino, 1982, 1992; Klaus et al., 1995; Lerner et al., 2002). Barr (1990) argued, for example, that infant behaviors such as excessive crying or early sleep problems can create tension among family members and have a negative effect on family functioning. They can lead to the development of parents' negative perceptions of their infant, and can in turn undermine parents' confidence in their ability to parent. The NBO can be used to address this issue within the context of the family.

With single-parent families or families who feel isolated or have no support system, the NBO can be used by the clinician to serve as a bridge between the family and the broader community and increase the availability of informal community support for the family on the one hand and more formal family resource services and early intervention in the community on the other hand (e.g., Hauser-Cram, 2006; Mahoney & Perales, 2005; Meisels, Dichtelmiller, & Fong-Ruey, 1993; Sameroff & Fiese, 2000; Shonkoff & Meisels, 2000; Weissbourd & Kagan, 1989; Wolke et al., 1994). This can best be achieved by a long-term partnership between the clinician and the family, as illustrated by the Touchpoints model, which is based on the assumption that helping parents identify and expect bursts and regressions in child behavior (the "touchpoints") can reduce parental frustration and self-doubt while fostering their parenting and enjoyment of their child (Brazelton, 1992, 1995; Stadtler, O'Brien, & Hornstein, 1995). The use of home visitors to provide this kind of support is especially common in Europe and in federally mandated early intervention programs in the United States, while certain innovative programs in North America involve grandparents (Crockenberg, 1986), foster grandparents' making home visits to isolated young mothers during these first months (Anisfield & Pinkus, 1978), or peer-support groups (Boger & Kurnetz, 1985). (See Sweet and Applebaum, 2004, for a meta-analytic review of home-visiting programs for families with young children.) The NBO is being increasingly used in early intervention environments from birth to the third month as part of the weekly home-visiting program, where the findings are integrated into the individualized family service plan (IFSP; Levine, 2006). In such environments, the NBO-based intervention sessions not only can serve to strengthen the relationship of the clinician and the family but also can be used to strengthen the relationship between the family and community support systems.

## Fifth Clinical Principle: The NBO Is Based on a Positive-Adaptive Model

For entering into a partnership with the parents, using a model that is positive-adaptive rather than pathological is proposed (Brazelton, 1982). This positive approach may be particularly difficult for some mental health clinicians, as Cramer (1987) pointed out, because of the nonadaptive bias of the psychoanalytically inspired intervention models. This is reflected in the persistence of the notion of the young infant as helpless and in the emphasis on the parents as the solitary contributors to the infant's development.

Although the NBO philosophy is built on the recognition and appreciation of the integrative capacities of newborn infants, this positive-adaptive approach in turn is extended to respect and acknowledgment of the caregivers' abilities to meet the needs of their young infant. The recognition of parents' capacities for nurturing is reinforced by a series of microanalytic analyses of early parent–infant interactions that were conducted at the Child Development Unit at Children's Hospital, Boston (Brazelton et al., 1974; Lester, Hoffman, & Brazelton, 1985; Tronick, Als, & Brazelton, 1980; Weinberg, Olson, Beeghly, & Tronick, 2006; Weinberg & Tronick, 1996). These data demonstrate that the social stimulation provided by caregivers is rich, multimodal, and reciprocal. Papousek and Papousek (1987, 2002) assigned these behaviors the position of intuitive behaviors because they seem to assume an intermediate position between categories of innate reflexes and responses that require rational decisions. The idea that human parental behaviors may be selected during evolution and that parents have endogenous parenting capacities demands that clinicians who work with parents have a respectful, nondidactic, and nonjudgmental attitude toward parents. Belsky's (1985) reanalysis of his previous data and the authors' own work with infants who are small for gestational age and their families (Nugent et al., 1987) suggested that the efficacy of behavior-based interventions is mediated by parental involvement and interest and lies as much in the quality of the clinician–parent relationship as it does in the demonstration of newborn behavioral capacities.

The quality of the clinician's relationship with parents is crucial because it is intended to have a transforming effect on the parents' relationship with their child. The parameters of respect, concern, accommodation, and basic positive regard become crucial as the envelope of the entire *treatment* process. The more concerned or anxious the parent is, the more crucial this reliable emotional context becomes. Although the nature of the relationship will change over time, the quality of respect and mutuality must remain to withstand the unanticipated problems that inevitably occur. This aspect of the parent–clinician relationship can provide parents with what Lieberman (1991) referred to as a "corrective attachment figure" that contrasts with the criticisms that they may be experiencing from other sources in their lives. By valuing the parents' attempts to reach out and understand their child, the clinician provides the parents with an experience and a model of a more nurturing and supportive relationship.

## Sixth Clinical Principle: The NBO Promotes the Development of a Positive Clinician–Family Partnership

The establishment of a relationship of trust between the clinician and the family is the cornerstone of the development of a therapeutic alliance, as Greenspan (1981), Harrison (1993), Stern (1995), and Stewart (1995) pointed out. The infant-focused nature of the NBO-based intervention is well suited to developing a partnership with parents. This infant-focused intervention, in contrast with an exclusively parent-centered, verbally mediated approach to intervention, may be particularly effective in working with families in the newborn period.

The clinician's predominant attitude toward parents, therefore, is both respectful and nonjudgmental. The clinician must be able to listen empathically to parents' questions and observations (Boukydis, 1986; Cowan & Cowan, 2000; Heinicke, Feinman, Ponce, Guthrie, & Rodning, 1999; Hirschberg, 1993; McDonough, 1993). In Cramer's (1987) view, paying attention to a mother's verbal reports and what she thinks about her infant is crucial, because these attributes play a significant role in determining the unfolding of the mother–infant relationship. The NBO environment should always provide parents with an opportunity to share their perceptions of their infant and to relate their experience of becoming a parent, in what Zeanah and McDonough (1989) referred to as the *family story.*

In high-risk environments where families are under stress, however, parents may be unable to respond contingently to their newborn's eliciting behaviors. When there is maternal depression or when parents are affectively unresponsive or unavailable, interactive disturbances may occur (Field, 1987; Murray, 1994; Murray & Cooper, 1997). However, results of a recent study on the effects of the NBO showed that parents who participated in the NBO were less likely to have postpartum depressive symptoms as compared with a matched group of first-time parents who did not participate in the NBO (Nugent, Valim, Killough, Gonzalez, Wides, & Shih, 2006). Helping parents read their infant's cues or merely confirming the validity of their own observations and providing parents with feedback on how their infant responds to them can help mobilize confidence in their efforts to communicate with their young infant. During the NBO session, clinicians try to give parents an opportunity both to observe and to interact with their infant. Parents have a chance to elicit these behaviors from their own infant, and, in this way, they have an opportunity, with the facilitation and support of the clinician, to experience the sense of efficacy in eliciting these responses (Munck, 1985; Munck, Mirdal, & Marner, 1991).

## Seventh Clinical Principle: The NBO Is Designed to Be Used to Bridge the Clinician–Family–Community Gap

It must be recognized that the newborn infant enters into a social network that may be made up of parents, grandparents, siblings, and friends, all of whom can exercise a significant influence on the infant. Although the newborn period often provides the clinician with a unique opportunity to develop a relationship with the infant's father or mother, the effectiveness of the NBO session can benefit from the inclusion of the siblings, grandparents, or other important elements of the infant's social network, because they all need to adjust to the presence of the new family member (Cowan & Cowan, 2000; Lerner et al., 2002; Minuchin, 1985). Expanding the scope of the intervention to include a broader range of potentially supportive allies is particularly important when working with families under stress, such as economically disadvantaged families, migrant families, single-parent families, adolescent parents, families with preterm infants or infants who are small for gestational age, or families with infants who are behaviorally irritable and difficult to handle (Nugent, Blanchard, & Stewart, 2007). In this way, the NBO can be used to try to bridge the gap between the family and the support networks within the community.

This means that the traditional transactional view of development with its emphasis on the bidirectional nature of parent–infant relations must be complemented by an understanding of the newborn as an active participant in a larger social network (Bronfenbrenner, 2002; Lerner et al., 2002). The application of systems theory to parent–infant relations demands that clinicians extend their focus from the mother–infant dyad to the family system to understand better the transforming effects of the infant on the family system and the effects of the various elements of the family system on the infant's adaptation and development. Although the infant is necessarily at the center of this approach, the NBO is done best in a family context, which provides an opportunity to focus on the potential role of the infant in influencing mother, father, grandparents, neighbors, or whoever makes up the informal network of relatives or friends who have an investment in the growth and well-being of this new infant. The family and the entire network of family interactions becomes the focus of this approach in clinical environments. Although the infant and his behavior is the focus of the NBO session, it is the family that becomes what Stern referred to as the *port of entry* for the clinician (Stern, 1995).

From this systems perspective, the NBO approach attempts to assess the contribution of the new infant to family interactions and, at the same time, work with the family to learn what it has to do to incorporate this new element into their system. Using the NBO in such environments requires what Emde (1987) referred to as *systems sensitivity*, which he defined as "the empathic registration by the therapist of the quality of functioning of complex personality subsystems and their interactions" (p. 1314). Within the context of the NBO, this means that the clinician must be able to understand and assess ongoing interactions with the family system—between parent and infant as well as between the parents themselves.

The NBO intervention takes place at different levels, so for the clinician it requires an appreciation of the simultaneous operation of multiple systems within the intervention environment. At one level, the clinician is interacting with the infant as he or she attempts to assess the infant's interaction capacities and potential influence on the parents' caregiving. At another level, the clinician is interacting with the parents in an effort to develop a supportive and trusting relationship with them around their infant. The systems-sensitive clinician is equally aware that the quality of the parents' own relationship and their extended family and community supports, their attitudes toward the infant, and their relationship with the clinician all affect the emotional climate of the session and will play a role in influencing the outcome.

## SUMMARY

The period from birth to 3 months can be considered a major transition period in the newborn's adaptation and development and in the parents' own psychological development. It is a period that is defined by specific developmental challenges for both the infant and the parents as the newborn attempts to make a successful transition to his or her new, extrauterine environment and the parents attempt to respond to their infant's needs. What the NBO can teach is that this process is highly individualized and that there is a wide range of variability in how newborn infants adapt to their new environment during these first 3 months and how caregivers respond to their infants. It has become clear that this transition period provides the clinician with a remarkable opportunity to play a supportive role in promoting the infant's self-regulation on the one hand and facilitating the mutual affective regulation process between the parents and the infant on the other hand.

In sum, the NBO is an individualized, infant-focused, family-centered observational system that was designed to be used by pediatric practitioners to elicit and describe the infant's competencies and individuality, with the explicit goal of strengthening the relationship between the parents and the child and promoting the development of a supportive relationship between the clinician and the family. The NBO consists of a set of neurobehavioral observations that need to be interpreted or reframed in a way that enables parents to understand the meaning of the behavior and thereby support them in their efforts to get to know and become attached to their infant. Because it is short and designed to be flexible, it can be used by a wide range of professionals in a variety of clinical environments, both in-hospital and outpatient. It is important that clinicians understand the theoretical principles that inform its use and that they are able to interpret the observed behavior in terms of the infant's and the parents' developmental and caregiving agenda.

# 2

# TRANSITION TO PARENTHOOD:
## *Promoting the Parent–Infant Relationship*

Sarah A. Birss

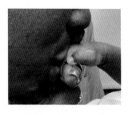 very infant is born to a mother, and every mother once was an infant. The newborn experience is common to every human being, and nonverbal memories of that experience are stored in the cells and synapses of the brain, however unconsciously. The memories of this experience come back when new mothers or fathers are surprised at the depth of feeling and tenderness that they feel in holding or feeding their new infant or in the moments when they find themselves repeating behaviors of their own mother or father that they wished not to repeat: "I can't believe I sound like my mother!" Sometimes there is an assumption that when a woman has a baby, "maternal instinct" will provide the necessary motivation to become a successful parent, but is there a maternal instinct? Mothers and fathers do not necessarily instinctively love their infants. Maternal (and paternal) behavior often emerges slowly and develops in response to external cues from the infant and the environment. "Nurturing itself needs to be nurtured" (Hrdy, 1999, p. 174).

How and by what processes do women become maternal, fathers become paternal, and parents become parental? Of course, there are biological processes of conception, pregnancy, parturition, and lactation. Beyond the biological, what are the psychological changes and behavioral changes that accompany this transition to parenthood? What changes in thinking and feeling and behaving in parents promote healthy development in infants and children? How can the parent be supported in this transition? How does the infant participate in this process?

This chapter explores the nature of parents' experiences in transition to parenthood and the emergence of maternal, paternal, and parental behavior. The caregiving environment, made up of primary caregivers (usually parents) and extended family and social networks as well as the wider community and cultural environment, provides a supportive matrix for the development of the newborn infant and for the new parent. This social environment, particularly the parents' adaptation to the new infant, will contribute to the infant's emotional and behavioral adaptation.

This chapter explores the physiological and, with special attention, the psychological aspects of becoming a parent, and it examines the specific psychological reorganization that the mother faces when she becomes a mother and how this psychological reorganization is similar and different for fathers. It examines the nature of the early interactions between parents and infant—the earliest foundations of the parent–infant relationship—and explores the ways in which the Newborn Behavioral Observations (NBO) system can be used to support the parent–infant relationship from the beginning. In addition, the chapter discusses some of the challenges that parents face when there are difficulties with their own or their infant's adaptation and how professionals who work with parents of newborns can recognize these difficulties and provide help and support.

## CONCEPTION: BIOLOGICAL AND PSYCHOLOGICAL

An infant is conceived—and conceived of. Union of ovum and sperm leads to biological conception. The infant as an idea or fantasy, however, also has a psychological existence in the minds of the parents.

### Biological Conception

The actual conceptus, the fetus, has a biological existence, and the biology of a pregnancy produces physiological and physical changes that progress in an orderly and predictable manner. An embryo is conceived by the union of ovum and sperm; the fertilized egg travels down the fallopian tube to the prepared endometrial lining of the uterus, where it implants, stimulates a host of hormonal and physical changes, and begins to grow. The initial act that leads to conception may be sexual intercourse between a woman and a man or the result of artificial insemination or in vitro fertilization. The pregnancy may be planned and desired or accidental, unexpected, or unwanted. Raphael-Leff (2001) emphasized that the circumstances of conception—

the timing, the partner, whether planned or unplanned, whether wanted or unwanted—set the stage for acceptance of the pregnancy. This is true for fathers as well as mothers.

## Psychological Conception

Although there is the actual conceived baby, there also is a conceived of, imagined, or fantasized baby. Raphael-Leff (2001) wrote of "conceived fantasies":

> The inside story differs for each pregnancy; every mother infuses it with her personal feelings, hopes, memories, and powerful unconscious mythologies. An imaginary baby is juxtaposed on the embryo expanding in her fertile womb. Even before conception, the unknown baby is drawn into an expectant woman's psychic reality, invested with illusion and ascribed a place among the many images of significant primary figures in her internal world (p. 8).

Fathers also have wishes and fantasies about their baby-to-be (Gurwitt, 1976, 1988). Although pregnancy often is thought of by society as an unequivocally joyful and fulfilling time, mothers- and fathers-to-be experience intense wishes and fears about their unborn child and about the huge changes on which they are about to embark in both their external and internal (psychological) lives. "[E]ven the most joyfully anticipated conception entails some ambivalence, since creation of a new life also signifies loss of the old" (Raphael-Leff, 2001, p. 15).

## PREGNANCY: INNER AND OUTER CHANGES

A pregnant woman experiences change at many levels that prepares her for the new role of parent. Some change is invisible and internal, such as the physiological hormone surges and the psychological shifts. Other changes are external and visible, such as the physical changes in her body shape.

## Physiological Changes

With the onset of pregnancy, a biological cascade of physiological processes begins, with hormonal effects playing a significant role. Estrogen (estradiol) levels increase to 100 times and progesterone levels rise to 10 times the prepregnancy levels, and both decline to low levels in the first week postpartum. The placenta produces during pregnancy corticotrophin-releasing hormone, which produces increased cortisol (stress hormone) levels. Oxytocin increases significantly in the third trimester. Prolactin increases during pregnancy and declines during the period of lactation. Beta endorphins, which regulate pain and pleasure, increase with the stress of labor and then decrease. Each of these hormones has both physiological and behavioral effects. These hormones "likely work in concert to prepare a woman for the actual physical process of childbirth as well as complex activities associated with child care" (Epperson, 2002, p. 19).

Animal studies have shown that estrogen, prolactin, and oxytocin all act to stimulate maternal caregiving behavior. Whereas estrogen and progesterone sustain the pregnancy, prolactin is involved in milk production, and oxytocin stimulates the uterine contraction during labor and milk ejection during nursing. Oxytocin also induces sleepiness, mild euphoria, an increased threshold for pain, emotional calm, and feeling of closeness with the infant (Klaus & Klaus, 1998, p. 98). Cortisol likely also is involved in stimulating maternal behavior (George & Solomon, 1999). Hormones exert their effects through actions on neurotransmitters, which then influence behaviors. Genes that regulate these hormones have been identified.

Biological factors can affect maternal behavior. Animal studies have shown that alterations of genes that interfere with the function of these reproductive and lactation hormones can produce decreases in certain maternal behaviors (Hrdy, 1999, pp. 150–151; Mayes, 2002, p. 7). In addition, experience affects maternal behavior. Animal studies also show that virgin females, with no hormonal preparation to display mothering behavior, will develop maternal behaviors when repeatedly exposed to infants of their species (Hrdy, 1999, p. 151). It is apparent that there is a complex interplay of physiology, genetics, and experience that prepares a mother for parenting.

## Physical Changes

The physical experience of the pregnancy belongs solely to the mother (although fathers may experience reactions to the physical changes in the mother's body and even some physical reactions themselves [see Gurwitt, 1976, 1988]). When a woman becomes pregnant, her body undergoes physical changes. Initially, in the first trimester, as she misses her period and gains some weight in her abdomen and breasts, she may have morning sickness and mood changes. She becomes aware that her body is changing, that there is a baby growing inside of her. In the second trimester, while morning sickness and mood changes usually decrease, her body begins visibly to change in shape. For some mothers, this is welcomed, but for others, even when a pregnancy is very much wanted, the showing of the pregnancy (and therefore of their sexuality) and the sense of lack of control over their body produce anxiety (Cohen & Slade, 2000; Notman & Lester, 1988; Raphael-Leff, 2001).

Quickening, the sensation of fetal movement that appears in the fourth to fifth months, along with ultrasound pictures of the fetus, make the existence of the baby all the more real. This often is greeted with excitement and aids the psychological transition toward becoming a mother. Although the mother's bodily changes, the ultrasound images, and the baby's movement make the baby real for the mother and the father, it is important to realize that many mothers, even those who are pleased with their developing pregnancy, can have ambivalent feelings about what this transition to motherhood will mean. In the third trimester, the baby primarily is increasing in size, and the mother may be physically uncomfortable, having difficulty moving around and sleeping. Some mothers require bed rest because of late pregnancy complications such as premature contractions, placenta previa, gestational diabetes, or preeclampsia.

## Psychological Changes

With the increasing reality of the baby, the mother in the third trimester becomes preoccupied with the impending birth. Winnicott (1975) suggested that there is a period of time in late pregnancy and during the first weeks after the birth of the child during which a mother has a heightened sensitivity to her infant that he calls "primary maternal preoccupation." He suggests that this would be considered an illness if it were not for the state of pregnancy. Brazelton and Als (1979) described this state from prenatal interviews with normal first-time mothers. The interviews:

> " . . . uncovered anxiety which seemed at first to be of almost pathological proportions. The unconscious material was so loaded and so distorted—so near the surface—that before delivery the interviewer felt inclined to make an ominous prediction about each woman's capacity to adjust to the role of mothering. Yet, when we saw each in action as a mother, this very anxiety and the distorted unconscious material seemed to become a force for reorganization, for readjustment to an important new role. We began to feel that much of the prenatal anxiety and distortion of fantasy was a healthy mechanism for bringing a woman out of the old homeostasis which she had achieved to be ready for a new level of adjustment." (p. 350)

Men and women enter into this intense preoccupation. A study at the Yale Child Study Center (Leckman & Mayes, 1999, cited in Mayes, 2002) showed that men think about becoming fathers: how he will be seen in the world, whether he has fathered a healthy infant, and whether he will be able to provide for the mother and their infant. Women worry about bringing the baby successfully to term, about the health of the infant, about surviving the birth and delivery, about being able to provide milk and nurturance to their infant, and about being a "good enough" mother. Winnicott (1975) suggested that this sensitization is a necessary state to enable the new mother to "feel herself into her infant's place, and so meet the infant's needs." (p. 304)

It is as though the mother, with her altered physiology, changed body shape, and disrupted sleep states, and both parents, with their heightened emotional and affective arousal at the end of pregnancy, are physiologically and emotionally dysregulated. This state of dysregulation in the parents may act in such a way as to prepare them to be open to their own new roles, open to the infant's more immature states of regulation, and able to engage more readily with the infant in his or her first task of self-regulation.

# CREATING A PSYCHOLOGICAL SPACE FOR THE NEW INFANT

The psychological work of pregnancy involves significant changes in a parent's view of him or herself, accompanied by often intense feelings, both positive and negative. This "ambivalence" is a result of the parent's necessary psychological identity reorganization, as the parent makes mental room for the coming baby.

## Identity Disruption and Ambivalence

A new mother, or mother-to-be, is filled with feelings: joy at anticipating a new infant; anxiety and fear about the birth process and the health, survival, and normality of the infant; frustration at the things that are out of her control; fear about her own neediness; and even sadness about the loss of her previous, self-sufficient identity. Although pregnancy and motherhood are expected to be experienced as happy (Cohen & Slade, 2000), in fact, a mixture of feelings, both positive and negative, is common, not only during pregnancy but also once the infant has arrived (Raphael-Leff, 2001; Slade, 2002). This is true for fathers as well. The new or expectant father also may worry about the health of the infant, feel envious of his wife's capacity to bear a child, fear loss of his autonomy, fear his own neediness and dependence, and feel out of control of the whole process. Fathers also may distance themselves to defend against these intense feelings (Gurwitt, 1988) and feel excluded and responsible (Brazelton & Cramer, 1990). Although all new parents have ambivalent feelings and expressing these feelings in a supportive context can be helpful, intense ambivalence with serious anxiety or predominantly negative feelings in a mother or a father may be seen as a warning sign of potential difficulties in adjustment to parenthood (Barrows, 1999).

## Identity Reorganization and Acceptance of the Role of Parent

As noted above, this cauldron of intense feelings about the anticipated or new infant is a challenge to and disruption of the previous internal psychological organization of both parents. This disorganization can be seen not as pathological but rather as being in the service of a reorganization of the sense of self to make way for a new conception of the self as parent. Arriving at this new self-concept is a journey that begins with the work of pregnancy and the postpartum period. For the mother, it requires a shift in identity from being the daughter in a mother–daughter relationship to becoming the mother in a mother–infant relationship, from being an independent woman to becoming a mother with a dependent child, from being a wife to becoming a partner in parenting. This shift is not a simple giving up of the old identity; it is a reorganization that requires creating a new space in her mind to being daughter *and* mother, independent adult *and* mother, wife *and* mother. The father has a similar shift in identity, from being a son to his parents to being father in a father–infant relationship, from being a husband to becoming a husband and father, requiring him both to support his wife emotionally and to share her body, her attentions, and her attachments. For him, too, this is a reorganization to become son *and* father, independent adult *and* father, husband *and* father.

For the mother, this period of disruption and reorganization, brought on by the birth of an infant and called by Winnicott (1975), as noted above, primary maternal preoccupation, was described by Stern (1995, p. 171) as "a new and unique psychic organization," which he called "the motherhood constellation." Stern suggested that the mother is preoccupied with four themes. First, she is concerned for the life, growth, and survival of her infant. Can she mother on a biological level? Can she provide the milk, if breast-feeding, and the care necessary to keep the infant alive? Second, she worries about her ability to relate to and love her infant and feel that her infant loves her. Can she psychologically nurture her infant? Third, she searches for a support system, particularly the support of her mother or other experienced mothers. Can she make connections with supportive (m)others? Fourth, she is challenged to rework her own identity. Can she successfully incorporate her infant and her view of herself as mother in a way that expands her self-identity without losing herself? (See Chapter 4 for further elaboration.)

As a new mother contemplates her new role and shifting identity, she is drawn to her conscious and unconscious memories and feelings about her own childhood and her own mother, feelings of neediness and dependence, competition, merger, and separation (Cohen & Slade, 2000; George & Solomon, 1999; Notman & Lester, 1988; Raphael-Leff, 2001; Stern, 1995). Fathers, too, rework their childhood relationships. For a father, this task involves reexamining his relationships with his mother, father, and siblings, with conscious and unconscious feelings around dependence and rivalry being at the forefront (Barrows, 1999, 2004; Gurwitt, 1976, 1988).

Stern (1995) drew attention to three particular preoccupations in a new mother's thinking: 1) a reworking of her relationship with her own mother and her relationship to her in her early childhood; 2) a reworking of her internal view of herself, especially herself as a mother; and 3) a growing set of thoughts and feelings about her new infant. Stern called these three internal conversations the motherhood trilogy (1995, p. 172). Fathers, too, rework their relationship to their mothers and fathers, their relationship to their wife, their own identity, and their feelings and fantasies about the new infant.

One mother, aware of her overwhelming intense feelings in this early emotional period after the birth of her daughter, said, "Sometimes I don't know if I am my mother, my daughter, myself as a helpless child, or myself now as a mother." The degree to which a new mother (or father) can differentiate and consciously sort out these feelings has implications for promoting the infant's healthy emotional development, yet, as explored next, a parent's ability to use his or her feelings to *feel with* his or her infant in the earliest phases of development, when communication is nonverbal, is of great importance (Furman, 1992).

# INTERGENERATIONAL TRANSMISSION OF PARENTING

A parent's early experiences with his or her own parents will have an effect on parenting. Parents who felt loved and cared for as children will expect to love and care for their own children. Parents with a difficult, perhaps abusive or depriving, childhood often are determined to be better parents to their own children. Often they succeed. However, both positive and negative parenting behaviors may be passed from one generation to the next. The field of attachment research, testing Bowlby's (1982) attachment theory, has provided a wealth of information about the intergenerational transmission of parental caregiving. Parents' experiences in and feelings about relationships, especially with their parents, can have an effect on the way they interact with their own children (for review, see Lyons-Ruth, Zeanah, & Benoit, 2003).

## Learning from Attachment Studies

Bowlby (1982), after becoming interested in the emotional and behavioral responses of young children to separation from their mothers, developed a theory of attachment. He proposed that there is an attachment system that is biologically based and promotes survival. Infants have attachment behaviors (e.g., clinging, crying, smiling, gazing, crawling) that function to keep themselves in proximity to the caregiver. Many of these behaviors are present at birth and are observable using the NBO (see Chapter 3).

Bowlby (1982) postulated that the goal of these attachment behaviors could be observed in the infant's achieving proximity to the caregiver. Sroufe and Waters (1977; cited in Kobak, 1999) proposed an internal emotional goal of "felt security," or a feeling of security, that motivated the proximity-seeking behavior. In other words, infants and children would seek access to the caregiver to feel secure and comforted. Caregiver behaviors such as emotional availability, nurturance, protection, and providing comfort (Zeanah & Boris, 2000) promote a sense of felt security, and multiple repetitions of such caregiving interactions over time lead to an "internal working model," or internal representation of the attachment relationship. Both the infant and the child develop an internal representation of the relationship, and an infant has a specific attachment relationship with each caregiver (van IJzendoorn & De Wolff, 1997).

Attachment research has shown that attachment behavior can be classified into secure and insecure (avoidant, resistant, or disorganized) attachment patterns (Ainsworth, Blehar, Waters, & Wall, 1978; Main & Solomon, 1990). Security of attachment has been shown to be correlated with sensitive and consistent caregiving in the home in the first year of life (Ainsworth et al., 1978). An Adult Attachment Interview (George et al., 1985; Main, 2000; Main & Kaplan; 1985) was developed to classify security of attachment in parents on the basis of narrative coherence in response to questions about the feelings of these adults in regard to their experience of their parents' caregiving behaviors when they were children. Adults could be classified as autonomous with regard to attachment, or dismissing, enmeshed, or disorganized, corresponding to infant classifications of secure, avoidant, resistant, or disorganized. Studies of parents using the Adult Attachment Interview have shown an 80% correspondence with the classification of their infant's attachment (Hesse, 1999, p. 406). Some longitudinal studies were done by administering the Adult Attachment Interview to adolescents and young adults who originally were given attachment classifications in infancy using the Strange Situation procedure, (Ainsworth et al., 1978, pp. 31–43). Several longitudinal studies have shown significant (70% to 80%) correspondence of secure/insecure classification in infancy with coherent/incoherent classification in adolescence or young adulthood if the individual did not have an attachment-related trauma (e.g., parental death, divorce, parental mental illness, physical or sexual abuse) in the intervening years (Hamilton, 2000, p. 690; Main et al., 2005, p. 272; Waters, Merrick, Treboux, Crowell, & Albersheim, 2000, p. 684). Although some studies have not found such continuity based on attachment measures (Grossman, Grossman, & Kindler, 2005, p. 129; Weinfield, Sroufe, & Egeland, 2000, p. 695), Grossman et al. (2005) found that "[s]ensitive and supportive experiences with both parents during childhood contributed very significantly to the child's later attachment representation." (p. 120)

Attachment research demonstrates that caregiving behaviors in the parent, such as sensitivity and consistent availability, influence security of attachment in the infant. Research using the Adult Attachment Interview has shown that the infant's security of attachment predicts to a large degree his or her adult state of mind in relation to attachment and that the adult parent's state of mind in relation to attachment predicts his or her infant's attachment security. This intergenerational transmission, however, is not 100%. Intervening negative experiences can influence attachment security, and adults can be classified as secure even when they describe their childhood relationships as neglecting or abusive. Adults who were from difficult backgrounds and were found to be secure may have experienced some supportive relationship experience outside the early family, such as a coach, teacher, marital partner, or therapist (Hesse, 1999).

It has been seen that the early relationship experiences of parents can affect their own parenting. Parents' state of mind in relationship to *their* early attachment figures predicts the attachment behavior of their own children. The next section explores how early internal working models from a parent's past may influence interactions with his or her new infant.

## The Birth of a Parent

Early attachment relationships are stored in the infant's memory as representations of early repeated interaction patterns between infant and parent. These representations create expectations for similar and continued social and emotional interactions as the infant grows and develops. As these interaction experiences continue, the infant develops an attachment to his or her caregivers (Stern, 1985; Zeanah & Boris, 2000).

These early experiences of the infant are remembered, but not as consciously recalled, narrative stories or visual images. Rather, these early memories are laid down as sensory, somatosensory, behavioral, implicit memories, and they are recalled as feelings in the here and now. These early feeling memories literally are reexperienced and return without the sense that they are "a memory" (Siegel, 1999). Why speak of the infant's early memories when thinking about a parent's transition to parenthood? There is tendency for an intergenerational transmission of attachment patterns: Parents who have a secure sense of their attachment to their own parents are more likely to have infants with a secure attachment.

It is likely that part of the reason for this transmission comes from the parent's unconsciously recalled sensorimotor experience of his or her own infancy. From the earliest moments of life, if not before, the infant forms representations of his own and his caregiver's behaviors and emotions. For example, sometimes a parent, while rocking his or her infant, may suddenly remember a long-forgotten lullaby that was sung by his or her own mother and begin to sing. Lack of experience can have an effect as well: Animal studies show that rhesus macaques that are separated from their mothers in the first year of life do not show the normal maternal behaviors of "play mothering" that usually are seen in the young macaques (George & Solomon, 1999).

The infant, who is nonverbal, is a powerful generator of affective, sensorimotor signals. Stern (1995) referred to the importance of "the present remembering context." He drew attention to the presence of the infant's bundle of behaviors and emotional, visual, auditory, olfactory, and tactile signals and cues as triggers in the present moment of emotional memories from the past (see also the section Angels and Ghosts in the Nursery).

With all of these factors in mind, when one speaks of a parent of a newborn, one could say literally that the person is a "newborn" parent: a person who is awash with hormones that create a disrupted internal biological milieu, a person who is filled with feelings that are triggered by the momentous appearance of a new infant, a person who is making a transition to a new role in life as a parent. This parent, who is responsible for a new, helpless infant, also may be a person who is reexperiencing, in the presence of the infant's powerful emotional and nonverbal signaling, his or her own deep emotions of early childhood.

The disruption of the mother's experience at the physiological, psychological, and emotional levels primes her to be in tune with a newborn infant. A new mother who is in touch with her own feelings and needs is well situated to be able to feel herself into the infant's position, to imagine what the infant is feeling, and to provide sensitive care before the infant has the capacity to communicate. Fonagy (2002) suggested that parents who have the capacity for self-reflection—

able to understand the self and others as being motivated by mental states such as beliefs, intentions, and feelings, which he called mentalization—are more able to be empathic and respond sensitively to their child's emotional signals. Such parents are able to differentiate their feelings from their child's feelings yet to "feel with" their child in such a way that they can respond to the child's emotional needs (Furman, 1992). As a new parent feels his or her way through his or her own transition to parenthood and feels with his or her infant, with attention to the uniqueness of this new infant and with the help of supportive others, a new parent is born.

## THE CENTRALITY OF SELF-REGULATION IN INFANT AND PARENT

The newborn infant is immature and unregulated physiologically and emotionally and must develop the capacity to self-regulate. This capacity develops through parental caregiving behaviors that help to regulate the infant. A parent's own self-regulatory capacity and sense of self contribute to his or her ability to promote the infant's developing sense of self. In addition, the infant's needs and developing capacities create an opportunity for parents to experience new aspects of themselves.

### The Parent's Role in Infant Self-Regulation

As was described in Chapter 1, the first developmental task of the newborn infant is self-regulation as he or she adapts to life outside the womb. The infant must learn about a whole new animate and inanimate environment from the moment of birth. The newborn's nervous system is still immature and requires outside help with aspects of regulation. The infant must achieve regulation of his or her physiologic or autonomic system, motor system and state changes, and affective interactive behavioral system during the first few months of life (Nugent, Blanchard, & Stewart, 2007). The basic developmental task of achieving homeostatic neurophysiological regulation is essential for the infant to be able to begin to engage in the affective and interactive social exchange with his or her caregiver (Brazelton & Als, 1979; Sander, 1961; Tronick, 2003).

The parent is instrumental in helping the infant learn to regulate his physiological and emotional arousal to help him to calm and focus. By providing necessary holding and feeding in a sensitive manner and by learning and responding to the infant's cues, the parent helps the infant become physiologically regulated and enables him to begin to engage with the world. At the same time, the parent develops as a caregiver and social partner. Parents—and unrelated adults—have a repertoire of affective and behavioral responses to the infant. These behaviors include behaviors that will help alert a drowsy, waking infant, such as jiggling the infant, or that will help the tired, irritable infant go to sleep, such as rocking the infant. A parent also positions the infant in a face-to-face position at a distance of approximately 10 inches between his or her face and the infant's face—the optimal distance for an infant's visual focus, not an adult's focus. In addition, parents exaggerate facial and vocal expressions, repeat behaviors and sounds with variation, and encourage matching expressions and vocalizations (Emde, 1983; Papousek & Papousek, 1987). In analyzing films of these behaviors, Papousek and Papousek described the parent's responsiveness as slower than purely innate reflexive behaviors and faster than behaviors that require cognitive appraisal; they referred to these responses as "intuitive behaviors." Papousek and Papousek suggested that these responses are biologically based and produce behaviors that teach infants about social and emotional interaction in just the ways that infants are biologically prepared to learn.

## Mutual Regulation of Parent and Infant

Although these parental behaviors initially serve to help regulate the infant physiologically and emotionally, emotional interaction also consists of emotional communication and produces emotional experience. Emde (1983) drew attention to the continuity of emotional experience. He suggested that our "affective core . . . guarantees that we can understand others who are human." (p. 165) Tronick (2003) described the process of "mutual regulation [as] a co-creative process that generates unique ways in which the mother and infant, or the infant and any other individual, are together." (p. 35) This interaction over time "allows for the co-creation of shared meaning." (p. 36) As the infant and the parent interact, the parent attempts to maintain the infant's alert state without overstimulating or to bring the infant into an alert interactive state from either an understimulated state (drowsiness) or an overstimulated state (fussiness). If the parent is successful and the infant is prepared for interaction, then both experience pleasure. Beebe and Lachman (2002) suggested that the ability of the parent–infant pair to negotiate these state transformations "makes a crucial difference to the emerging organization of the infant's representations." (p. 88) The interaction between parent and infant, the behavioral and affective matching, underlie the development of empathy and the "participat[ion] in the subjective state of the other" (Beebe & Lachman, 2002, p. 109). The infant is representing the interaction, the parent's action and emotion, and the feeling state and action of the infant's self. Fonagy (2002) stated, "The mother, in mirroring the infant's affect, does more than express sympathy— she provides a stimulus that may organize the child's internal experience and provide a label, or symbol, for what he or she is feeling." (p. 64) Fonagy (2002) suggested that the ability to think about others' mental states and to empathize grows out of the interaction between mother and infant.

It can be seen that the earliest and ongoing interactions of the parent with the infant help to regulate the infant physiologically and emotionally. This emotional, behavioral, nonverbal interaction functions not only to regulate but also to communicate. The interaction produces emotional experience and memory, and the representation of the interaction contributes to the development of empathy and the development of the self. This is true not only for the infant but also for the parent. Emde (1983) wrote of the self as a process, a developing aspect of the personality (see also Stern [1985] and Erikson [1963]). Schore (1994) explored the neurobiology of affect regulation as central to the development of the self. Whereas self-awareness does not begin until the second year, the early process of interaction between infant and parent provides the foundation for representation of the self, representation of the object/other, and the development of attachment and empathy.

This process of mutual regulation in the relationship—in the interaction of infant with parent and of parent with infant—leads to development of the infant and to development and change within the parent. Certainly, the time of transition to parenthood is an opportunity for expanded self-awareness and self-growth. The interactive capacities of the infant can capture the new parent, and both can grow and develop.

## NURTURING THE NURTURER

Knowing the important role the primary caregivers have in infant development and in helping the infant with the primary task of physiological and emotional regulation, one can see how important it is that the new parents have social supports. The father's role is multifaceted: Not only is he a new parent himself, but also his support for the new mother is crucial. In modern societies in which families live at a distance from families of origin, fathers often are called on not only for caregiving but also for emotional support of the mother (Stern, 1995). In addition, the father often has the traditional role of economic support and protection from the outside world (Brazelton & Cramer, 1990). New mothers often turn to their own mothers, to experienced mothers, and to other new mothers.

New parents may have a range of needs, and a range of services are available to them. For example, in the period before birth, childbirth classes offer support. Some mothers engage a doula for additional support during delivery and the postpartum period. A doula is a woman who accompanies a pregnant woman continuously throughout childbirth and the early postpartum period and provides emotional support. Some studies have shown a positive effect of the presence of a doula on breast feeding and mother–infant interaction (Langer, Campero, Garcia, & Reynoso, 1998; Stein, Kennell, & Fulcher, 2004). The support of a doula may be especially helpful if the new mother has no extended family available or is isolated.

Lactation consultants offer support for breast feeding and provide general support. Visiting nurses and pediatric nurses or nurse practitioners also play a helpful role. Some community agencies offer weekly home visits by community volunteers (e.g., Spielman, 2002; Visiting Moms program). Mothers' groups are helpful in providing community support and developmental guidance and connecting new mothers to other new mothers (Mayes, 2002; Slade, 2002). When an infant is at risk developmentally or because of concerns about the parent's risk for depression, mental illness, or abuse, early intervention services are available.

## Establishing and Assessing Relationships

The clinician's every contact with new parents—on the obstetric floor in the hospital, in the newborn nursery, in the pediatrician's office, or in home visits or early intervention centers—whether performing an evaluation for specific concerns, making observations during routine interactions, or during administration of the NBO, is an opportunity to assess not only the infant but also the parents' adaptation to the new role of parent to this child and to assess the new relationship. "Throughout the assessment and intervention process, diagnostic and therapeutic aims are inextricably intertwined: Even in the earliest stages of the evaluation, relationship building and information gathering are interdependent" (Seligman, 2000, p. 80). This section covers general aspects of assessment. For a more detailed description of the psychiatric assessment of infants and parents, see Seligman (2000) and Thomas (1998).

When meeting with parents, much can be observed with close attention to the parents' emotions, behavior, and verbalizations. Explicit questions can be asked to follow up on spontaneous statements or to obtain additional information. For specific *probe* questions, see Chapter 4. For specific indicators of postpartum depression or psychosis, see the section Postpartum Difficulties.

The clinician may observe the parents' current emotional states, the parents' behavior with the infant, and the attributions that the parents make about the infant. Regarding the emotional state, the clinician observes whether a parent is happy, calm, exuberant, sad or tearful, depressed, withdrawn, anxious, irritable, angry, or hostile. Is this emotion directed toward the infant or toward others? Is there a lot of change in a parent's emotional state? How do the parents behave with the infant? Is the infant held in the parents' arms (and in which parent's arms), in a bassinet nearby, or in the nursery—and for what reason? Is the mother comfortable feeding the infant? What sort of attributions do the parents make about the infant? Are the comments about the infant's appearance positive—"He's so small and cuddly"—or do they have a negative edge—"Look at that ugly face!" Is the baby's behavior interesting—"Look at the way she moves her fingers!"—or burdensome—"All she does is eat and cry." Are the interpretations of behavior appropriate—"He's just figuring out how to suck"—or is there some projection of the parents' interpretation that seems out of proportion to the behavior—"He's angry at me that I'm not feeding him enough."

Areas of inquiry might include the parents' childhood history and important relationships. For example, what were their early family relationships like—relationships with their mother, father, siblings, and grandparents? Were there any family members with difficult personalities, anxiety, depression, bipolar disorder, psychosis, or alcohol or substance abuse? Is there a history of abuse or neglect? Were there any losses of significant attachment figures, and what are the current emotions regarding any losses or difficult past experiences? Were any sibling relationships particularly difficult? Past relationships may influence current expectations, both positively and negatively.

It also is useful to listen for or elicit anything about this particular infant that connects him or her to the parents' past. For example, is the infant said to be like or look like someone else in the family, and what was the relationship with this other person? Was that person loved (or not)? Is the infant named for someone, and does this naming create a legacy of connection? Characteristics of the infant in the present may trigger positive and/or negative feelings from the past.

It is important to ask about the current relationships. Is there a partner in parenting, and is the marital or partner relationship supportive? Are there grandparents or other extended family, and are these relationships positive and supportive? Sensitive attention to the mental state, history, and current social setting of new parents is helpful to the clinician both in establishing a relationship with the parents and in assessing any risk and need for referrals.

## Managing Intense Emotions

Many parents will be happy and excited and will enjoy talking about their infant. Other parents may be overwhelmed with all the change, with a stressful delivery, or with concerns about an infant who is ill and in the special care nursery or the neonatal intensive care nursery. Even with a healthy infant, some parents will be filled with emotion, may become tearful, or may ask anxious questions. In such early encounters, parents may bring up difficult material, such as past losses or lack of support. Often, just the presence of a listening ear is helpful (see Chapters 4 and 5 for further discussion). When parents believe that their concerns are being taken seriously, they feel valued in the relationship with the clinician, and their sense of competence as a parent is increased. In early and brief contacts, it is important to emphasize the strengths and competencies of the infant and the parent (see the section Angels and Ghosts in the Nursery).

Sometimes, however, even when a clinician responds, the parents may remain anxious, continually seek reassurance, or may be angry that the response is not sufficient. Sometimes the parents' concerns seem to be out of proportion to the situation (e.g., getting upset about small things, being distressed without an apparent cause). Or a parent may make inappropriate remarks about the infant or negative remarks about him- or herself (see the section Postpartum Difficulties for specific symptoms of postpartum blues, depression, or psychosis).

A deeper exploration of parents' difficult past emotional experiences is something that will take time in the context of an ongoing supportive and therapeutic relationship. It does not need to be—nor can it be—resolved in brief encounters. It is important to remember that when a parent continues to be anxious and overwhelmed and when the clinician begins to feel overwhelmed by that parent's emotions and needs, the clinician does not need to handle the situation alone. A clinician's own sense of feeling pressured, worried, or overwhelmed often is a clue to a parent's own state of mind and a good indicator of the need for a consultation with a colleague or a referral to a mental health clinician.

## POSTPARTUM DIFFICULTIES: WORKING WITH DISTRESSED RELATIONSHIPS

When postpartum difficulties are a significant concern (e.g., a clearly distressed relationship, maternal depression, significant anxiety), referral can be made for mental health services. Parents may need psychiatric evaluation for medication and/or referral for psychotherapy. Infant mental health services also are available in the form of parent–infant psychotherapy during which the parents and the infant are seen together. Parent–infant psychotherapy may take many forms. The clinician may help the mother attend to and read the infant's cues, and the NBO can be an important part of this process. The parents can be helped to see the way the infant responds to them and the way they respond to the infant. Sometimes videotape feedback is used to help the parents see the interaction (McDonough, 2000a). At other times, particular attention is paid to the parents' history; psychological state; and representations of their own parents, of themselves as parents, and of their child (Fraiberg, 1980; Stern-Bruschweiler & Stern, 1989). Interpretations are made to help the parents understand the impact of their past experiences on the present relationship (see the section Angels and Ghosts in the Nursery).

Parents often seek help when symptoms of crying or sleep disturbance occur in the infant, because they can be seen as symptoms of dysregulation. There also may be similar dysregulation in the parent. In Chapter 1, signs and symptoms of dysregulation in the infant were described (e.g., difficulties in autonomic and state regulation, emotional arousal, and motor regulation). These aspects of dysregulation can affect crying, sleeping, and feeding in infants, and difficulties in the infant such as colic and excessive crying, hypersensitivities, and feeding problems can affect the parent–infant relationship. In parents, dysregulation can involve emotional arousal, with mood changes or anxiety, and difficulty with sleeping and eating. In fact, many of the symptoms of peripartum and postpartum mood changes such as "baby blues," postpartum depression, and postpartum psychosis involve dysregulation. It is important to recognize these mood changes because of their effect on the mother and infant and on the parent–infant relationship and subsequent child development (see Table 2.1). Infants of depressed mothers have shown lower rates of positive behaviors in early face-to-face interaction, higher rates of insecure attachment (see Seifer & Dickstein, 2000, for review), and increased childhood aggression (Hinshaw & Lee, 2003). In addition, postpartum psychosis is considered a psychiatric emergency. (For a summary of treatment options for postpartum disorders, see Table 2.2.)

## "Baby Blues"

Mood changes with sad mood or emotional ups and downs, crying spells, irritability, anxiety, and sleep difficulties are common, occurring in 25% to 85% of new mothers in the early postpartum period. Onset of the blues usually occurs in the first 2 weeks after delivery and lasts from hours to a few days or weeks. Occasionally, antianxiety or sleep medication is useful, but many women respond to support from family and friends, education, and reassurance (Epperson, 2002; National Mental Health Association, 2005).

**Table 2.1.**   Recognizing postpartum disorders

"Baby blues"
- Common: 25%–85% of new mothers
- Early onset in first week; lasts a few hours to days
- Mood changes with emotional ups and down; crying

Postpartum depression
- Incidence: 10% of postpartum women
- Onset in the first months postpartum
- Diagnosis: depressed mood or lack of interest or pleasure in activities
  *and* four of the following (three if both depressed mood and lack of pleasure):
  - Change in appetite or weight
  - Oversleeping or difficulty sleeping
  - Agitation or slowing of behavior
  - Fatigue or loss of energy
  - Feelings of worthlessness or guilt
  - Difficulty concentrating
  - Recurrent thoughts of death or suicide or fear of harming the baby
  *also:*
  - Withdrawal from friends
  - Inability to cope
  - Fear of being alone
  - Lack of interest in or overconcern for the baby
  - Poor self-care
  - Uncontrollable mood swings

Postpartum psychosis
- Incidence rare: 1 to 2 in 1,000 new mothers
- Onset usually in the first 2 to 4 weeks postpartum
- Symptoms: delusions, hallucinations, bizarre behavior and feelings, agitated behavior

*Source:* American Psychiatric Association (1994), Epperson (2002), National Mental Health Association (2006).

**Table 2.2.** Treating postpartum disorders

"Baby blues"
- Usually responsive to psychosocial support by
  - Family
  - Friends and community
  - Pediatrician
  - Lactation consultant
  - New mothers' groups
  - Home visiting programs
- Medication usually not necessary
  - Anti-anxiety and sleep medication if needed

Postpartum depression
- Requires psychiatric evaluation
- Treatment usually includes one or both of
  - Antidepressant medication
  - Psychotherapy
    - Individual psychotherapy
    - Parent-Infant psychotherapy
      - Home-based
      - Office-based
  - Mothers' groups, lactation consultants, home visiting

Postpartum psychosis
- Requires emergency psychiatric attention
  - Potential risk for
    - Suicide
    - Infanticide
    - Child abuse
- Treatment includes
  - Medication for
    - Treatment of psychosis
    - Mood stabilization
  - Hospitalization often required
  - Psychotherapy
    - Individual psychotherapy
    - Parent-Infant psychotherapy
  - Mothers' groups, lactation consultants, home visiting

## Postpartum Depression

Postpartum depression is a major depressive episode (American Psychiatric Association, 1994) that occurs in the first year after a woman gives birth. Approximately 10% to 15% of women develop postpartum depression, and previous depression is a risk factor for recurrence. Diagnosis of a major depressive episode is made when there is either a depressed mood or a loss of interest or pleasure in usual activities for a period of 2 weeks as well as at least four additional symptoms (three if both depression and lack of interest or pleasure are present) from the following list: increase or decrease in appetite or weight not related to the care of the infant, oversleeping or difficulty sleeping, agitation or slowing down of behavior, fatigue or loss of energy, feelings of worthlessness or guilt, hopelessness, decreased ability to concentrate, and recurrent thoughts of death or suicide. The symptoms must cause significant distress or impairment in function-

ing. Symptoms also may include uncontrollable mood swings, withdrawal or isolation from friends and family, a feeling of being overwhelmed or unable to cope,
or a lack of self-care. Some mothers have physical complaints such as headaches,
hyperventilation, heart palpitations, or chest pain. Mothers may fear being alone
or harming their infant or themselves or they may show a lack of interest in or be
overly concerned about the infant. Postpartum depression requires psychiatric
evaluation and often is treated with antidepressant medication and/or individual
psychotherapy (American Psychiatric Association, 1994; Epperson, 2002; Gavin et
al., 2005). Parent–infant psychotherapy can be very important in helping a depressed mother engage with her infant. General support from new mothers'
groups and home visitors, and specific support from lactation consultants also are
useful.

## Postpartum Psychosis

Postpartum psychosis is rare, occurring in 1 to 2 of every 1,000 women who give
birth. There usually is a rapid onset of symptoms in the first month after delivery.
Symptoms are those of a manic episode, such as grandiose and racing thoughts,
increased activity, insomnia without tiredness, pressured speech, unusual or
bizarre behavior, delusions, and in severe cases suicidal or infanticidal thoughts
or behavior. Postpartum psychosis is a psychiatric emergency because judgment
is impaired and the safety of the infant and the mother may be in jeopardy.
Immediate psychiatric evaluation is needed, and treatment often requires hospitalization and antipsychotic and mood-stabilizing medication. A history of bipolar disorder is a predisposition (Epperson, 2002; National Mental Health
Association, 2006). In addition to the immediate stabilizing treatment, both individual and parent–infant psychotherapy can be helpful. General supportive measures as listed above are also important.

## ANGELS AND GHOSTS IN THE NURSERY

Parents draw on their own early family experiences as they relate to their infants,
wanting to give their infants the best they can. Even so, parents are sometimes unconsciously affected by difficult experiences in the past.

## Painful Past Influences ("Ghosts")

Fraiberg (1980), in working with parents who had great difficulty parenting,
described how traumatic, neglectful, or abusive experiences in a parent's past
could haunt the relationship of a new parent with a new child. For example, in
the "present remembering context" of the infant's cry, some parents with very
sad or painful past experiences may hear the infant's cry as their own. Many
parents will empathize with the infant, of course, and respond with comfort,
but if a parent's own adaptation to his or her difficult past is to defend against

those emotional memories, then he or she may wall off the infant's cries and not hear them or respond to them, or he or she may be annoyed and irritated by the cries. Fraiberg and her group developed in-home parent–infant psychotherapy using psychoanalytic principles to help parents talk about their past and connect their current painful emotions with their past experiences. This had the effect of freeing the infant from the "ghosts in the nursery," allowing the infant to be seen as who he or she is in the present, not as an emotional reminder of a painful past.

## Helpful Influences: "Angels" and "Good Fairies"

Lieberman, Padron, Van Horn, and Harris (2005) expanded on this concept. They drew attention to the availability of "angels in the nursery," positive experiences and figures in a parent's past that can be accessed to help parents make positive emotional connections with their new infant. They suggested that "we might think of the ability to retain loving memories as one of the building blocks of psychological health." (p. 514) Bruschweiler-Stern (2004) also wrote of "good [ghosts] too, and even good fairies" and emphasized that by looking for and helping a new parent see the positive attributes and strengths in the infant and him- or herself, the clinician can support the parent in making links to positive representations in his or her experience (p. 196).

Angels in the nursery can take many forms. Supportive figures from many environments may function as positive models for new parents. There may have been grandparents, aunts or uncles, foster parents, teachers, coaches, mentors, or friends in the past. There may be friends, therapists, siblings, or partners in the present who provide support and positive modeling. Zuckerman and Zuckerman (2005) described how pediatricians can help elicit both ghosts and angels when they work with parents. As noted previously, pediatricians, nurses, early intervention specialists, lactation consultants, leaders of mothers' groups, and mental health providers when making positive, connecting relationships with new parents function in the here and now as these benevolent influences whose presence can be felt as "angels" in the current generation.

## CLINICAL VIGNETTES

The following case examples illustrate the use of the NBO to help new parents recognize the unique characteristics of their new infant, and to guide sensitive interventions that promote the emerging infant–parent relationship:

✳

### Case 1: Feeding Disturbance

Anna, a 4-week-old girl who was born at term after a normal pregnancy and uncomplicated delivery and had been breast-fed, was brought to the physician with poor weight gain. The mother, holding the infant awkwardly, said that Anna seemed hungry but would nurse for a only few sucks and then stop and avert her gaze. The mother was beginning to wonder whether there was something wrong with Anna or with her own milk supply and her ability to mother.

Anna looked malnourished, and although many possibilities were considered in the differential diagnosis, including metabolic disorders and gastrointestinal disturbances, questioning about sensitivities revealed useful information. Anna had been observed to avert gaze and withdraw when approached by an emotionally effusive and loud family member.

The physical examination was normal. When the NBO was administered, responsiveness to stimulation in the habituation items showed a high degree of sensitivity to the light and the rattle. Whereas she was normally responsive to stimulation with face alone, she became overstimulated when presented with face and voice together and became irritable with the louder sound of the bell compared with the softer sound of the rattle. She was difficult to console unless swaddled, becoming aroused with eye contact and talking.

The pediatrician suggested an intervention that consisted of Anna's being fed in a quiet, darkened room without extraneous stimulation and without the mother talking to or looking at Anna to decrease overall stimulation beyond the necessary touch, taste, and smell sensations that are attendant to feeding. Anna began to gain weight over the next several weeks and to mold to and look more comfortable in her mother's arms. Gradually, she made more eye contact during feeding and, although she remained somewhat hypersensitive, continued to develop normally. Only after the intervention had succeeded did the family tell us that their apartment, on an upper floor of a triple-decker, was right next to the elevated interstate expressway with round-the-clock traffic. The intervention had led them to understand something about their infant daughter, to hear a noise from her point of view—a noise that they no longer noticed—and to place her in a quieter room in the house. By learning about her sensory and emotional experience, they were able to change the environment and their responses to help Anna become more regulated, which in turn helped her to internalize a representation of sensitive and responsive caregivers and to develop an ability to regulate her emotional experiences and eventually to comfort herself.

* * *

## Case 2: Sleep Disturbance

Hector, an 8-week-old boy, was brought to the doctor's office because of continued waking every 2 hours at night to feed, and both parents were exhausted. The term pregnancy had been normal, but there had been an emergency cesarean section for fetal distress. At birth, Hector had been healthy, with good Apgar scores, and the neonatal course had been unremarkable. He had been healthy at home and nursing well but waking continually to feed at night and reportedly irritable when not feeding during the day.

The physical examination had been normal. When parts of the NBO were administered, Hector was found to have moderate crying and was easy to soothe and console.

However, his state regulation was not well organized, with irritability in state transitions, although he was well organized in his response to stress.

What was remarkable during the administration of the NBO was the distress of the parents, particularly the father, at their son's cries. The father was anxious to have his wife pick up their son and nurse him to stop the crying. In obtaining more history, it was discovered that the father was sleeping in Hector's room and bringing Hector to the mother to nurse as soon as Hector woke up and started to cry. Further history revealed that the father had had significant separation anxiety as a child. For several years, he had difficulty separating from his mother when he went to school, and he also had a period of depression when he went to college. It seemed that it was difficult for this father to hear his son's cries without feeling the anxiety that he had experienced as a child separating from his own mother. Because Hector was so easily consoled, especially when given to his mother for feeding, a pattern had been set up, possibly interfering with his development of state regulation. At the same time, Hector could have a somewhat difficult temperament that was contributing to the parents' anxiety, and the emergency cesarean section had set the stage for the parents to see Hector as a "vulnerable child."

The pediatrician suggested an intervention that would demonstrate Hector's competencies: how robust he was in his motor development and in his response to social and other stimulation and to soothing. In particular, it was possible to demonstrate that he had a relatively high stimulation threshold of response to stress, and so the pediatrician talked to the parents about helping Hector learn to regulate his state by letting him cry a bit to see whether he could settle himself before picking him up at night for feeding. The father was encouraged to return to the parental bed, both to reinforce the parental relationship and to allow more time between the infant waking and being picked up for feeding.

This intervention was successful in enabling the parents to help their son lengthen his nighttime sleep periods. However, in situations such as this, in which one of the parents has an identified emotional difficulty in his or her own life, careful monitoring and anticipatory guidance are essential. For example, alerting the family to anticipate that normal stresses of separation such as child care may be distressing but manageable may be helpful. If monitoring and anticipatory guidance are not enough and symptoms that suggest lack of regulation of emotions continue, then further evaluation of the infant and the family by a mental health professional may be warranted. In such cases, work may involve parent–infant psychotherapy, family or couples therapy, individual psychotherapy for one or both parents, or a combination of the interventions.

✳

## SUMMARY

Just as there is a developmental process in a fetus becoming a newborn infant, there also is a developmental process in expectant parents becoming actual hands-on parents. In addition to the physical changes of pregnancy and childbirth, there are significant psychological changes. Parents have fantasies and ambivalent feelings, hopes, and fears about the new infant and about their new role and identity as parents. Whereas the newborn is unregulated at birth because of the immaturity of its nervous system, the parents are physically and emotionally dysregulated. This state of disequillibrium may prepare the parents to be open to the infant's way of being and to be able to engage more readily with him or her in the task of self-regulation. The intensity of psychological changes leads the parents to reexamine their past family relationships and to identify with their parents as well as with their newborns.

Parental representations of early attachments have been shown to be intergenerationally transmitted to infants through the sensitivity and consistency of caregiving. Early interactions between parents and infants involve not only caregiving and regulation of the infant's physiology but also regulation of the infant's affective arousal and emotional communication. The reciprocal back-and-forth interaction between parent and infant is a sophisticated, emotionally charged system of mutual regulation. As parents enter into this way of relating, they recall powerful feelings of their own childhood and become sensitively attuned to their new infant. These early interactions form the foundation on which early representations of self and other are built and lead to the development of attachment and empathy, much of what makes people human. Early interactions promote this new self-development in parents as well as in infants, and each birth is an opportunity for new growth and development in infants, parents, and families. Clinicians can play a key role in providing support and intervention at this crucial time. By nurturing the nurturer and helping the parents to understand and respond appropriately to their infant's cues, they can help promote the development of a healthy relationship between parents and infant.

# 3

# THE NEWBORN BEHAVIORAL OBSERVATIONS SYSTEM MANUAL

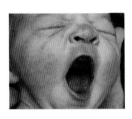 This chapter, first, presents recording and administration guidelines for the Newborn Behavioral Observations (NBO) system (see Figures 3.1 and 3.2), and, second, presents information on how to interpret each of the behavioral items in terms of its adaptive and developmental significance and implications for caregiving.

## THE MANUAL

Clinicians need to be trained to use the NBO appropriately; that is, how to conduct an NBO session and how to administer each NBO behavioral item. Whereas the specifics of how to conduct the NBO in different environments or with different groups, and guidelines on how to communicate with and interact with parents, are discussed in detail in the chapters that follow, this section describes how each behavior is elicited so that the clinician can capture the full richness of the infant's repertoire and describe the infant's individuality to the parents. It goes on to describe how each of the items is recorded on the NBO recording form and how the findings can be summarized for parents in terms of the infant's strengths and challenges. It also presents interpretative material for each observed behavior, providing information on the developmental significance of the behavior. Because the NBO is designed to help parents read their infant's communication cues to help

# Newborn Behavioral Observations (NBO) System
## RECORDING FORM

Name of infant _____ Gender _____ Date of birth _____

Today's date _____

Gestational age _____ Weight _____ APGAR _____ Parity _____

Type of feeding _____ Setting _____

Others present _____ Practitioner _____

| BEHAVIOR | OBSERVATION RECORD | | | ANTICIPATORY GUIDANCE CHECKLIST* |
| --- | --- | --- | --- | --- |
| | 3 | 2 | 1 | |
| 1. Habituation to light (flashlight) | with ease | with some difficulty | with great difficulty | ☐ Sleep patterns |
| 2. Habituation to sound (rattle) | with ease | with some difficulty | with great difficulty | ☐ Sleep protection |
| 3. Muscle tone: legs and arms | strong | fairly strong | very high/ very low | ☐ Muscle tone |
| 4. Rooting | strong | fairly strong | weak | ☐ Feeding cues |
| 5. Sucking | strong | fairly strong | weak | ☐ Feeding cues |
| 6. Hand grasp | strong | fairly strong | weak | ☐ Touch and contact |
| 7. Shoulder and neck tone (pull-to-sit) | strong | fairly strong | weak | ☐ Muscle tone |
| 8. Crawling response | strong | fairly strong | weak | ☐ Sleep position and safety |
| 9. Response to face and voice | very responsive | moderately responsive | not responsive | ☐ Social interaction |
| 10. Visual response (to face) | very responsive | moderately responsive | not responsive | ☐ Vision |
| 11. Orientation to voice | very responsive | moderately responsive | not responsive | ☐ Hearing |
| 12. Orientation to sound (rattle) | very responsive | moderately responsive | not responsive | ☐ Hearing |
| 13. Visual tracking (red ball) | very responsive | moderately responsive | not responsive | ☐ Communication cues |
| 14. Crying | very little | occasionally | a lot | ☐ Crying and soothability |
| 15. Soothability | soothes easily | soothes with some difficulty | soothes with great difficulty | ☐ Self-soothing |

**Figure 3.1.** The NBO recording form.

(continued)

**Figure 3.1.** *(continued)*

| BEHAVIOR | OBSERVATION RECORD | | | ANTICIPATORY GUIDANCE CHECKLIST* |
|---|---|---|---|---|
| | **3** | **2** | **1** | |
| 16. State regulation | well-organized | somewhat organized | not organized | ☐ State regulation |
| 17. Response to stress: color changes, tremors, startles | not stressed | moderately stressed | very stressed | ☐ Stimulation threshold |
| 18. Activity level | optimal | moderate | very high/ very low | ☐ Needs support |

**SUMMARY PROFILE AND RECOMMENDATIONS**

Strengths _____

_____

_____

_____

Challenges/areas in need of support _____

_____

_____

_____

Additional comments _____

_____

_____

_____

\* Use the checklist to specify areas that may require discussion, guidance, or continued follow-up.

# Newborn Behavioral Observations (NBO) System
## RECORDING GUIDELINES

### 1. Habituation to light (flashlight) and
### 2. Habituation to sound (rattle)

| | |
|---|---|
| 3: With ease | Habituates to stimulus with ease (after 1 or up to 5 presentations) |
| 2: With some difficulty | Habituates with some difficulty (after 6 or more presentations) |
| 1: With great difficulty | Still unable to habituate to the stimulus after 10 presentations |

### 3. Muscle tone: legs and arms

| | |
|---|---|
| 3: Strong | Well-modulated tone in legs and arms; good flexibility observed |
| 2: Fairly strong | Mixed or uneven tone |
| 1: Very high/ very low | Little or no tone or hypertonicity or rigidity observed in legs or arms |

### 4. Rooting response

| | |
|---|---|
| 3: Strong | Turns to stimulated side |
| 2: Fairly strong | Turns after latency |
| 1: Weak | Minimal or no head turning |

### 5. Sucking response

| | |
|---|---|
| 3: Strong | Initiates and maintains a modulated rhythmic suck |
| 2: Fairly strong | Sluggish sucking movement |
| 1: Weak | No sucking movement |

### 6. Hand Grasp

| | |
|---|---|
| 3: Strong | Clear-cut grasp-like movement |
| 2: Fairly strong | Moderate response; slight finger grasp observed |
| 1: Weak | No response observed |

### 7. Shoulder and neck tone (pull-to-sit)

| | |
|---|---|
| 3: Strong | Infant brings head to midline with minimum head lag and maintains it for at least 3 seconds |
| 2: Fairly strong | Infant has head lag, can bring head through midline; no ability to maintain it at midline |
| 1: Weak | Infant is unable to bring head to midline |

### 8. Crawling response

| | |
|---|---|
| 3: Strong | Coordinated crawling movement involving arms and legs and freeing of face |
| 2: Fairly strong | Some attempts to flex arms and legs |
| 1: Weak | No flexion of arms and legs and no freeing of face |

### 9. Response to face and voice

| | |
|---|---|
| 3: Very responsive | Focuses and follows with smooth head and eye movements |
| 2: Moderately responsive | Stills and focuses with moderate amount of visual tracking |
| 1: Not responsive | Very brief focus and/or no tracking with eyes |

### 10. Visual response (to face)

| | |
|---|---|
| 3: Very responsive | Focuses and follows with smooth head and eye movements |
| 2: Moderately responsive | Stills and focuses with moderate amount of visual tracking |
| 1: Not responsive | Very brief focus and/or no tracking observed |

### 11. Orientation to voice and
### 12. Orientation to sound (rattle)

| | |
|---|---|
| 3: Very responsive | Stills and brightens; turns and locates sound |
| 2: Moderately responsive | Stills and brightens; may turn eyes but unable to locate sound |
| 1: Not responsive | Eyes remain closed or dully alert; minimal or no reaction to sound |

### 13. Visual tracking (red ball)

| | |
|---|---|
| 3: Very responsive | Focuses and follows with smooth head and eye movements |
| 2: Moderately responsive | Stills and focuses with moderate amount of following; often "loses" the stimulus |
| 1: Not responsive | Very brief or no following |

*(continued)*

**Figure 3.2.** The NBO recording guidelines.

*Figure 3.2.* (continued)

## 14. Crying

| | |
|---|---|
| 3: Very little | Hardly cries or fusses |
| 2: Occasionally | Cries or fusses intermittently throughout the session |
| 1: A lot | Cries consistently throughout the session |

## 15. Soothability

| | |
|---|---|
| 3: Soothes easily | Easily soothed and/or consistently self-soothes |
| 2: Soothes with some difficulty | Soothed only after rocking or swaddling |
| 1: Soothes with great difficulty | Very difficult to soothe or never self-soothes |

## 16. State regulation

| | |
|---|---|
| 3: Well-organized | States are well defined, robust, and easy to read, and/or state transitions are smooth and predictable |
| 2: Somewhat organized | States are somewhat well defined, and state transitions are fairly smooth although not predictable |
| 1: Not organized | Unable to maintain well-defined states; transitions are unpredictable, abrupt, and difficult to read |

## 17. Response to stress (color changes, tremors, startles)

| | |
|---|---|
| 3: Not stressed | No tremors, no more than one startle, minimal color change; high threshold for stimulation |
| 2: Moderately stressed | Moderate color change, some tremors and startles; can tolerate moderate levels of stimulation |
| 1: Very stressed | Very tremulous; many startles and extensive color changes present; very low threshold for stimulation |

## 18. Activity level

| | |
|---|---|
| 3: Optimal | Well-modulated activity level |
| 2: Moderate | Moderate level of activity |
| 1: Very high/ low levels | Either persistently high or extremely low level of activity all the time |

them better understand their child, the clinician must be able to interpret even the most subtle forms of behavior in terms of the infant's strengths and the kinds of support the infant may need to adapt successfully to her [1] new environment.

## The Clinician

The clinician's ability to elicit, observe, and describe the behavior of the newborn infant is at the heart of the NBO session. It is the sensitivity and the appropriateness of the clinician's handling techniques and his or her ability to observe and describe these behaviors that constitute the effectiveness of the NBO as a teaching tool. For that reason, clinicians who use the NBO must be trained and certified in its use. While the handbook in general and the manual in particular are presented here as resources to help clinicians with this process, users must complete the NBO training program and become certified in its use before using the NBO in their clinical practice (training information is available at www.brazelton-insti-tute.com). For refining their observation skills, it is also recommended that clinicians become familiar with the rich, detailed descriptions of behavior that are provided by the Neonatal Behavioral Assessment Scale (NBAS; Brazelton & Nugent, 1995), which describes the wide range of behaviors and behavioral patterns that make up the behavioral range of the newborn infant. (In clinical environments, it is extremely helpful when a clinician who is trained in the NBAS is available as a resource for beginning trainees.) The clinician should have the ability to enable the newborn infant to demonstrate the full range of her behavioral repertoire. The clinician's handling skills are important because he or she can serve as a model for parents in demonstrating the kinds of facilitating and handling techniques that respect the infant's thresholds of responsiveness. (The NBO training program provides both real and virtual demonstrations of the NBO to prepare clinicians to administer it appropriately, but previous clinical experience with infants is extremely important for all practitioners who plan to use the NBO.)

For the clinician to use the NBO effectively, he or she must also have a deep understanding of the principles of infant and parent development so that he or she can interpret the infant's behavior in terms of the infant's developmental agenda and in terms of the developing parent–child relationship. In the hands of a developmentally informed clinician, the NBO enables the parents to understand better the meaning and the developmental significance of their infant's behaviors and of their own feelings about themselves as parents and the implications of the observations for caregiving. Providing the developmental information to parents, in turn, will help parents better appreciate the importance of each individual behavior as it relates to the infant's overall functioning. Parents may not be aware of the significance of the more subtle signs of stress (e.g., color change, gaze aversion,

---

[1]To eliminate the excessive use of "him or her" and "she or he" in this chapter, we are in some instances alternating the use of both.

hiccoughs, yawns), so the clinician can help parents understand their significance in terms of the infant's development. These observations can serve as the basis for guiding parents in identifying the appropriateness or inappropriateness of various levels of stimulation for their infant's development. The clinician thereby will sharpen the parents' awareness of their infant's threshold of responsiveness, enabling them to observe the handling techniques that promote the infant's overall organization. This level of interpretation requires that examiners have a thorough understanding of the theoretical framework of the NBO so that the discrete behaviors will be meaningful within the broader context of the infant's adaptation to his newly experienced extrauterine environment.

Because the NBO is a relationship-building tool, the clinician must have well-developed clinical skills in working with parents. The best way for pediatric professionals to communicate to parents the information that is derived from the NBO is by including them as partners in the NBO session. The clinician, therefore, must be ready to acknowledge and respond sympathetically to the concerns or questions of the parents throughout the session, eliciting their participation to the degree with which they feel comfortable. It is this clinical openness that can set the stage for successful communication around the observation of the infant and set the collaborative tone of the session. Because the NBO is an interactive system, the clinician needs to have the therapeutic skills to provide caregiving information in a nonjudgmental way and such that the parents develop insight into themselves and their infants (deGangi, 2002). Although the NBO training program includes a mentoring component and the chapters in this handbook provide guidelines on relationship building, the value of the kind of ongoing reflective supervision described by Costa (2006); Fenichel (1992); Gilkerson and Shahmoon-Shanook (2000); McDonough (2000); Pawl, St. John, and Pekarsky (2000); and Weatherston (2000) cannot be underestimated. Because relationship-building work with infants and parents tends to evoke complex emotional responses in professionals, it is important, as Fenichel (1992) pointed out, that clinicians have the opportunity for reflection on their practice within the context of an ongoing supervisory relationship.

The clinician who uses the NBO must have a keen awareness of the importance of cultural differences in child-rearing philosophies and practices so that he or she uses the NBO in a way that is nonjudgmental and nonprescriptive. In this way, the NBO can be used with parents from any cultural background and in a way that can allow them to integrate the observations about their infant into their own child-rearing philosophy and practices. (This is described in detail in Chapter 8.)

## Administration, Interpretation, and Caregiving Guidelines

Although the ability to elicit and describe the full range of the infant's behavior for parents is essential for the administration of the NBO, the clinician's ability to interpret these observations in terms of the infant's current developmental agenda is the hallmark of the skilled clinician. The material that is presented in this manual

is designed to provide not only information on administration and scoring guidelines but also background developmental and clinical information to help clinicians interpret each behavior and to discuss with the parents the implications for
caregiving, but this information will need to be complemented and deepened by
material from the other chapters in this book and other sources to prepare the clinician adequately to meet the needs of infants and all families. This manual provides a summary of the background information on the underlying research and
theory behind the items of the NBO behaviors so that the clinician can help parents
understand the meaning of these discrete behaviors in terms of the overall developmental challenges that the newborn infant faces. Interpreting the behavior in
terms of its developmental significance will enable the parents to see the discrete
behaviors as part of a whole, as part of the infant's unique style of interacting, or
as part of the infant's struggle to adapt to this new, extrauterine world. Observations of hand-to-mouth movements, for example, can be interpreted as reflecting a
high level of motor organization but also, in context, may be an index of the infant's
self-regulating or self-consoling capacities. Sharing such an observation with parents and asking parents to share their own observations and interpretations of this
behavior confirms the parents' own observation skills and respects the parents'
values on the one hand and helps the parents reframe their observations in light of
the new information that is proffered by the clinician on the other hand.

The individual items of the NBO are presented under the following headings:

1.  Administration: Guidelines on how to elicit and describe each behavior to par-
    ents are presented.

2.  Recording: Each of the observed behaviors is coded on a three-point scale,
    from "weak" to "fairly strong" to "very strong," or from "not responsive" to
    "moderately responsive" to "very responsive," for example.

3.  Interpretation: The infant's behavior is explained and interpreted in terms of
    its adaptive and developmental significance.

4.  Developmental sequence: The developmental sequence of the behavior from
    embryonic appearance through the first months of life is described.

5.  Implications for caregiving: The possible implications of this behavior for
    caregiving are discussed with the parents.

The nature and amount of material that is presented to parents during any one
session will be shaped by salient issues of the session and will always depend on
factors such as the relationship between the parents and the clinician, the emotional availability of the parents, the health and well-being of the mother, the
health and behavior of the infant, and the degree of the parents' knowledge about
child development. The amount of information presented and how it is presented
will be different for clinicians who are likely to see the parent in a follow-up visit,

as opposed to a one-time encounter with the parents and their infant. In addition, the importance of information on feeding issues, for example, may be more immediate and pressing in the early days of life, whereas parents may have more questions about sleep–wake states at the 2-week or 1-month visit than at the initial session, or there may be more pressing questions about crying at the 2-month follow-up visit. No individual session could hope to include information on all of the behavioral areas that are covered by the NBO, so each clinician has to respect and respond to the parents' individual needs and then judge the depth and the range of the interpretive material to be presented.

The goal of the clinician is to share the observations and interpretations with the parents in a way that is supportive and collaborative and that acknowledges the role of the parents as the primary caregivers in the infant's life. Many clinicians invite the parents to elicit some of the behaviors and provide them with appropriate facilitation to do this appropriately. Some of the social interaction items, such as observing the infant's response to the human voice, are often best elicited by asking the parents to call the infant's name; the response to face and voice can also be elicited by the parents. The habituation items can easily be elicited by parents with guidance from the clinician, while parents already know how to elicit behaviors such as rooting, sucking, and hand grasp.

The recording takes place afterwards, so as not to interfere with the flow of the session, take the focus away from the infant's behavior as it unfolds, or interfere with communication with parents. Each behavior is coded on a three-point scale, from optimal (3) to nonoptimal (1), to capture the infant's level of adaptation across behavioral domains. However, it must be pointed out that this recording scheme is designed to describe behavioral variability and individuality. The "1" rating does not imply pathology; it is simply a descriptor that can be integrated into the overall summary of the infant's behavior. Clinicians must train themselves to remember what they have observed when moving through the NBO items, so that the behavior can be reliably recorded when all the items have been administered and then summarized for the parents. Recording an observation on the NBO recording form can help clinicians refine their own observations skills.

## Newborn Behavioral Observations System: Contents

The NBO is a brief neurobehavioral scale that consists of 18 behavioral and reflex items designed to describe the newborn's physiological, motor, state, and social capacities. On the basis of the assumption that the developmental agenda of the newborn infant involves the integration of the autonomic, motor, state, and interactive systems, the NBO items include startles, lability of color, and tremulousness; muscle tone, activity level, sucking, and rooting; habituation to sound and light; crying and soothability; and attentional-interactive behavior.

> The NBO is not a diagnostic scale; it is not designed to describe or assess the parameters of typical or atypical behavior.

The following are the NBO items and the modal sequence of administration that are used in the introduction and initial observation of the infant state:

1. Habituation to light (flashlight)

2. Habituation to sound (rattle)

*Uncover and undress (optional).*

3. Muscle tone: legs and arms

4. Rooting

5. Sucking

6. Hand grasp

7. Shoulder and neck tone (pull-to-sit)

8. Crawling response

9. Response to face and voice

10. Visual response (to face)

11. Orientation to voice

12. Orientation to sound (rattle)

13. Visual tracking (red ball)

14. Crying

15. Soothability

16. State regulation

17. Response to stress: color changes, tremors, startles

18. Activity level

## Administration Sequence of the NBO

The administration of all 18 items, with description and discussion, may take approximately 5 to 10 minutes to complete. However, because it is designed to be used flexibly, some sessions will take less time, whereas others will last much longer, depending on the goals of the session and the nature of the clinical issues that emerge in the course of the observation. This chapter presents guidelines for the sequential administration and interpretation of all 18 behaviors. This will serve as the basic model, although, as already pointed out, the sequence of item presentation will vary according to the needs and vicissitudes of each clinical environment, and each NBO session will be shaped by the goals of the clinician and the nature of the clinical contract between the clinician and the family.

## The Introduction

The clinician should use the initial phase of the session to create an open, warm, nonthreatening atmosphere for the parents and the family. It is important that parents understand that the NBO is not a diagnostic examination designed to identify pathological or atypical signs or assess the infant's typicality. Rather, it is a competency-based approach designed to describe the infant's behavioral capacities and to join parents in identifying the kinds of caregiving strategies that are best suited to the infant's needs. The clinician therefore invites parents to become involved as partners in the observation and conveys to them that he or she is ready to acknowledge their questions and concerns and values their expertise. In this way the clinician and the parents know what to expect from the session. The position of the bassinet or the crib and where the parents and clinician sit should be considered, because these seemingly small "choreographic" preparations convey the clinician's underlying assumptions about the nature of this encounter and how participants can be expected to relate to each other. (This is discussed in more detail in Chapter 4.) When the clinician has established the tone of the session and is about to begin, it is useful to introduce the session with a general description of its aims. For example:

> "Over the next few minutes, we would like to learn as much as we can about your infant—what she is able to do and what she finds difficult or challenging at this time. Above all, we want to find out what makes her unique so that you can learn what she needs from you to help her grow and develop." Or, "Together, let us observe your infant's behavior. In this way, we can learn how he is responding to his new world to see what attracts him and to learn what is stressful for him and how he would like you to help him." Or simply, "Let's see what she would like to tell us about herself through her behavior."

This kind of introduction will vary from environment to environment and, above all, will reflect the clinician's specific professional goals and the goals for this particular family. After the introduction, it can be helpful to ask parents what they have already observed about their infant, which can serve as a baseline for the subsequent observations. Questions such as "What have you noticed about your child so far?" allow parents to share their own experiences and perceptions of their infant. (This subject is addressed in subsequent chapters in terms of different disciplines and environments.) It also may be helpful for the clinician to explain to parents before the session begins that although nothing that is done in the NBO is painful, most infants cry during some portion of the session. This may be an opportunity to ask parents how they feel about their infant's crying. It may be reassuring to explain that infants often cry in response to changes in their environment and to give examples of these changes that are familiar to parents, (e.g., waking up, having diaper changed, being dressed). It also may be helpful to tell parents that the NBO is designed to enable parents to observe how well the infant can quiet himself or be soothed and to listen to the quality of the cry. This explanation may reduce the parents' anxiety if or when the infant does cry during the session. Describing the purpose of the NBO can reduce parents' anxiety and provide a realistic goal for their expectations, because some parents may assume that it is a test that will produce a pass/fail result.

The clinician then may describe briefly the sequence of observations as it is likely to proceed or, alternatively, give a description of the major areas of functioning—the autonomic, motor, organization of state, and responsivity (AMOR) sequence (described in detail in Chapters 1 and 6)—and explain that the NBO will examine the infant's thresholds of responsivity to the various levels of stimulation.

### Overall Administration Sequence Summary

After the introduction, the clinician invites the parents to quietly observe their infant's behavioral state. If the infant is in a sleep state, the clinician can begin with the habituation items. The habituation items can provide an excellent environment for the clinician and the parents to share observations and to establish rapport. If the infant is in the father's arms, for example, it is preferable to leave him there and begin the administration of the habituation items. There is as yet no tactile manipulation of the infant, so together the parents and the clinician can observe the infant's responses and discuss the implications of what they see for the development of his sleep behavior. The clinician now shines a light into the infant's closed eyes at 5-second intervals, up to 10 times, to see how the infant responds and whether he can *shut out,* or habituate to, the stimulus. "Shut out," or habituation, takes place when the infant is no longer responding to the stimulus for at least two consecutive presentations of the stimulus. Then the clinician shakes the rattle at the same pace, up to 10 times, to see whether the infant can shut out the sound. This will show how well the infant is able to protect his sleep states in the face of unpredictable, disturbing stimuli and provides the clinician and the parents with a forum to begin a discussion of the development of the infant's sleep–wake states and, above all, to discuss the kinds of handling techniques that can best promote the infant's development in this area. By the third week, management of sleep and decision making about how to promote the infant's sleep usually are central issues for parents.

The infant then is uncovered and undressed (if deemed necessary). Observing the infant's adjustment to being uncovered, to being undressed, and to being placed supine provides important information for parents about the infant's response to various levels of tactile stimulation.

Moving on to the infant's reflexes and muscle tone by observing the infant's tone in the arms, legs, shoulders, and neck, the clinician and the parents can begin to formulate approaches or strategies to meet the infant's motor needs. Does he need to be swaddled more? Does he need more shoulder and neck support? How can the parents help him develop hand-to-mouth, self-quieting abilities? Is he cuddly or hypertonic? How does he like to be held? In this way, the clinician engages the parents for a search of the underlying causes of the behavior and allows them to suggest strategies to support the infant. As the clinician moves through the rooting, sucking, pull-to-sit, hand grasp, and crawling maneuvers, he or she describes the infant's response and continues to observe the infant's response to stress and how much he cries, how easily he is upset, and how easily he can be soothed. Throughout the session, as the infant is exposed to the various levels of stimulation or handling, the clinician and the parents observe the infant's threshold for stimulation and the amount of crying. Does the infant move easily from sleep to wake states, or does he remain in an insulated crying state? Again, by the 3-week visit, management of crying is a matter of concern for many parents because they may see that the onset of colic and much of the attention in the session is addressed to the state organization items. All the while, particular attention is paid to the infant's threshold levels to ascertain what may be overstimulating for him or what kind of handling he prefers. The infant's autonomic functioning is ascertained by observation of the number of color changes, tremors, and startles or variations in the respiratory patterns.

Finally, the clinician examines the infant's attentional interactive capacities and his response to the face and voice and sound of the rattle and his ability to track a red ball. As the infant's capacity for alertness expands as the weeks go by, the clinician and the parents learn how to promote the infant's attention and read his communication cues and how to interact with him.

## Summary Profile and Recommendations

After the session, the parents and the clinician together construct a profile of the infant's behavioral repertoire, identifying her strengths and the areas in which she needs support. The clinician can begin either by asking the parents questions such as, "What did you notice about your infant's behavior?" or, "What struck you about your infant's behavior?" or, "Was there anything that surprised you?" This can provide a base for a joint summary and integration of the observations. Some parents find a narrative of the session helpful so that the clinician and the parents can share their recollection from the beginning of the session; for example, "Remember what happened when we shined the light in her eyes when she was asleep?" The clinician can frame the discussion by emphasizing the infant's responses to the graded levels of stimulation over the whole session, thereby enabling parents to identify more readily with the infant's thresholds of responsiveness and the levels of stimulation that were either overstimulating or appropriate.

This is especially effective in the case of preterm infants. Some clinicians use the four behavioral dimensions described in Chapter 1 as the basis for summarizing what they have observed. This allows the clinician and the parents to talk about the infant's 1) autonomic, 2) motor, 3) organization of state, and 4) responsivity (AMOR) dimensions and how they are being integrated by the infant at this time.

Then, the clinician and the parents together fill out the final section of the NBO recording form (Figure 3.1). This serves to confirm the parents' role as partners in the observation of their infant. This joint endeavor, in which parents classify the infant's behavior in terms of the infant's strengths as well as the challenges with which she needs special support should give the parents a sense of efficacy and confirm for them their central role as observers. Working from the anticipatory guidance checklist, the clinician can then discuss the kinds of strategies that will enhance the infant's behavioral organization, on the one hand, and promote an interactive match between the parents and their infant, on the other hand. This guidance is future oriented in that it is designed to help parents prepare for the next stage of their infant's development.

In summary, the NBO examines the newborn's behavioral repertoire by describing the infant's strengths as well as the challenges or difficulties she faces in her efforts to adapt to her extrauterine environment. The NBO items yield a profile of the infant's behavioral capacities in a way that does justice to the full richness of her behavioral repertoire and that can capture her individuality or uniqueness. Because it also is an interactive scale, the parents' own observations and feelings should always be integrated into the session. Moreover, whenever possible, the parents should have an opportunity to elicit some of the items. This is especially true of the interactive items, such as soothability, or the social interactive items. The clinician merely guides the parents in eliciting the infant's response to the voice, for example, by describing the best distance and the kind of tone that is most likely to engage the infant's interest. In general, the clinician maintains a collaborative stance toward parents throughout. Finally, the clinician and the parents discuss the newborn's strengths and challenges and identify the kinds of caregiving strategies they believe will enhance the infant's growth and development and facilitate the parents' efforts to help their infant meet the challenges of the next stage of development.

## ADMINISTRATION, RECORDING, INTERPRETATION, AND CAREGIVING GUIDELINES

The NBO is applicable for healthy term infants, from 36 weeks' gestational age up to 3 months post-term, but in the hands of an experienced clinician, it can be used with younger, more fragile infants under certain optimal conditions, as described in Chapter 6. It can be administered in hospitals, clinics, doctors' offices, early intervention centers, or the home. The NBO kit consists of a rattle, a red ball, a flashlight, and the NBO recording form (Figure 3.1) and the NBO recording guidelines

(Figure 3.2). Although it may not be possible, especially in the case of home visits, it is recommended that the NBO be carried out in a semidarkened room and that the room temperature be between 72°F and 80°F. It is preferable to begin midway between the infant's feedings.

## Observing Behavioral States

Begin the NBO session with a brief observation of the infant's state. If the infant is in a sleep state, then proceed with the two habituation items. If the infant is not asleep, uncover, and, if appropriate, undress him. Assess the tone in the legs and the arms or do the orientation items. If the infant is crying, observe soothability, but if the infant is asleep, observe the regularity or irregularity of breathing, the presence or absence of eye movements under closed eyelids, and the presence or absence of movement, including startles or tremors. This will reveal whether the infant is in a deep sleep state with no rapid eye movement (non-REM sleep) or a light sleep state with rapid eye movement (REM sleep), and the infant's sleep organization and his capacity to protect his sleep from negative or obtrusive external stimulation to the visual system can be observed.

This may be a good time for the clinician to categorize newborn behaviors for the parents by first pointing out that certain behavioral patterns or behavioral states have similar characteristics, tend to recur, and can be recognized and identified easily in newborns. These are referred to as *behavioral states* (Brazelton, 1973; Prechtl & Beintema, 1964; Wolff, 1959). These behaviors tend to co-occur and can be observed and identified reliably. The clinician needs to be able to translate this concept in a way that parents can understand easily, adding, perhaps, that being able to identify these states is indispensable in helping them get to know their infant. The clinician can begin by asking parents what they have noticed so far about their infant's wake and sleep patterns and then, building on that, describing the following six behavioral states of the infant as he or she begins the NBO administration:

1. Deep sleep state: regular, shallow breathing, eyes closed, no spontaneous movement, and no rapid eye movement; startles may appear approximately every 5 minutes (see Figure 3.3)
2. Light sleep state: eyes closed, irregular respirations (in depth and rate), and more modulated motor activity; rapid eye movement is present along with facial expressions, even half-smiles, and sucking (see Figure 3.4)
3. Drowsy or semi-alert state: eyes may be half-open or open and closed; activity levels are variable (see Figure 3.5)
4. Quiet alert state: bright look and minimal motor activity (see Figure 3.6)
5. Active alert state: eyes open and considerable motor activity; fussing may or may not be present (see Figure 3.7)
6. Crying state: This prolonged intense crying may be referred to as "State 6 crying" in the material that follows to differentiate it from the kind of indeterminate fussing that can appear in the active alert state, State 5 (see Figure 3.8)

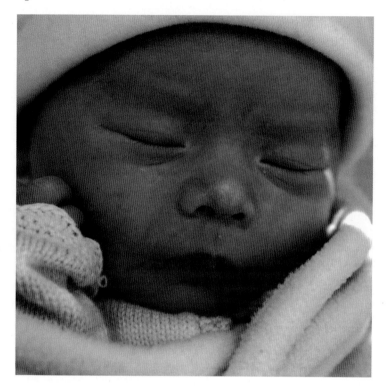

**Figure 3.3.** Deep sleep state.

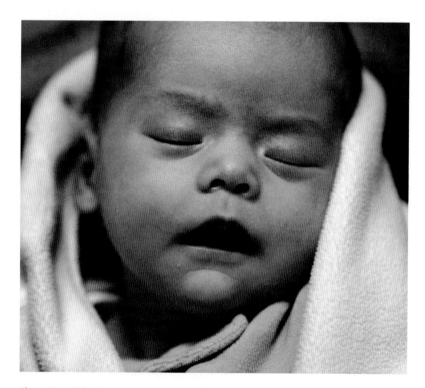

**Figure 3.4.** Light sleep state.

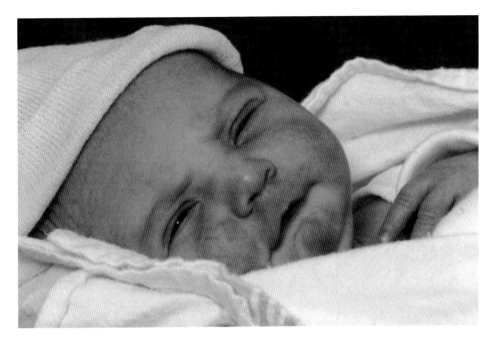

**Figure 3.5.** Drowsy state.

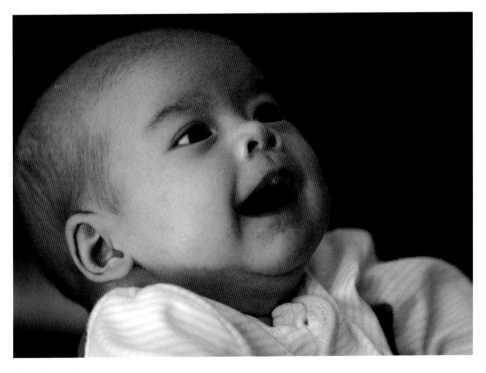

**Figure 3.6.** Quiet alert state.

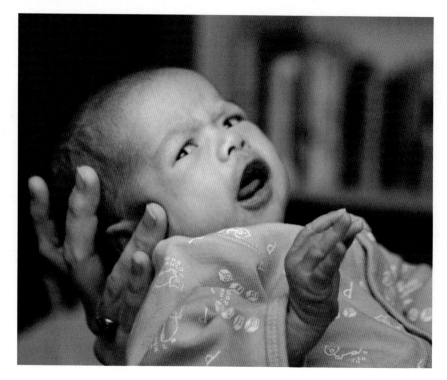

**Figure 3.7.** Active alert state.

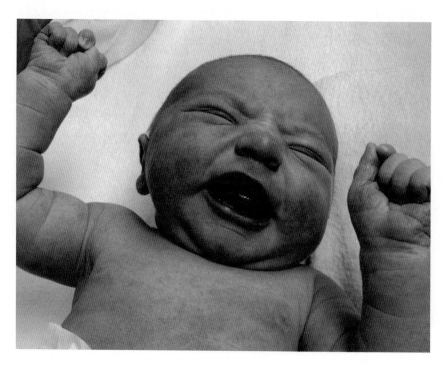

**Figure 3.8.** Crying state.

By recognizing that infants have different states, parents can begin to understand the temporal structure of the newborn's life and thereby are better able to predict the infant's behavior. Although many parents have observed these behaviors, naming them and categorizing them can serve to heighten the parents' awareness that there are defined, predictable periods when the infant is asleep or awake. Moreover, the concept of *behavioral states* provides parents with a frame or a lens to enable them to organize their own observations about their infant and learn to read their infant's behavioral cues. In addition, *state* is a powerful concept for parents to help them understand their infant's behavior and to recognize the appropriateness of their handling techniques or the quality of the stimulation they need to provide to meet the needs of their infant. They will begin to recognize that certain activities are more appropriate in one state than in another (e.g., an infant who is in a deep sleep state will not respond to feeding, and the mother's attempt to feed will not be beneficial for the infant). The notion that feeding is more likely to be rewarding for both infant and mother in the awake states is an important point that can be emphasized at this time.

At this stage, the clinician takes out the flashlight and presents a series of aversive or disturbing stimuli to the sleeping infant and describes what he or she is doing. The clinician should mention to the parents at the outset that this next maneuver is not a test of hearing or vision but, rather, examines the infant's capacities to defend himself from disturbing, negative visual and auditory stimulation while asleep; it examines the infant's ability to protect his sleep. As such, the next two items attempt to replicate the unpredictability of the extrauterine environment to which the newborn must adapt in the neonatal period. This is an opportunity to observe how he copes with these stresses by observing closely his responses and the decrement in response to the following visual and auditory stimuli:

1. Habituation to light (response to flashlight)

2. Habituation to sound (response to rattle)

## Administration

The light stimulus (flashlight) first is presented. If the infant is still in a sleep state, then the clinician shines the light from a distance of approximately 10 to 12 inches (25–30 cm) across the infant's eyes for no more than a second (see Figure 3.9). The clinician observes the infant's response and continues to shine the light every 5 seconds until the infant's responses have shown a clear decrease in the level of responsivity. If the infant is not able to decrease his level of responding or shut out the stimulus entirely and return to a lower state, then the clinician discontinues after 10 presentations. The aim of this observation is to see how well the infant is able to deal with or shut out this negative, obtrusive visual stimulus. The infant may respond with a startle, body movement, change of position, or merely a grimace. The clinician notes the first response carefully because this is the baseline against which

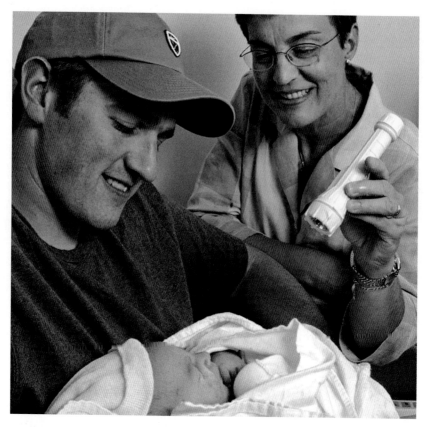

**Figure 3.9.**  Habituation to light (flashlight).

"shut down" will be measured. The clinician waits for 5 seconds and then shines the light again and continues every 5 seconds until a clear-cut decrease in response level is observed. This may happen even after one or two presentations. The infant may respond initially with a startle, and by the second presentation, she may merely show a grimace. Some infants will find it difficult to tolerate this level of stimulation and may continue to respond. The clinician observes the infant's movements during this exercise and watches for any signs of stress, such as color change, tremors, or startles, which will give an insight into the quality of the infant's response decrement. Up to 10 presentations may be performed if there is no "shut down." Some infants may not be able to shut out the light and may wake up or begin to cry. The clinician can point out the increase or decrease in responses to the stimuli in terms of the infant's gross body movements, startles, tremors, changes in respiration, REM, facial movements, mouthing, color changes, and so forth.

If the infant is still in a sleep state, then the clinician proceeds to administer the habituation to sound maneuver and follows the same administrative guidelines as in the previous item. The clinician shakes the rattle approximately 10 to 12 inches (25–30 cm) from the infant's ear, using a brisk, repetitive (two to three

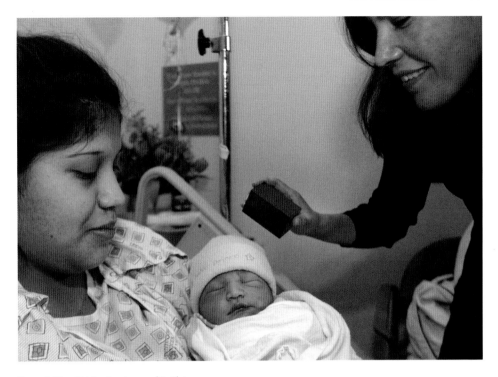

**Figure 3.10.** Habituation to sound (rattle).

times) staccato shaking movement that lasts approximately 1–2 seconds (see Figure 3.10). Again, the clinician observes the infant's response and continues to shake the rattle every 5 seconds until the infant's responses have shown a clear decrease in the level of responsivity. As in the case of the light, the clinician waits for 5 seconds and then shakes the rattle again. The clinician continues to shake the rattle every 5 seconds until a clear-cut decrease in response level is observed. Again, up to 10 presentations may be performed if there is no "shut down."

## Recording

With ease: Habituates to stimulus with ease (after one or up to five presentations)

With some difficulty: Habituates with some difficulty (after six or more presentations)

With great difficulty: Still unable to habituate to the stimulus after 10 presentations

It should be pointed out that each NBO item is recorded on a 3-point scale, with 3 being optimal, 2 being moderate or in between, and 1 being less optimal.

## Interpretation

As the clinician and the parents observe the infant's behavior, the clinician can point out that the infant's ability to maintain extended sleep states and eliminate responses to irrelevant or disturbing stimuli are major factors in caloric conservation and thermal homeostasis. The clinician can interpret this behavior in terms of its adaptive value, the infant's self-regulation, and the infant's ability to protect her sleep. Habituation also can be seen as a primitive form of learning, with the presumption that the newborn infant can store an integral representation of a stimulus and compare subsequent inputs with the one already stored. The capacity to habituate in the newborn period can be depressed as a result of obstetric medication. Similarly, nutritional status, gestational age, intrauterine exposure to drugs, and other perinatal variables will affect habituation behavior (Als, 1982, 1984; Lester & Zeskind, 1978).

The habituation item highlights the infant's self-regulatory capacities and capacity to protect sleep (Bornstein & Suess, 2000; Porges, Doussard-Roosevelt, Stifter, McClenny, & Riniolo, 1999). The infant's capacity to maintain sleep in the face of such disturbing environmental stimulation is an index of the contribution she is making to her own growth and development. This item also presents a unique opportunity to observe the infant's stress signs as she attempts to cope with this essentially negative stimulus. The obvious global stress signs (e.g., crying, startles, tremors, rapid color change, spitting up, apneic spells) can be interpreted easily. The more subtle signs of stress (e.g., grimaces, mouthing movements, changes in respiration, slight color changes) may be less obvious to the parents but are important stress cues. They may be interpreted accurately as the "cost" to the infant of maintaining a sleep state in the face of an intrusive stimulus.

It is the selective nature of the newborn's capacities to deal with stimuli that is a major focus for the interpretation to the parents. Whereas the alert newborn will choose to orient selectively to these stimuli when presented in an appropriate state, the well-organized sleeping infant will be able to shut out these same stimuli and protect his sleep. (Later in the session, the clinician and the parents may be able to see how the infant responds to this same auditory stimulus when he is in an awake state.) The infant's remarkable self-protective mechanisms are pointed out and his self-regulating capacities are highlighted in these items as he attempts to maintain himself in a sleep state despite the increasingly invasive nature of the stimulation.

## Developmental Sequence

In the newborn period, the parameters of habituation show wide variation and individual differences. Some infants have difficulty in shutting out the stimuli. Hypersensitive reactions may occur when the infant's level of tolerance to stimulation is low (low threshold) or the central nervous system (CNS) does not habituate efficiently to sensations (Miller, Reisman, McIntosh, & Simon, 2001). As result, the sensitive infant may display excessive crying and/or withdrawal from sensory stimuli.

This discussion of habituation may lead to a more in-depth examination of sleep behavior in newborns. In terms of the developmental sequence of state regulation and the development of sleep–wake patterns in particular, the first 3 months of life can be called a period of transition as the infant's behavior and physiology shift from intrauterine to extrauterine regulation and her developmental agenda centers on the regulation of her states (Mirmiran & Lunshof, 1996). During this period, there are marked changes in many aspects of infant functioning, stemming from the electrical patterns of brain activity (Emde et al., 1979) and influencing the regulation of visual attention and sleep (Rothbart, Posner, & Boylan, 1994). Infants in the newborn period are beginning to develop individual sleep–wake cycles as they try to acquire day–night, wake–sleep patterns, but the length of sleep–wake cycles changes with age (Barr, 1998; DiPietro, Hodgson, Costigan, & Hilton, 1996).

Newborns sleep from 16 to 18 hours a day, or approximately 60% to 70% of the time, and rarely sleep for longer than 4½ hours at a time (Davis et al., 2004). The extended sleep states of the newborn are associated with lower metabolic rates and comprise the infant's major energy conservation strategy. Conversely, crying or excessive wakefulness increases metabolism and depletes the infant's energy levels, which is particularly costly for small or preterm infants. In term infants, active sleep (REM sleep) occupies 45% to 50% of total sleep time, whereas indeterminate sleep occupies 10% and quiet sleep (non-REM) occupies 35% to 45% of total sleep time. That infants spend most of their time in REM sleep has led researchers to speculate that REM sleep stimulates the growth of the neural systems (DiPietro, Hodgson, Costigan, & Hilton, 1996). This may explain why preterm infants spend nearly all of their sleeping time in quiet REM sleep. Although stimulation of REM sleep may safeguard the growth of the CNS, others have argued that as the brain cycles through REM-sleep periods, REMs stir up the vitreous (gelatin-like substance within the eye), ensuring that the eye is fully oxygenated (Blumberg & Lucas, 1996).

The greatest change is that the sleep–wake pattern conforms to a circadian rhythm, or a 24-hour schedule (Goodlin-Jones et al., 2000). As Anders et al. (1992) pointed out, newborns do not seem to know night from day, so one of the key tasks for the newborn infant during the first 2 to 3 months is to establish a predicable day–night rhythm (Ikonomov, Stoynev, & Shisheva, 1998). Some may sleep through the night after only a few months, whereas others will take much longer. By 3 months, the infant needs only 14 hours of sleep per day, and periods of a quiet alert state become longer and more robust (Anders et al., 1992). In general, the task of state regulation must be negotiated successfully before the infant can maintain prolonged moments of mutual gaze with her caregiver and develop the capacity for shared mutual engagement that constitutes the major task of the next stage of development (Adamson, 1996; Brazelton et al., 1974; Stern, 1995; Trevarthen, 1993; Tronick, 1989, 1998).

In general, the ease with which infants can develop sleep–wake regulation increases with age, although there are great differences that distinguish the development of infants' sleep–wake patterns (Stern, 1977). During the first months of life, the organization of sleep and wakefulness and the length of sleep–wake cycles will change substantially. In general, the ability of the infant to maintain uninterrupted sleep cycles increases with age, so that by 6 or 7 months of age, the infant may sleep for up to 10 hours at a time and may begin to sleep through the night.

## Implications for Caregiving

Many newborns, in the face of routine or unpredictable stimulation, show a remarkable resistance to being disturbed: They shut out the stimuli and maintain a prolonged sleeping state. This enables parents to appreciate better that their infant may not be as fragile or vulnerable as they may have thought. Even when there are siblings present or the family is living in a crowded space, this will be a good indicator of how well the infant effectively can shut out the noise and light and maintain prolonged sleeping periods. This ability, in turn, promotes the infant's adaptation and growth. The ability to adapt to the steady stream of stimulation that is experienced in a typical household is essential for an infant to maintain calm, organized internal states and regular sleep/feeding rhythms and to be able to engage in successful interactions with caregivers (Ayres, 1979; Dunn, 1977). There are data to suggest that ineffective habituation to stimulation can compromise the parent–child relationship (DeGangi, Craft, & Castellan, 1991; Maldonado-Duran & Sauceda-Garcia, 1996).

Some infants whose sleep protection is less well developed may need more environmental support to help them develop better sleep regulation. Setting aside a quiet dark or shaded space in the home might be less stressful for the infant and may make it easier for him to protect his sleep and to develop more robust sleep–wake patterns at his own pace and with support from the caregiving environment. If parents learn to recognize the sleep–wake patterns, they can prepare the newborn more easily for feeding at appropriate times.

Finally, questions of where the infant should sleep may come up at this juncture. It is important for clinicians to remember that sleeping practices reflect a culture's socialization goals, or what parents want for their children, and therefore is strongly influenced by cultural values (Barr, 1991; Kawasaki, Nugent, Miyashita, Miyahara, & Brazelton, 1994; Lozoff, Wolf, & Davis, 1984; Nugent & Brazelton, 2000). Parent–infant co-sleeping is the norm for 90% of the world's population, whereas it has been reported that 89% of infants in the United States sleep alone. On the basis of studies of sudden infant death syndrome (SIDS), the American Academy of Pediatrics officially recommends that the safest sleep environment for young infants is in a separate crib/bassinet with a firm mattress in the same room as the parents. The most recent edition of Dr. Spock's *Infant and Child Care* (Spock & Needleman, 2004) advised parents to move their infants into their own rooms by 3 months of age. On the other hand, McKenna (2000) and McKenna and Moskol (2001) cited the low incidence of SIDS in countries where co-sleeping is the norm (usually with light covering on hard surfaces or with the infant in a bas-ket next to the parents), and a recent longitudinal study showed no differences in infants who had bed-shared in their early years in terms of their psychosocial ad-justment at 18 years (Okami, Weisner, & Olmstead, 2002). Researchers point out that many factors, including maternal cigarette smoking during and after preg-nancy, prenatal abuse of drugs, preterm birth, and low birth weight, increase the risk for SIDS (Hauck et al., 2003).

In general, it should be emphasized that there are wide variations in the sleep–wake patterns in newborns. It is reassuring for parents to know that some infants seem to require more sleep than others and that whereas some may sleep through the night after a few months, others will take much longer to do that.

## Uncovering, Undressing (Optional), and Placing Supine

Uncovering and placing the infant on her back provides an opportunity to ob-serve tone, posture, and activity level and to see how the infant responds to being handled or moved. Removing the cover may stimulate a state change in the infant, especially if she had been well swaddled. Removing the infant's clothing makes it possible to observe color change across the whole body. However, room tempera-ture and cultural concerns should guide the clinician in making this decision in collaboration with the parents.

### Administration

The infant is uncovered and undressed (if deemed appropriate). The clinician places the infant supine, head in midline. The infant's responses can be described in terms of state change, postural adjustments, and movements of the extremities. Some infants may find this very stressful because they may need the support of the clothes to inhibit their random arm movements, and tight swaddling may be necessary to help these infants maintain solid sleep and alert states. If the infant is alert, then this is a good opportunity to observe her level of activity.

If the infant begins to cry at any time during these items, then the clinician should wait no more than 10 seconds before beginning the consoling maneuvers, which are described in the Soothability section. If, however, the infant comes to an alert state, then the clinician proceeds to observe the physical/motor items or the social interactive items.

### Recording

This is not recorded because it is not an item, per se, on the NBO.

### Interpretation

Observing the infant's adjustment to being uncovered, to being undressed, and to being placed supine provides important information for parents about the infant's response to various levels of tactile stimulation. These procedures may be stressful for some newborns and may result in decreases in body temperature and disturbance of the infant's sleep period. Observing how easily infants readjust their posture to this item will reveal the quality of their self-organizing abilities. Many infants use the asymmetric tonic neck response to regain their motoric and state equilibrium, whereas others may use hand-to-mouth maneuvers. The infant's activity level can be observed at this time: Some infants may show a high degree of spontaneous movement, whereas others may remain quiet with minimal motor activity. This also may be a good time to observe the quality and the robustness of the infant's motor system. Some infants may become jittery and emit spontaneous startles, whereas others will be able to maintain a "tucked" posture with minimal motor activity. The influence of primitive reflexes may be observed: The asymmetric tonic neck reflex may influence the position of the head and the extremities; the tonic labyrinthine reaction may manifest itself by setting off extension and kicking in the lower extremities; the rooting reflex may be elicited if the infant brings her hand close to her mouth. In general, this transitional item can provide the clinician and the parents with a unique opportunity to observe the infant's movements when she is in a supine position and can allow the clinician and the parents to identify the infant's individual self-regulation strategies.

## Developmental Sequence

The newborn's typical posture is one of *physiological flexion*, whereby the head is turned to one side, the hand is kept close to the mouth, and the legs are tucked in flexion. The infant will show random arm and leg movements—*stretching*—which may trigger startles or a change of state. The emergence of balance reactions in supine thus can be observed from the first day of life as the infant responds to the displacement of her center of gravity that is caused by her own movements.

By the end of the first month of life, movements become smoother and less random. The infant now can maintain a quiet posture while supine, with arms relaxed along the trunk (Piper & Darrah, 1994). The infant's ability to remain supine without stress improves over time as her ability to maintain a semiflexed posture in the arms and legs improves and as tone and motor organization develop during the first months of life. She will demonstrate reciprocal kicking movements by 2 months and will be able to control voluntarily the position of her arms and legs. The arm movements gradually relax, and by approximately 2½ months, the infant is able to lay her hands on her abdomen, tuck in her chin, and look at objects that are placed in front of her. The infant now can maintain her head firmly in midline, and she will begin to reach with more accuracy and grasp objects that are placed within reach. By 4 months of age, the infant can reach and play with her knees and be able to roll over to her side when lifting her legs.

## Implications for Caregiving

For some infants, being placed in a supine position can be stressful—for sleep or even during routine daily care (e.g., diapering). Parents can learn to minimize the level of stress by swaddling, tucking in the infant's arms, and inhibiting the infant's arm movements. Similarly, parents will be able to identify the infant's self-regulating strategies as the infant attempts to return to sleep.

## Muscle Tone: Legs and Arms

The next behavior to be observed is the quality of the infant's muscle tone—first in the legs and then in the arms.

### Administration

While the infant is supine and preferably in a relaxed alert state, the clinician holds each of the infant's legs in his or her hands, holding them firmly but gently between the ankle and the knee. The clinician flexes the legs at the knee by gently pushing them upward toward the trunk (see Figure 3.11). The clinician will observe how much consistency and resistance there is in the tone as he or she presses the legs and the quality of muscle elasticity or flexibility. Then, in one smooth movement, the clinician extends or stretches both legs as far as they can go and releases them to observe the quality of the recoil, or what Andre-Thomas and Dargassies (1960) referred to as *elasticité* or *extensibilité*. The clinician does the same with the arms—pressing and extending them to assess their level of flexibility and observing the quality of the retraction as they are released (see Figure 3.12).

### Recording

Strong: Well-modulated tone in legs and arms; good flexibility observed

Fairly strong: Mixed or uneven tone

Very high/very low: Either little or no tone or hypertonicity or rigidity observed in legs or arms

A recording of 3 means that the infant has excellent tone, while a recording of 1 means that the infant is either hypertonic or hypotonic. This should be recorded only if the infant is in a quiet alert state.

### Interpretation

These items examine the infant's tone while in a passive, relaxed state, as opposed to tone while being handled. This component of tone is related to muscle elasticity. Very tense, jittery infants may show extremely strong resistance to having their arms or legs extended; at the other end of the continuum, floppy infants show a complete lack of resistance. The infant who has typical passive tone shows moderate resistance against passive movement, with some variability ranging from high to low resistance and moderately brisk snapback in the arms and legs.

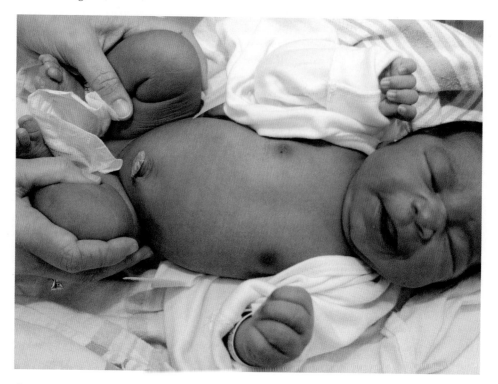

**Figure 3.11.** Muscle tone: legs.

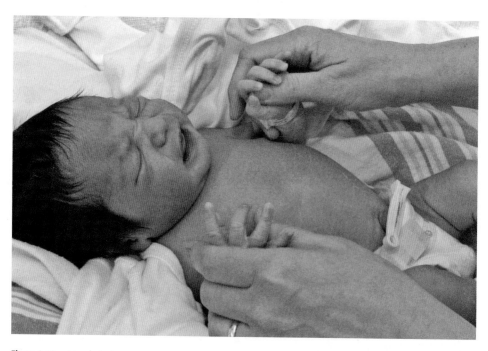

**Figure 3.12.** Muscle tone: arms.

## Developmental Sequence

The first isolated movements of the arms and legs can be seen in the eighth week after conception. Fetal movements peak at approximately the fifth month as many spontaneous movements come under the control of higher brain centers. By the time the infant is born, he has been exercising the kinds of arm and leg muscle movements needed for life outside the womb, and this muscle activity is critical for refining the infant's neural circuits.

The motor tone response is stronger in the first few days of life, when flexion postures predominate, but is present throughout the neonatal period. Dubowitz, Dubowitz, and Mercuri (1999) pointed out that the overall flexor tone of preterm infants at term is less marked than in term infants, and this reduction is more marked in the arms than in the legs. Although preterm infants show a recoil response to passive stretching of arms and legs, their response can be based on the quality of their overall flexor tone. They tend to show a more extended posture than term infants and show only a partial flexed posture, which often is accompanied by the asymmetrical tonic neck reflex. However, there is no evidence to conclude that hypertonic or hypotonic infants will continue to be so during the first year (Amiel-Tison & Grenier, 1986). Most infants who exhibit moderate signs of hypertonicity or hypotonicity in the neonatal period have typical passive tone by 3 months. In the case of persistent hypotonicity or excessive floppiness in the neonatal period, when these are accompanied by other clinical signs such as poor sucking, general hypotonia, poor interaction, and so forth, the observations of poor passive tone may be indicative of developmental problems. Nevertheless, it can be said that the evolution of passive tone varies considerably during the first year of life (Dargassies, 1977), so typical development falls within a very broad range.

## Implications for Caregiving

It has been pointed out that whereas extreme cases of high or low tone may have diagnostic significance (Prechtl, 1977), variations within the typical range do not have clear implications. Normal tone gives reassuring feedback to parents about the infant's typicality as they routinely handle their infant, and good tone may be considered important by parents as an indication of health and strength.

If, conversely, their infant is floppy or hyperextensible, there are many ways in which parents can facilitate their infant's motor development. Parents whose infants are hyperexcitable and extremely sensitive to stimulation, such as those who are withdrawing from narcotics or other medications, also can be taught to recognize how excessive proprioceptive or vestibular stimulation can overload their infants and how certain postural adjustments such as providing frontal inhibition through swaddling or placing the infant prone can facilitate tonal adjustment. Of singular importance is that whatever intervention is provided be individually tailored to an individual infant's needs (Denhoff, 1981). Similarly, in the case of floppy, unresponsive infants, parents can be encouraged to provide tactile-kinesthetic experiences as well as appropriate social stimulation during routine feeding and play episodes.

Gentle stroking of the infant and flexion and extension of the limbs have positive effects on the infant's behavioral development and enhance the parent–infant relationship itself (Field et al., 1986; Onozawa, Glover, Adams, Modi, & Kumar, 2001; Scafidi et al., 1993). However, it should be pointed out that each infant experiences sensory input in a unique way (Williamson, Anzalone, & Hanft, 2000), so parents have to be aware of their own infant's threshold for touch. Although there is no conclusive evidence that handling techniques such as these will modify motor outcome (Ferry, 1986), parents whose infants are eligible for early intervention services are taught to induce facilitatory postures during the routine care of their infants so that they can play a role as active participants in their own child's development. Preterm infants who were supported in their efforts to maintain a tucked posture during their hospital stay have been shown to develop tone that is closer to that of the term infant (Mouradian & Als, 1994). By participating in the NBO, these parents will be able to recognize their child's strengths and foster the infant's overall development, including social adaptive capacities, without being wholly preoccupied with the child's motor behavior. (See Vergara and Bigsby, 2004, for further information on developmental and therapeutic interventions with preterm infants.)

## Rooting

The rooting reflex is now elicited.

### Administration

The rooting response is elicited by gently stimulating the perioral skin at the corners of the mouth to see if the head or lips/mouth will turn to the stimulated side (see Figure 3.13).

### Recording

Strong: Turns to stimulated side

Fairly strong: Turns after latency

Weak: Minimal or no head turning

This means that a good optimal response is coded as 3, while little or no head turning is coded as 1. This response will be influenced by the infant's state, so that if the infant is in a sleep state, it should not be coded.

### Interpretation

The probability of the newborn infant's locating her mother's breast is increased by the ability to root toward stimuli that touch the cheek or oral area. The rooting

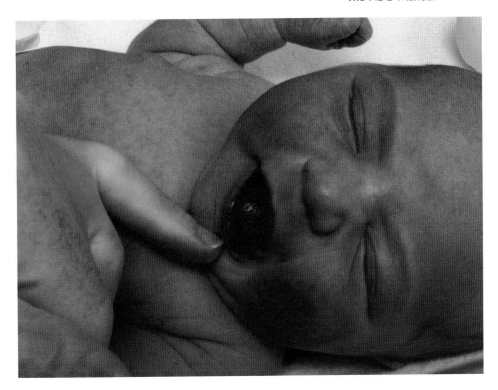

**Figure 3.13.**   Rooting.

reflex, which propels the infant to search for her mother's nipple, is displayed most intensely when the infant is hungry (Rochat & Hespos, 1997). Newborn infants are sensitive to touch. The infant's touch sensations are connected directly to the primary somatosensory region of the cerebral cortex. This well-developed sense of touch, which can be observed clearly in the rooting response, has clear-cut survival value. The rooting reflex facilitates the newborn's search for her mother's breast as a solution to this highly specific but critical problem.

The rooting will be more intense before a feeding when the stimulus is warm (Peiper, 1963). However, olfaction also seems to play a role in the newborn's capacity to find her mother's nipple (Macfarlane, 1975). Breast-fed infants show a preference for the smell of their own mother's breast scent over that of an unfamiliar lactating mother (Cernoch & Porter, 1985).

*Developmental Sequence*

Although simple reflexes such as head or limb withdrawal from a touch emerge early in gestation, the rooting reflex emerges at around the 24th week, when the infant turns her head and opens her mouth to a light stroke of the cheek. Most preterm infants who are 32 to 34 weeks old and are without medical or respiratory complications can be fed orally (Dubowitz et al., 1999). Rooting is present in preterm infants even before sucking is effective (Prechtl, 1977). However, immediately after birth, term infants who are placed face down between their mother's breasts spontaneously latch onto a nipple and begin sucking within an hour (Varendi & Porter, 2001). The rooting reflex begins to fade by the end of the first month, as voluntary head turning becomes more established.

## Implications for Caregiving

Touch is a fundamental means of interaction between parents and infants, and the rooting response is how the infant shows her readiness for feeding. In general, the positive effects of touch have been well documented. Infants experience a light touch and a firm touch differently, just as a touch on the face may be more intense than a touch on the arm. In the case of rooting, the stroking or touching of the area around the mouth stimulates the search for the breast, so mothers should be aware of the communicative meaning of this behavior and be ready to respond accordingly. Understanding this behavior as a set of purposeful movements helps mothers direct the infant's search efforts. They learn to see the head shaking that often appears as part of the infant's search and not as something negative, and they learn to avoid extraneous touch of the cheek (e.g., by blankets) that may interfere with turning to the correct side.

## Sucking

Moving from the observation of rooting, the sucking response is now elicited.

## Administration

The clinician places his or her index finger (gloved) into the infant's mouth with the pad toward the palate and attends to the strength and the rhythmicity of the suck (see Figure 3.14). The clinician then describes the responses to the sucking in terms of two components: strength (degree of negative pressure) and rate (regular or irregular). Obstetric medication levels will influence sucking rates, and responses are highly influenced by state.

## Recording

Strong: Initiates and maintains a modulated rhythmic suck

Fairly strong: Sluggish sucking movement

Weak: No sucking movement

A strong, well-organized sucking response merits a score of 3, while a weak, slow poorly organized sucking response merits a score of 1.

## Interpretation

A major task of the newborn is to obtain enough food to help him grow. The infant presses the nipple against the roof of his mouth and pushes out the milk. A

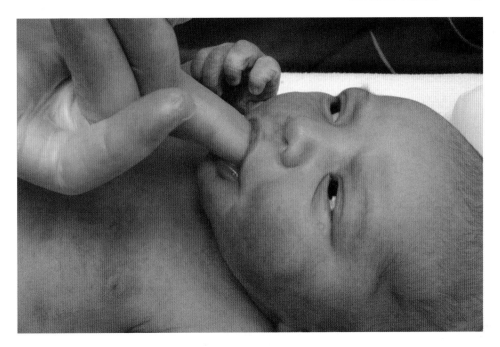

**Figure 3.14.**    Sucking.

major task for the newborn is to integrate sucking and breathing in a smooth pattern without having to release the nipple to breathe. Infants soon discover that they can swallow between inhaling and exhaling and begin to develop their own sucking rhythms. They begin to suck in bursts and then take a pause (Kaye & Brazelton, 1971; Kaye & Wells, 1980). This burst–pause pattern is even clearer during nonnutritive sucking and usually is accompanied by a high level of arousal and social availability. It is important to note that infants develop their own individual sucking styles (Dunn, 1977; Kron, Stein, & Goddard, 1966); turning away from the stimulated side may be observed in satiated infants.

Studies that have compared the sucking behavior of term infants and infants born at less than 34 weeks' gestational age indicate that maturation of the feeding apparatus occurs during the last months of gestation (Medoff-Cooper, McGrath, & Shults, 2002). Compared with term infants, the feeding bouts for preterm infants are shorter in duration with significantly lower sucking pressures, lower average sucking rates, and shorter bursts of sucking. A cross-sectional study by Medoff-Cooper et al. (2002) revealed that infants who are between 37 and 40 weeks, although considered term equivalents, have less mature sucking responses and do not feed as effectively as term infants. They have fewer sucks per feeding episode, decreased within-burst suck frequency, shorter sucking bursts, and lower sucking pressure than term infants. Even in term or near-term infants, the suck/swallow/breathe pattern may be uncoordinated, resulting in poor latch and inadequate milk transfer (Wolf & Glass, 1992).

Although sucking is a reflexive behavior, it is clear that it is modified through learning. There is evidence to show that infants can adjust their sucking pressure to how easily the milk flows from the nipple (Craig & Lee, 1999). Indeed, research has demonstrated that newborns can learn to adjust their level of sucking to produce interesting sights or sounds. For example, newborns suck faster to be able to see visual designs or hear music and human voices; therefore, sucking behavior can be seen as a powerful index of visual attention or auditory attention (Floccia, Christophe, & Bertoncini, 1997).

## Developmental Sequence

Embryos at just 5½ weeks after conception can sense touch to the lips or nose, and this rapidly extends to the rest of the body. In this early stage of fetal development, thalamic axons begin to form synapses onto their mature cortical targets and only after these connections are in place does the fetus begin to have clear perceptions of touch experiences. Sucking and swallowing can be observed during the first trimester, and by 28 weeks, they become coordinated. However, infants who are born before this time cannot integrate sucking and swallowing with breathing and need to be nourished intravenously or through a feeding tube. The newborn sucking reflex tends to be replaced by voluntary sucking after approximately 4 months. As reaching develops, infants frequently mouth novel objects, running their lips and tongue over the surface. This exploratory mouthing peaks at approximately 6 months, as eye–hand coordinated reaching becomes more accurate.

## Implications for Caregiving

Both waking and feeding cycles seem to be controlled by an endogenous rhythm (Meier-Koll, Hall, Hellwig, Kott, & Meier-Koll, 1978). The infant's state of arousal is a key to successful feeding because the infant must be actively involved if the feeding is to be successful. If the infant is drowsy or stressed, for example, it will be important for the caregiver to help the infant return to a quiet alert state before feeding can begin. Feeding the infant when he is in an alert state facilitates the continuous feedback between mother and infant, which has consequences for each and for the development of their interactive patterns of behavior. Mothers can learn to identify their own infant's sucking patterns and hunger and satiety cues. Sensitivity to the infant's cues during feeding will facilitate the infant's nursing and at the same time promote positive mother–infant interactive experiences. The infant's individual burst–pause–sucking pattern provides mothers with an exquisite opportunity for the earliest mother–infant dialogue.

Observing the infant's sucking response can give the clinician an opportunity to discuss mother–infant feeding and the importance of reading and responding to the infant's communication cues as a key to positive feeding interactions between mother and infant. Asking questions such as "How do you know she is ready to feed?" or "How does your infant show you he has had enough?" or "What seems to distract him from feeding?" are the kinds of open-ended questions clinicians can pose as a way to discuss communication cues as part of anticipatory guidance. The clinician can point out that proximity and touch also foster good feeding interactions and that, especially in preterm infants, affectional maternal touch during feeding not only promotes better feeding but also results in an increased sense of efficacy in the mother (Feldman, Keren, Gross-Rozval, & Tyano, 2004).

The clinician can point out the importance of sucking as a regulatory response. As an infant builds up to crying, self-regulatory efforts can be seen when the infant attempts to get his finger or hand into his mouth and suck on it. The sense of achievement or gratification at having reached this level of self-regulation appears as the infant's face softens and he becomes alert. A pacifier can achieve this same kind of quieting in an upset infant but may not serve the self-regulatory feedback system as well as the infant's own self-initiated sucking maneuver. Indeed, recent research suggests that being held and breast-fed can minimize the pain of heelsticks and other painful medical procedures (Gray et al., 2002).

## Hand Grasp

The hand grasp is now elicited to examine its presence and strength.

### Administration

While the infant is supine with the head in midline and the arms semiflexed, the clinician places his or her finger in the infant's hands and presses the palmar surface. The clinician describes the response in terms of the infant's ability to sustain a strong grasp (see Figure 3.15).

### Recording

Strong: Clear-cut grasp-like movement

Fairly strong: Moderate response; slight finger grasp observed

Weak: No response observed

A strong grasp is coded as 3, while a weak or nonexistent grasp is coded as 1. This response is best observed when the infant is an alert state.

### Interpretation

Touch is the very first sense to emerge in utero, so it is not surprising, therefore, that the infant's sensitivity to touch is well developed at birth. Touch encompasses various sensory abilities, each with its own neural pathway. Touch, temperature, and pain sensations each begin in the skin, where specialized receptors for each modality are located. It has been well documented that touch and physical contact are essential to the infant's sensorimotor development and to the infant's emo-

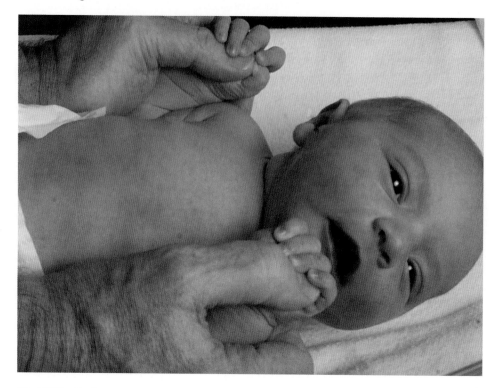

**Figure 3.15.** Hand grasp.

tional and physical growth. It is clear that touch seems to enhance the infant's responsiveness to the environment.

The hand grasp may be less intense during the first few days and is seen best
in the awake states. Some infants are able to use the hand grasp reflex to maintain
a pacifier or a bottle in position, and this seems to facilitate sucking.

## Developmental Sequence

The human embryo responds to touch, particularly around the mouth and the
soles of the feet, from the second month of life. By the 11th week, the fetus can
open and close her hands and suck on her thumb. In general, touch sensitivity develops in a head-to-toe sequence, and the mouth is the first region to become sensitive. Preterm infants as young as 25 weeks' postconception exhibit electrical activity in the somatosensory context in response to touch stimuli. At approximately
37 to 38 weeks' gestational age, the grasp reflex can be strong enough to allow the
infant's shoulders to be lifted off the mattress (Dubowitz et al., 1999).

Although newborns are able to feel through their mouths, they have better
developed touch sensitivity in their hands. Infants often use the hand grasp to
maintain the nipple during sucking or feeding. Newborns can even use touch to
distinguish object shapes and are able to reach out and grasp objects if given an
opportunity (Bower, 1974). These poorly coordinated swipes or swings at an ob-

ject that is dangling in front of them are referred to as *pre-reaching*. By 2 months of age, the hands are open most of the time, and at approximately 3 months, the hand grasp reflex is replaced by active, voluntary grasping. The infant will grasp the mother's index finger purposefully by this time and will reach for objects that are placed in front of her, but she will miss and be unable to grasp them. By approximately 4 months, however, infants will be able to retain a toy that is placed in their hands and at approximately 5 months can grasp a block precariously and can transfer objects from hand to hand (Rouchat & Goubet, 1995). Sensory axons that enter the spinal cord are not fully myelinated until 6 months of age, but electrical response to touch in the somatosensory cortex grows stronger and faster throughout the first year of life.

## Implications for Caregiving

Most mothers become aware of the strength of the hand grasp from the beginning and spontaneously integrate this awareness into their routine feeding and play periods by providing their fingers for the infant to grasp. Sucking will facilitate the hand grasp reflex if it is weak during the first few days (Prechtl, 1977). More important, perhaps, in terms of the parent–child relationship is that the hand grasp provides an opportunity for physical contact between caregiver and infant and may be used in soothing or helping the infant inhibit random motor activity. It often becomes part of the more robust infant–parent play interactions during the first few months (Yogman, 1982). Feeding, or rather the pause period in the infant's sucking, seems to be the time when mothers' tactile behavior tends to occur (Kaye & Wells, 1980). Mothers seem to adapt their tactile behavior to the burst–pause pattern of their infant's feeding (Alberts, Kalverboer, & Hopkins, 1983).

The positive effects of touch in general have been well documented. Infant massage, for example, which involves gentle stroking of the infant's entire body and flexion and extension of all limbs, has positive effects on weight gain and on the infant's behavioral development (Ferber, Kuint, et al., 2002; Ferber, Laudon, Kuint, Weller, & Zisapel, 2002). It also has been demonstrated to enhance the parent–infant relationship itself (Field et al., 1986; Onozawa et al., 2001; Scafidi et al., 1993). For preterm infants in particular, skin-to-skin contact, or *kangaroo care*, which provides tactile stimulation and support, helps infants regulate their temperature, improves their overall weight gain, and promotes positive interactions between mother and infant (Ohgi et al., 2002). Finally, studies of infant pain reveal that in preterm and term infants, gentle holding by the parent can help lessen pain. Research on infant mammals indicates that physical touch releases endorphins, which are painkilling chemicals in the brain (Gormally et al., 2001).

## Shoulder and Neck Tone (Pull-to-Sit)

The pull-to-sit maneuver is now elicited to enable clinician and parents to observe the infant's shoulder strength and head control. It is administered only when the infant is in a quiet alert state and should be administered with great care and sensitivity, particularly in the case of infants who are still frail.

## Administration

The clinician holds the supine infant's wrists and pulls him slowly into a sitting position (see Figure 3.16). The clinician watches for head lag and how well the infant can pull his head toward or through midline. The clinician may need to hold one hand protectively behind the infant's head if significant head lag is noticed or if there is parental concern about this maneuver. The clinician describes to the parents the infant's resistance to extension of the arms and how flexed they are at the elbows throughout the procedure. The clinician also describes the degree to which the infant is able to maintain an upright head position and the strength of the shoulder and neck muscles.

## Recording

Strong: Infant brings head to midline with minimum head lag and maintains it for at least 3 seconds

Fairly strong: Infant has head lag and can bring head through midline; no ability to maintain it at midline

Weak: Infant is unable to bring head to midline

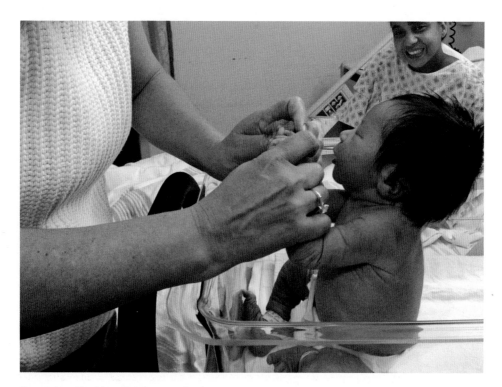

**Figure 3.16.**   Shoulder and neck tone (pull-to-sit).

The infant who has good head control and is able to maintain the head at midline is best described in the 3 category, while the infant for whom this is too difficult or impossible merits a recording of 1 and will need a great deal of support from the parents to support his head.

## Interpretation

In general, the pull-to-sit maneuver is seen as a measure of 1) traction, 2) head control, and 3) strength of neck muscles. The head control is a joint function of the strength of the neck muscles and the activity of the labyrinth, whereas the traction response examines the infant's arm flexion and resistance. During the first month, the infant's head control will increase; however, parents can be reassured that there is a great deal of variability in infants' ability to maintain their head at midline. The clinician also can point out that cultural differences have been observed in response to this maneuver. Among the Gusii in Kenya, for example, newborn infants were able to maintain their head in midline for up to 60 seconds with no apparent signs of distress (Keefer, Tronick, Dixon, & Brazelton, 1982). In preterm infants, the clinician usually will need to support the head with one hand and pull the infant to sit with the other. By 40 weeks' gestational age, many healthy preterm infants will be able to maintain some head control and shoulder and neck tone.

## Developmental Sequence

Whereas many coordinated motor movements appear during the first trimester, by the second half of pregnancy, many spontaneous movements come under the control of higher brain centers and strengthen the infant's muscles and refine the developing motor circuits. Mastering control of the head is the first challenge newborn infants face before they progress to rolling over, sitting, crawling, standing, and finally walking by the end of the first year. Although the head and neck control may be weak during the first 2 or 3 days, it increases during the first month. The infant's ability to maintain the head constantly and without support in the upright position with only minor oscillations will improve during the next few months. By 3 months, the head is almost completely steady, and between 3½ and 4 months, most infants will tuck their chin while being pulled to sit and may assist the movement with their abdominal muscles and arm flexion (Piper & Darrah, 1994). Finally, by 4 or 5 months, the infant can sit supported by a cushion, using his arms for support, although, if not firmly supported, the infant tends to slump forward. By 6 or 7 months, many infants can sit up without support.

## Implications for Caregiving

Parents will be able to notice the level of their infant's strength and robustness. However, the clinician can point out that it is not advisable to leave the infant without head support when held upright. For many first-time parents, the pull-to-sit item typically elicits some combination of concern ("What is the doctor doing to my infant?"), surprise ("She's much stronger than I thought!"), recognition ("I notice that she does this when I am holding her on my chest"), or understanding ("Yes, I can see that she needs support; she's not yet ready to hold up her head"). The pull-to-sit item, therefore, can be used by the skillful clinician to help parents address their concerns about how careful they need to be when holding or handling their infant.

During the first few months at least, infants need head support while feeding or when placed in an infant seat. The infant's increasing ability to maintain her head without support will facilitate the ability to maintain interaction with and exploration of the world. Supporting the infant's head and placing her on the shoulder can facilitate visual alertness and exploration (Korner & Thoman, 1972).

## Crawling Response

The infant is now picked up and placed gently on her stomach to observe the crawl response.

### Administration

The clinician places the infant on her stomach, making sure that her arms are not underneath her trunk. Observing the infant on her stomach, the clinician describes the infant's response in terms of her ability 1) to raise her head, nose, and chin off the surface; 2) to turn her head to one side; and 3) to crawl spontaneously using her arms and legs (see Figure 3.17). The crawl is difficult to elicit in sleep states and may not be observable clearly in the first few days of life (Prechtl, 1977).

### Recording

Strong: Coordinated crawling movement involving arms and legs and freeing of face

Fairly strong: Some attempts to flex arms and legs

Weak: No flexion of arms and legs and no freeing of face

The recording of 3 suggests that the infant has demonstrated a clear-cut crawl response, while the infant who does not move her legs or move her head is best described under 1. This should be coded only if the infant is in a quiet alert state.

### Interpretation

The crawl response shows the infant's capacity to protect herself from any interference with the breathing capacity when placed on her stomach. In addition, the prone response facilitates the infant's motoric equilibrium, because it may stimulate hand-to-mouth activity and enable the infant to self-quiet and become alert. Preterm infants also may use the crawling movements to *search out* the protective

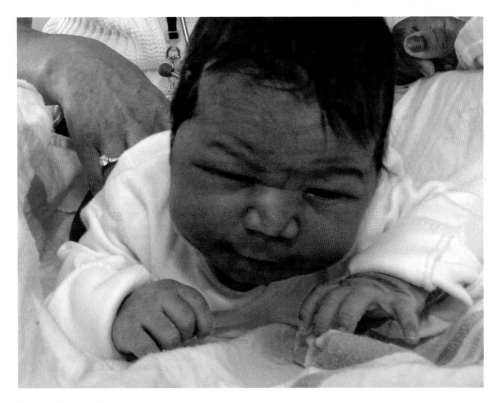

**Figure 3.17.** Crawling response.

boundaries at the corners of the bassinet, which seem to help them inhibit their spontaneous motor behaviors and conserve their energy, thereby serving their recovery. Although more attention is directed to the dangers of infants being left on their stomach because of the dangers of SIDS, this observation of the infant in prone highlights the survival value of this response.

## Developmental Sequence

Within 6 weeks after conception, the first spontaneous fetal movements can be observed, and coordinated movements such as stretching and grasping emerge during the first trimester. By the third trimester, as motor circuits mature in the higher areas of the brain, fetal movements become more purposeful and coordinated and serve to strengthen muscles. Whereas the newborn infant is able to move her arms and legs in a coordinated crawling pattern, her ability to raise her head while prone will continue to improve during the next few weeks. By 2½ months, this position can be held firmly, and infants are able to raise the upper trunk and support themselves on their forearms, and by 6 months, they can rest on the palm of their hands and shortly thereafter initiate voluntary crawling, using the arms to pull body and legs. Not until the second half of the first year will the transition from being an obligatory response to what could be called a voluntary behavior take place, when the full-fledged crawl begins to emerge. The course of head and shoulder tone and the crawl response are influenced by genetic factors and by environmental factors such as imitation, handling practices, nutrition, and so forth, as Brazelton, Koslowski, and Tronick (1976) showed in the case of Zambian infants and as Keefer et al. (1982) demonstrated in the case of Kenyan infants.

## Implications for Caregiving

The crawling reflex can be reassuring in that it shows mothers that infants have the capacity to free their airway and have built-in protection against smothering during sleep or when placed on the stomach. Given the emphasis on the importance of placing infants on their backs for sleep, parents may be afraid of ever placing their infant in the prone position. This item provides the clinician and the parent with an opportunity to discuss the potential value of "tummy time" for the development of extensor motor strength. As long as parents stay with the infant, the infant can be placed prone. The prone response facilitates the infant's motor development and may stimulate her efforts at self-regulation. In general, parents should keep in mind that there are advantages to upper body exercise in the early months and should give their infants as much "tummy time" as possible during waking hours, as long as they are present with the infant.

> If the infant is in an alert state, the clinician can now administer the attentional-interactive items. If the infant seems to be frail or fragile, it may be best to begin with the least invasive or the least stimulating stimulus, such as the red ball or the rattle or with the face only (without the voice). However, if the infant is alert and seems to be ready to respond to interactive stimulation, then the clinician can proceed with the next item. Throughout the administration of these items, the clinician should try to avoid abrupt movements as he or she moves from visual to auditory items and should try to maintain a smooth, natural flow between these various presentations.

## Response to Face and Voice

Now the clinician moves into a face-to-face position with the infant and prepares to interact with him (see Figure 3.18). Some clinicians may feel more comfortable sitting down to better elicit the infant's best response. It is important that the clinician take a position where the parent is able to join him or her in observing the infant's responses and eliciting some of these behaviors.

## Administration

The clinician can begin the social orientation items by engaging the infant in a face-to-face position. The clinician begins to interact with the infant and when the infant is engaged—when he is in a quiet alert state and is looking at the clinician—

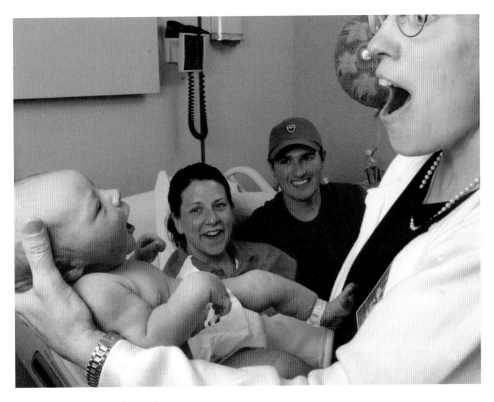

**Figure 3.18.**  Response to face and voice.

the clinician slowly moves to one side to see whether the infant follows with his eyes. The clinician should move slowly, so that the infant can maintain eye contact with him or her, and try to avoid jumpy or abrupt movements. If the infant is in a drowsy state, then it may be helpful to rock him gently, providing mild vestibular stimulation, to bring him to an alert state. If the infant is fussing or crying, it will be necessary to console him and bring him back to a quiet alert state before these behaviors can be administered. Once the item is begun, the clinician simply allows the infant to respond and then may describe the infant's behavior to the parents, pointing out the components of his responses:

1.  Respiration changes, such as pauses or slow- or fast-breathing patterns

2.  Increase or decrease in activity level

3.  Changes in facial expression, including brightening and widening of the eyes

4.  The ability to still and focus on the clinician's face

5.  The tracking with eyes and head, both vertically and horizontally, as well as the quality of the tracking responses

## Recording

Very responsive: Focuses and follows with smooth head and eye movements

Moderately responsive: Stills and focuses with moderate amount of visual tracking

Not responsive: Very brief focus and/or no tracking with eyes

The infant whose attention is prolonged and predictable is described in the 3 category, while the infant who is not ready or able to respond or become engaged is best described in the 1 category.

## Interpretation

The human face is the most important stimulus in the visual world of the newborn (Morton & Johnson, 1991). Newborn infants can focus and visually track stimuli, have certain scanning preferences, and are sensitive to eye gaze from the very beginning. Not only can the newborn visually track (Brazelton & Nugent, 1995; Dannemiller & Freedland, 1991; Laplante et al., 1996; Slater, Morison, Town, & Rose, 1985), but he also prefers the mother's face and can even discriminate his mother's face from that of a stranger (Pascalis et al., 1995). Farroni et al. (2004) showed that newborns looked significantly more at a face with direct gaze than at a face with averted gaze. There also is evidence to suggest that newborns are able to discriminate between different affective facial expressions (e.g., happy, sad, surprised) and are even capable of imitating expressions and gestures (Field et al., 1982; Meltzoff & Moore, 1994).

The infant's gaze behavior not only regulates his internal physiological state but also signals his readiness to engage in communication (Adamson, 1996). Gaze aversion, conversely, suggests the need to withdraw from a situation that is too demanding (Stern, 1985) or the need to recover from the excitement of the interaction (see Figure 3.19; Brazelton et al., 1974).

## Developmental Sequence

Visual development begins in the fourth week of embryonic life with the initial formation of the eye. In the visual cortex, the adult number of cells has been reached before birth (Rakic, 1977), but there is a striking increase in their size and connectivity between birth and 3 months. At birth, infants can see, and they depend on vision more than on any other human sense to explore the world around them. In fact, radical changes in visual behavior take place between the first and third months of life (Haith, 2004). One proposal is that the change at approximately 2 to 3 months marks the onset of cortical visual function and that the visual behavior of the newborn is controlled by subcortical pathways, particularly that of the superior colliculus (Bronson, 1974; Johnson, Slemmer, & Amso, 2004). Whereas many of the newborn's motor skills are limited, such that they cannot use their hands to explore the world around them, the oculomotor system—un-

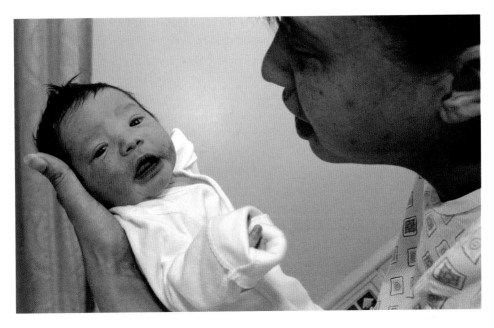

**Figure 3.19.** Gaze aversion.

like other motor systems—approximates its mature state during the weeks and months after birth. Indeed, by 1 month to 6 weeks, many infants spend 1 hour or more in an alert, socially available state.

Previous studies with the NBAS suggested that the increasing ability to be alert is the central evolving developmental agendum of the newborn. Als (1979) pointed out that the differentiation of the attentional-interactive system is the most rapidly changing subsystem in the newborn period. The issue that most newborns seem to get under control in the first weeks after birth is the increasing stabilization of the alert state, as they move from sleep to aroused crying states and back to sleep again. Whereas the 2-day-old infant's alert periods often are short and difficult to come by and are often interrupted by episodes of crying, by 2 to 3 weeks, these periods of alertness have become more reliable and consolidated.

As the ability to prolong the duration of the gaze improves during the first weeks of life, the infant is better able to explore the internal features of the face and to gather cues about the partner's emotions (Blass & Camp, 2003). Trevarthen (1993) demonstrated that by 6 weeks of age, during periods of attention to the mother's face, brow knitting precedes social smiles, which is followed in turn by relaxation of the brows, vocalizations, and hand gestures that occur in a predictable pattern. At this time, the infant begins to make cooing noises because the larynx now has descended into its adult position and he is better able to control breathing and the muscles of his tongue and mouth. This opens up a new possibility for face-to-face turn-taking interaction between infant and caregiver.

Indeed, the infant's open-mouthed smiling in response to his mother's gaze may appear as early as the first month and increases in frequency and stability from the second to the sixth month (Lavelli & Fogel, 2005). By then, infants show endogenous smiling in response to various forms of auditory, tactile, and visual stimulation (Wolff, 1987).

Lavelli and Fogel (2005) showed that the second month of life is a special period of developmental change and reorganization in the patterns of infant attention and emotion. Although there is a wide range of variability, simple attention seems to dominate face-to-face interactions during the first month (gazing at the face without any sign of emotional engagement). During the second month, however, infants show a wide range of facial expressions and emotional responses, from interest to concentration to astonishment and pleasure. From the fourth to sixth weeks of life, cheerfulness and excitement begin to predominate. The earlier simple gaze now is accompanied by more active positive emotional expressions, by expressions of effortful concentration, by smiling, and often by motor excitement. By the third month, the duration of smiles and cooing increases as smiles become more open and cooing becomes more playful. This more active approaching pattern of attention is accompanied by excited attention during face-to-face interactions. Clearly, the infant's response to the mother's face is emotional, so gaze/attention is not merely neutral or cognitive.

Indeed, by 10 weeks, when infants are scanning their mother's face, they seem to look mainly at her mouth and eyes, just at the time when the infant begins to take a more active part in mother–infant interaction (Hunnius & Gueze, 2004). The infant now can track the mother as she leaves, approaches, or moves about the room. Visual acuity increases steadily and reaches near adult level by 6 months (Slater, 2001). At approximately that time, the infant's preoccupation with gazing at the human face is partially replaced by a greater interest in reaching for and manipulating objects.

## Implications for Caregiving

The most important implication of caregivers' observing the neonate's visual capacities is the recognition that their infant not only can process visual stimulation but also can see a parent's face and is able to discriminate expressions. Parents intuitively seem to choose to stay centered in the infant's visual field in the face-to-face position in a range in which the neonate can visually accommodate the caregiver's face and thereby facilitate affective interchange.

The infant's visual system, therefore, serves to elicit a dyadic form of interchange, which helps a parent recognize that his or her infant indeed is a fully responsive human being—a person with an individual personality. Conversely, parents have the chance to identify skin color change or gaze aversion behavior as signs of the infant's need to withdraw from a situation that is too demanding. Often, the infant needs a *time–out* to recover from the excitement of the interaction.

It is within this environment that parents and infants begin to interact with each other, mutually responding to each other's facial, vocal, and proprioceptive cues. The infant's open-eyed alertness is greeted in turn by the parent's raised eyebrows, wide-open eyes, slight retroflexion of the head, smile, or verbal greeting. In response, the initial glance of the infant expands to wide eye opening, raising of the eyebrows, softening of the cheeks, and shaping of the mouth into an "ooh" configuration (Als, 1979; Papousek & Papousek, 1987, 2002).

Infants who see poorly have more difficulty in eliciting caregiver interaction. Their emotional responses are muted, and because they cannot gaze in the same direction as the partner, they have difficulty engaging their caregivers and their exploration may be stunted (Bigelow, 2003). Consequently, establishing a close emotional bond with the caregiver becomes critical, and by focusing on the infant's other communication strengths the NBO can serve as the first step in this process.

## Visual Response (to Face Only)

Now the infant's response to the face, without the addition of the voice, is observed.

### Administration

The clinician begins by merely looking at the infant and then slowly moving to one side to see whether the infant follows with her eyes (see Figure 3.20). The clinician must move slowly and try to avoid jumpy or abrupt movements, so that the infant can maintain eye contact.

### Recording

Very responsive: Focuses and follows with smooth head and eye movements

Moderately responsive: Stills and focuses with moderate amount of visual tracking

Not responsive: Very brief focus and/or no tracking observed

Infants who respond with bright-eyed alertness and can track the face are coded under 3, while the infant who is unable to respond to the clinician's face is coded as 1.

### Interpretation

The interpretative material for Visual Response to Face is the same as for Visual Response to Face and Voice; see above.

### Developmental Sequence

See Visual Response to Face and Voice above.

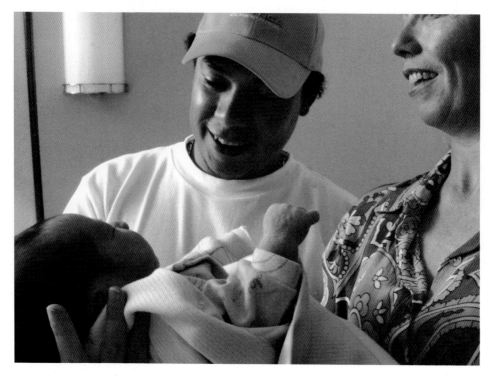

**Figure 3.20.** Visual response to face.

## Implications for Caregiving

See Visual Response to Face and Voice above.

## Orientation to Voice

Now, the infant's response to the human voice is observed.

## Administration

For observation of the infant's response to the clinician's voice, the clinician moves out of the infant's line of vision and calls the infant's name, maintaining a continuous, high-pitched voice. The clinician waits to see whether the infant turns toward him or her and gives the infant time to find his or her voice. This can be done on both sides. Again, the clinician should try to avoid abrupt movements as he or she moves from visual to auditory items and try to maintain a smooth, natural flow between these various interactive items.

This item can provide the clinician with an opportunity to engage the parents by inviting them to elicit this behavior by calling the infant's name (see Figure 3.21). The clinician's role is to facilitate this and guide the parent through it. The clinician may ask the parent to call the infant's name in a repetitive manner but,

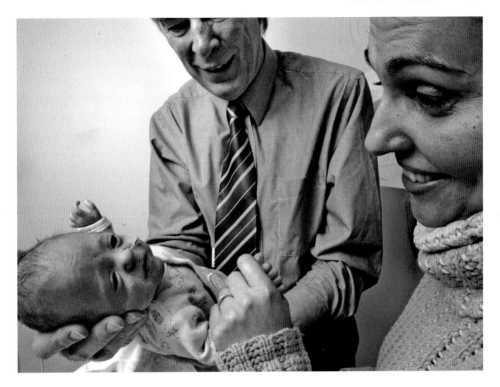

**Figure 3.21.** Orientation to voice.

as stated earlier, the parent should do this only when he or she is confident that the infant's ability to respond is robust and predictable.

## Recording

Very responsive: Stills and brightens; turns and locates sound

Moderately responsive: Stills and brightens; may turn eyes but unable to locate source

Not responsive: Eyes remain closed or dully alert; minimal or no reaction to sound

The infant who actively turns toward the voice and can locate it is rated as 3, while the infant who clearly responds to the sound but does not turn in that direction is coded as 2. The infant who does not respond to the sound is coded as 1. This set of responses is coded only if the infant is in an alert state.

## Interpretation

The neonate's auditory capacities are in an advanced stage of development at birth (Hecox & Deegan, 1985). The dimensions of the cochleas, which are the major factors in determining the frequency response of the ear, have reached adult values by the fifth month of gestation. Within the cochlea, all of the main anatomic features essentially are adult-like at birth, and the auditory nerve is said to be well myelinated (Bronson, 1974, 1994). For that reason, it should not be surprising that newborns are capable of auditory localization within minutes after birth (Brazelton & Nugent, 1995; Klaus et al., 1995). Research shows that newborns can hear and locate sounds (Muir & Field, 1979), and can even remember speech sounds (Swain et al., 1993). Newborns are more responsive to voices than to pure tones and can respond better when held upright than when supine (Muir & Field, 1979). They respond best to sounds in the range of the human voice (Eisenberg, 1976) and seem to prefer the mother's voice (DeCasper & Spence, 1991; Fifer & Moon, 1994; Moon et al., 1993; Morrongiello, Fenwick, Hillier, & Chance, 2004; Spence & Freeman, 1996). Indeed, they can detect the overall patterns of rhythm and pitch that differentiate one person's voice from another's (Clarkson & Clifton, 1995; Nazzi et al., 1998). Newborns also seem to be able to detect the sounds of any language and can make fine-grained distinctions between many speech sounds (e.g., between "ba" and "ga" and between "ma" and "na") and show a greater sensitivity to low-frequency sounds as compared with adults, who show maximum sensitivity to high frequencies (Aldridge et al., 2001). There also are data to suggest that newborns seem to prefer happy-sounding speech to speech with negative or neutral emotional qualities (Sansavini, Bertoncini, & Giovanelli, 1997, Trehub, 2001).

## Developmental Sequence

The underlying neural structures of hearing are present from early in utero and are functioning well before the end of gestation. By the end of the third trimester, sounds from the outside world penetrate the womb, and infants can hear the voices of both the father and the mother. In fact, by then, the infant is capable of sound discrimination. At birth, infants are not sensitive to quiet sounds and have a limited range of tones they can perceive, but DeCasper and Fifer (1980) showed that newborn infants could recognize their mother's voice and concluded that infants remembered the sound from their time in utero.

The child's hearing grows more acute as the cortical structures that are involved in hearing progressively myelinate and complete their synaptic refinement. As infants grow older, their auditory functioning continues to improve and differentiate, playing a major role in language development (Eisenberg, 1976). By 5 months, they have become sensitive to syllable stress patterns in their own language, and between 6 and 8 months, they begin to screen out sounds that are not used in their own language (Anderson, Morgan, & White, 2003; Weber, Hahne, Friedrich, & Friederici, 2004). From 6 months of age, an infant's ability to distinguish the full range of frequencies is almost fully developed, as is the ability to localize sound. (Whereas newborns can localize sounds on the horizontal plane, by 6 months they can localize sounds on the vertical plane as well.)

## Implications for Caregiving

Hearing may well be the infant's most important sense. Through it, infants experience language and music, both of which stimulate intellectual and emotional development. Although touch, smell, and vision all play a role in establishing the bond between parent and child, hearing permits a full form of communication. Mothers intuitively tend to use unusually high-pitched voices when speaking to their infants, as if they are predisposed to talk to infants at a tonal frequency and temporal pace to which the newborn is most likely to attend (Stern, 1977). This is referred to as *motherese*. Clearly, infants respond better to this high-pitched motherese than to any other kind of auditory stimulus and even to typical speech and seem to recognize and prefer the mother's familiar voice (Fifer & Moon, 1994). This mode of speech usually is accompanied by positive attention and affection, so it is the optimal form of auditory stimulation for the young infant. Young infants can hear their caregivers talk to them, and indeed this remarkable capacity would seem to serve one of the major developmental functions of the infancy period—namely, the promotion of mother–infant attachment. Specifically, it can be demonstrated to parents that infants are more responsive to higher pitches when awake but to lower pitches when drowsy. Lower tones will calm infants who are upset, whereas higher tones may arouse or even stress infants.

Fathers and older siblings also find that by raising the pitch of their voices and producing long, 5- to 15-second tone sequences, they are more likely to engage the infant's attention. Parents can be encouraged to talk to their newborns by attempting to match the frequency, utterance length, tonal pattern, and rhythm of such speech to the sensitivity of the infant. An adult who holds an infant at a range of approximately 18 to 38 cm (7–15 inches) and talks in a soft voice perhaps is an ideal stimulus for getting the attention of the newborn. Within this interactive environment, by 4 to 6 weeks of age, the infant and caregiver become involved in a vocal turn-taking temporal pattern that often develops into vocalizing in unison as the interaction becomes more animated (Stern, 1977). This vocal interchange would seem to serve optimally the development of the caregiver–infant relationship and in a secondary manner serve as a precursor to later turn-taking dialogue skills that typical conversation requires (Tronick, 2003).

## Orientation to Sound (Rattle)

The red rattle is used to observe the infant's response to an inanimate sound.

## Administration

The clinician usually holds the alert infant while supporting the head in midline and leaving him or her free to turn to each side (see Figure 3.22). The rattle is presented on each side while the clinician or the parent varies the sound in intensity and rhythmicity to elicit the infant's best response. The infant's responses are ob-

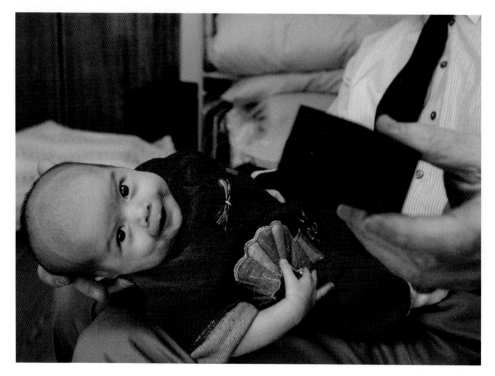

**Figure 3.22.** Orientation to sound (rattle).

served in terms of 1) respiration changes, 2) increase or decrease in activity level, 3) changes in facial expression including brightening and widening of the eyes, and 4) shifting of the eyes and head toward the sound.

To observe the infant's response to the rattle, the clinician moves it out of her line of vision and shakes it approximately 10 inches from her ear in a gentle, repetitive movement. If this does not seem to elicit a response, then the clinician changes the pitch or the shaking pattern. The clinician should always begin with a soft sound, because some infants are especially sensitive to stimuli and it may cause them to avoid the stimulus and turn away. The stimulus must be attractive to the infant. The clinician waits to see whether the infant turns in the direction of the rattle and gives the infant time to orient to the sound. This can be done on both sides.

## Recording

Very responsive: Stills and brightens; turns and locates sound

Moderately responsive: Stills and brightens; may turn eyes but unable to locate source

Not responsive: Eyes remain closed or dully alert; minimal or no reaction to sound

Infants who respond predictably to the sound of the rattle are categorized under the 3, while infants who do not respond to the sound are coded as 1. This is only valid if the infant is in a quiet alert state.

## Interpretation

The interpretive information follows the same information presented on auditory perception for the Orientation to Voice item above.

## Developmental Sequence

See Developmental Sequence in Orientation to Voice above.

## Implications for Caregiving

See Implications for Caregiving in Orientation to Voice above.

## Visual Tracking (Red Ball)

The red ball is used to observe the infant's ability to track and follow an inanimate object.

## Administration

By now, even before the clinician presents the red ball to the infant, he or she will be in a position to gauge the infant's threshold level and to identify the kind of visual stimulation that is appropriate for this individual child. The clinician will give the infant an opportunity to lock on to the ball at a distance of approximately 10 to 12 inches before moving it slowly to one side, making sure that the infant has locked on (eyes have focused on the stimulus and gaze is maintained for at least 1 to 2 seconds) before beginning to move the ball (see Figure 3.23). He or she then draws the infant along, like a magnet, ensuring that the ball is kept within the infant's visual range.

## Recording

Very responsive: Focuses and follows the ball with smooth head and eye movements

Moderately responsive: Stills and focuses with moderate amount of following—often "loses" the stimulus

Not responsive: Very brief or no following of the ball

The infant who tracks and follows with ease is described under the 3 rubric, while the behavior of the infant who does not track or follow is best described under the 1 rubric. This is only recorded if the infant is in a quiet alert state.

## Interpretation

At birth, newborn infants can actively scan and focus on a stimulus. They seem to prefer stimuli that contain curves over straight edges and attend mostly to points of highest contrast (Fantz & Miranda, 1975). They also seem to prefer face-like patterns to non-face patterns (Goren, Sarty, & Wu, 1975; Maurer & Barrera, 1981). Whereas typically seeing adults are said to have 20/20 vision, newborn infants

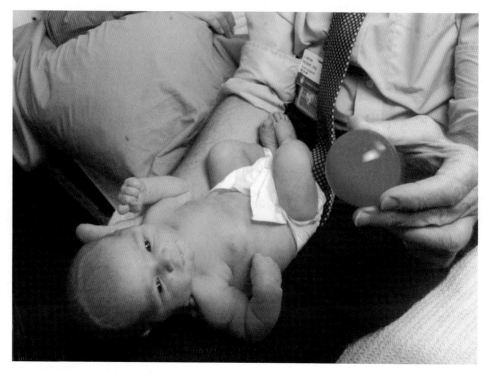

**Figure 3.23.** Visual tracking (red ball).

have approximately 20/200 vision; whereas objects that are distant from the infant appear fuzzy, newborns can focus much better up close. They are capable of accurately adjusting their accommodation to targets that are between 20 and 50 cm in distance (Banks, 1980). They can see the human finger at less than 23 cm (9 inches) and the human face at approximately 20 to 38 cm (8–15 inches). Farroni et al. (2004) showed that newborns have a rudimentary form of gaze following, although they may have difficulty shifting their gaze toward another, interesting stimulus (Hunnius & Geuze, 2004).

Research indicates that newborns are capable of *perceptual constancy,* in that they can recognize an object as being the same size despite changes in its distance (Slater, Morison, Town, & Rose, 1985; Turati, Simion, & Zanon, 2003). Turati (2004) demonstrated that infants are able to detect, extract, and recognize perceptual similarities between stimuli that belong to the same perceptual category, and they are capable of discriminating different shapes and recognizing the presence of common perceptual features that gather together stimuli into the same category.

## Developmental Sequence

Pathways that serve subcortical visual networks begin at approximately 2 months' gestation and are completed approximately 3 months after birth, arising from neural growth, increased myelination, synapse propagation, and pruning

(Johnson et al., 2004). Infants are capable of only very limited color vision at birth. Most newborns can discriminate successfully a broad band of red from white, but most fail to do so when presented with blue, yellow, or green (Adams, Courage, & Mercer, 1994). Whereas newborns prefer colored over gray stimuli, by the second month, infants can discriminate colors across the spectrum. Color discrimination then dramatically improves during the first 3 months of life (Brown, 1990; Teller, 1998).

By 2 months, infants scan more locations and various features of stimuli, and as they grow older, their scanning becomes more extensive, showing more brief fixations and more extensive scanning (Bronson, 1994). By 3 months, infants have gained more strategic control over their scanning behavior, and they can distinguish objects on the basis of actual size, not retinal image, and can attend to color, shape, and texture to identify objects (Johnson et al., 2004; Slater, 2001).

The first 3 months also are characterized by the infant's efforts to organize objects and events into coherent patterns and treat them as equivalent despite perceived differences. This is referred to as *perceptual categorization* and is a powerful adaptive process that helps the infant make sense of the environment. The accuracy of visual accommodation continues to improve during the first 3 to 4 months of life, a period when acuity also shows a rapid improvement. By that time, infants see about as clearly as adults or at least well enough to recognize a person across the room.

## Implications for Caregiving

Although it is clear that infants respond to visual stimuli and seem to have a special attraction to the human face, there is a limit to the kind and amount of stimulation that should be offered to the young infant (Cole & Frappier, 1985) . The clinician should help parents recognize both signs of availability and readiness and signs of disengagement or overstimulation. Too much stimulation can overwhelm the newborn's growing attentional system, whether from overstimulating interactions or too many toys or visual displays in the infant's line of vision. Infants still may find it hard to disengage and may fixate on the stimulus, which, in turn, may exhaust the neonate's system and compromise his or her ability to develop robust periods of social availability. This is described in detail in Chapter 6, when the use of the NBO with high-risk infants is discussed.

This is the end of the formal observation of items. With the infant now in the arms of his or her mother or father, the clinician can ask the parents whether they would like to try the face-to-face behavior and then guide the parents through it. This can provide the clinician with another excellent opportunity to engage the parents in eliciting their infant's responses. Once again, the clinician should do this only when he or she is confident that the infant's ability to respond is robust and predictable. The rest of the NBO items are summary items and are used to summarize the infant's behavior across behavioral domains and can be used to refine our understanding of the infant's temperament or individuality. Of these behaviors, crying may well be the most salient for new parents, and therefore clinicians need to have a clear understanding of the available research on the nature, range, and variability of crying in the first months of life and at the same time allow these interpretations to flow from the behavior of the individual infant as it is reflected in the NBO.

## Crying

Whenever the infant cries during the NBO, the clinician stops to listen to the cry and gives the infant a chance to self-soothe before initiating the soothing maneuvers (see Figure 3.24).

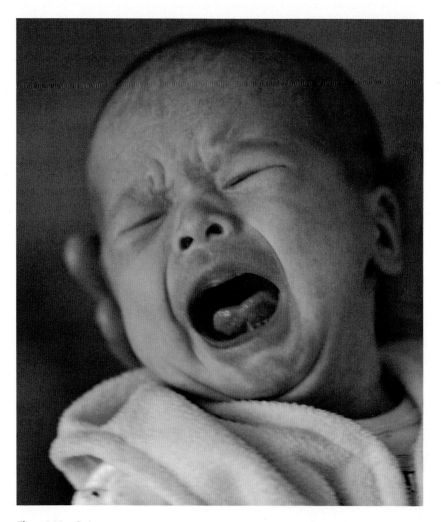

**Figure 3.24.**　Crying.

## Administration

A comprehensive NBO session ideally includes a crying episode because crying is one of the most important aspects of newborn behavior and has important implications for parenting. In other words, the clinician should welcome any crying or fussing that comes up during the course of the observations. This will give the clinician a chance to listen to the quality of the cry: Is it a good, solid, robust cry, or is it weak and frail? The clinician should take note of what may have led up to the cry: When did it take place? Was it early, when the environmental input was minimal, or was it only at the end of the session, when the infant had been handled quite a bit and had a lot of stimulation? One of the things the clinician wants to be able to identify during the course of the observation is the infant's threshold level (i.e., her tolerance for stimulation): How easily is the infant stressed, or how much handling can the infant tolerate without becoming stressed? Was the build-up to a crying state gradual or rapid? The clinician describes both brief fussing episodes and prolonged crying in terms of its 1) onset, 2) extremes in variability and pitch, 3) harmonic quality, and 4) pattern or rhythm.

## Recording

Very little: Hardly cries or fusses

Occasionally: Cries or fusses intermittently throughout the session

A lot: Cries consistently throughout the session

Crying behavior is coded as a continuum from little or no crying, which is coded as 1, to occasional crying which is coded as 2. A score of 3 is given when state 6 crying is consistent throughout the NBO session.

## Interpretation

Crying is a typical mechanism for discharging energy or tension and is tied to the regulation of state and physiological homeostasis as the newborn infant balances internal and external demands (Barr, 2002; Gustafson, Wood, & Green, 2000; Lester, 1984a). Crying can be a response to hunger, pain, or even too much stimulation when the system becomes overloaded. However, crying also is the infant's primary mode of communicating and expressing her needs. It usually has the effect of eliciting appropriate soothing intervention from the caregiver, which serves to reduce the infant's distress. There also may be periods of nonspecific fussiness or crying that occur throughout the day, after which the neonate may become alert or sleep more deeply. In this way, crying may contribute to state as well as physiologic dysregulation.

Several studies have suggested that sensory and behavioral regulatory difficulties may be underlying factors that perpetuate the infant's crying (DeGangi et al., 1991; Greenspan & Wieder, 1993; Maldonado-Duran & Sauceda-Garcia, 1996).

Sensory and regulatory problems may manifest as hypersensitivity to sensations, resulting in greater-than-typical irritability to sensory stimulation. The sensory-reactive infant's CNS may be inefficient in coordinating internal and external sensations. Other investigators have proposed similar underlying mechanisms for excessive crying, suggesting that an imbalance in the CNS, possibly sympathetic dominance, lowers the infant's threshold of arousal to various environmental stimuli and results in excessive motor activity and crying (Carey, 1999; Lester, Boukydis, Garcia Coll, & Hole, 1990).

The degree and frequency of irritable crying behavior in the newborn period may vary greatly from day to day (Bernal, 1972; St. James-Roberts & Plewis, 1996). Degree of fussiness in the perinatal period also may be influenced by factors such as maternal obstetric medication, mode of delivery, circumcision, degree of risk, temperament, and cultural differences. Chisholm (1989) suggested that irritability may result from reduced placental blood flow, possibly related to subjective stress. Standley, Soule, Copans, & Klein (1978) reported no sex differences in levels of irritability, while Lundqvist & Sabel (2000) reported gender differences in newborn behavior.

Almost all infants go through a fussy period during the day, but if crying lasts for longer than approximately 3 hours a day and is not caused by a medical problem (e.g., hernia, infection), then it is called *colic*. The timing varies, but colic usually affects infants beginning at approximately 3 weeks of age and peaking somewhere between 4 and 6 weeks of age. Wessel's *rule of 3s* defines a fussy infant as one who is otherwise healthy and well fed, but who has paroxysms of irritability, fussing, or crying lasting for a total of 3 hours a day and occurring more than 3 days each week and continuing to recur more than 3 weeks (Wessel, Cobb, Jackson, Harris, & Detwiler, 1954). Approximately 20% of infants cry enough to meet this definition of colic. Barr (1990) argued that early sleep and crying problems, for example, are understood best not as forms of infant pathology but as reflections of the typical range of individual differences. From this perspective, colic or excessive crying is merely the upper end of a spectrum of individual differences in typically developing infants.

Crying has been used as a measure of CNS integrity (Prechtl, 1977). The following dimensions could signify a compromised infant: 1) extremes in pitch, 2) extreme variability in pitch, 3) absence of harmonic quality, 4) lack of temporal patterning, 5) presence of nonharmonic disturbance, 6) extreme variation in length of each cry burst, and 7) short or long latency to cry (Lester, 1984a). The presence of one or more of these factors does not necessarily mean that something is wrong with an infant but may be used with other measures for differential diagnosis.

## Developmental Sequence

Across cultures, infant crying seems to follow a similar developmental sequence. All studies agree that crying is greatest in the first 3 months of life, although there is little agreement on how much crying is considered to be typical, and there is still little comparable data from non-Western societies (St. James-Roberts, 2001). However, there is evidence that even among Kung-San hunter-gatherers, for whom caregiving is characterized by physical closeness between mothers and infants, crying takes up more and more of the infant's day and peaks at approximately 6 to 8 weeks and then begins to decline (Barr, Chen, Hopkins, & Westra, 1996). There also is evidence to suggest that much of the crying that concerns parents is due to developmental processes that are part of the developmental agenda of the newborn. Barr maintained that excessive crying in the early months is a transient phenomenon and has no relation to later adjustment. Colic is "something infants do, rather than a condition they have" (Barr, St. James-Roberts, & Keefe, 2001, p. 89), so a lot of fussing and crying is typical. However, it should be acknowledged that cultural differences in caregiving also may influence the amount of crying: What is considered excessive crying may differ from culture to culture (Fox & Polak, 2002).

For infants who cry a lot, the question that remains is whether newborn characteristics persist. To what extent does irritability in the newborn period, for example, remain consistent over time? In a follow-up study of 28 clinic-referred infants with colic, excessive crying, or both at 4 to 12 weeks, Desantis, Coster, Bigsby, & Lester (2004) found that hours of fussing—but not crying—significantly correlated with inattention, emotional reactivity, touch processing, environmental coping, and externalizing behavior at 3 to 8 years. Children with more hours of early fussing showed less efficient sensory processing, poorer coping with the environment, and more attention/hyperactivity problems compared with those with fewer hours of fussing. Results suggest that hours of fussing rather than crying could be an early marker for infants who are at risk for these problems in sensory processing and regulation. A study by Nugent et al. (2006) demonstrated a relationship between some newborn behavioral profiles and behavioral profiles at 4 months of age. Highly reactive infants or infants who cried a lot and were difficult to soothe in the newborn period tended to be highly reactive at 4 months, while infants who were not easily disturbed and did not cry very much demonstrated the same profile at 4 months. Because the behavior at 4 months has been shown to have a strong association with later behavioral and biological features, specifically, infants who demonstrate a profile of high reactivity at 4 months may be biased to becoming fearful and shy, whereas those who are low reactive at 4 months, may be become more social and less behaviorally inhibited as school children (Kagan & Snidman, 2004). These data do not suggest that the newborn's ability to regulate distress combined with reactivity at 4 months of age inevitably results in later behavioral profiles, but the association between newborn behavior and temperament classification at 4 months reported in this study suggests the likelihood of biological bases for the later behavioral profiles.

Another approach to understanding the implications of excessive crying in the early months of life is based on the assumption that the developmental pattern of crying can be understood only within an interactional context. Sander, Stechler, Burns, & Lee (1979) showed that an infant's crying behavior is influenced from the earliest days by the caregiver's responses. The more quickly and frequently the caregiver responds to the infant's cries (i.e., the more individualized the attention), the less infants tend to cry. In Bowlby's (1982) view, crying and the mother's prompt attention tend to reduce crying and foster the growth of attachment. Bell and Ainsworth (1972) found that infants whose crying was ignored early on tended to cry more frequently and more persistently later in the first year of life, and that after 6 months, persistent crying discouraged mothers from responding. Nevertheless, it must be pointed out that individual differences in temperament must be taken into account before the effects of mother on infant and infant on mother can be untangled (Dunn, 1977; Garcia Coll, Kagan, & Reznick, 1984).

As infants develop during the first few months and their appreciation of the world expands, the causes of crying change and become more complex. Whereas newborns are likely to cry when their feeding is interrupted, 5- or 6-week-old infants are so interested in the world around them that they may hardly notice. At 2 or 3 months, they may cry when a toy is taken from them. Similarly, infants begin to cry more in response to strangers by 5 or 6 months or to being left in a strange situation by their primary caregiver (e.g., Ainsworth, Blehar, Waters, & Wall, 1978; Sroufe & Waters, 1977). Once again, however, there are marked individual differences in infant responses to strange situations at this time.

Work with the NBAS over the years suggests that the newborn infant is an open psychobiological system that needs environmental support to maintain its organization and development (Brazelton & Nugent, 1995; Buss & Plomin, 1984; Lerner et al., 2000; Tronick, 2003). Although Belsky (1993) maintained that infants who cry a lot and are difficult to soothe may be most susceptible to caregiving influences, and Van den Boom and Hoeksma (1994), for example, showed that these infants are more likely to receive inadequate caregiving and may be at risk for insecure attachment later, Bates (1986), Crockenberg (1986), and Kagan and Snidman (1998) concluded that this kind of temperament does not necessarily predispose a child to having adjustment problems. In summary, the developmental sequence of crying in infancy will depend on factors such as the infant's temperament, health, and age; parents' goals and parenting style; and environmental conditions such as nutritional adequacy and degree of physical comfort.

## Implications for Caregiving

There is evidence that the newborn cry induces anticipatory milk letdown and increased breast temperature in lactating mothers (Vuorenskoski, Wasz-Hockert, Koivisto, & Lind, 1969). This contributes to increased opportunities for social interaction for mother and infant. There is evidence to suggest that a certain amount of variability or unpredictability in state organization may be more adaptive for the newborn infant in that it ensures more facilitating involvement from the caregiver (Emde, 1987; Emde et al., 2000).

There is no doubt that caring for a child who cries a lot is extremely stressful for parents. Many parents may feel depressed or overwhelmed by the continuous and sometimes inconsolable crying of their infants. It has been demonstrated that parents tend to be more concerned about infant crying within the first 3 or 4 months of life, during what is called *the crying peak* (St. James-Roberts, 2001). It is especially important, therefore, for the clinician to recognize parents' need to talk about their feelings of frustration and inadequacy in the face of their infant's excessive crying.

Parents should not be made to feel responsible or guilty for crying behavior, so the clinician's approach to parents must be supportive and he or she must avoid blaming the mother. There is reliable evidence to show that infants can have prolonged bouts of fussing and crying even with sensitive and responsive parental care (Stifter, 2002). There also is evidence to suggest that providing an infant with prompt, appropriate responses to distress can enhance the parent–infant relationship (de Wolff & van IJzendoorn, 1997; Papousek & Papousek, 1990). It seems possible that a mother's effort to discover why her infant is crying and the relief of the two when she does find out may promote a mutually enjoyable relationship between mother and infant.

Helping mothers recognize the frequency of colic in young infants in general and its relative independence of caregiving strategies can help them tolerate continuous crying more easily. Clinicians can help mothers recognize that persistent infant crying, especially when it is high pitched and irregular, elicits negative emotions in most mothers. It is normal for mothers to feel angry and hostile toward infants who continue to cry despite the mothers' best efforts to quiet them. The clinician can help mothers acknowledge these feelings as normal and realize that this does not reflect on their parenting ability.

There is some evidence, as pointed out previously, that it is the child's threshold for responsivity, rather than his or her gastrointestinal system, that holds the key to supporting parents of infants who cry excessively (St. James-Roberts, 2001). The NBO can help parents understand that some infants are hypersensitive to stimulation and may cry more easily than others. The acknowledgment of the infant's individual repertoire and temperament will enable the parents to adapt their care to the needs of the infant. By observing the clinician's techniques, parents can try to identify the consoling techniques that work best for them and their infant.

In summary, crying is a normal mechanism for discharging tension, and there are great individual differences in the frequency and the duration of crying in newborn infants. The NBO can be used to help parents identify the kinds of consoling techniques that work best for their individual infant. The parameters of respect, concern, accommodation, and basic positive regard become crucial for the direction of the entire treatment process—from parent to infant and from practitioner to parent. The more concerned or anxious the parent is, the more crucial this reliable emotional context becomes. By valuing the parents' attempts to reach out and understand their child, clinicians provide parents with a safe and supportive relationship in which they can get to know and respond to their infant.

## Soothability

When the infant reaches an intense full-blown crying state, stop and observe her self-soothing efforts and then begin the soothing maneuver sequence.

### Administration

The clinician administers a graded sequence of maneuvers that are designed to bring the infant from crying to a quiet state. The infant's responses are described in terms of his responses to the sequence of interventions. When the infant cries, can he console himself, or what does it take to help the infant quiet? If the infant begins to cry, then the clinician should stand back for 10 seconds at most until the infant moves into a full-blown cry. The clinician then begins a series of steps to see how the infant can best be soothed (see Figure 3.25).

- The clinician begins by looking at and talking to the infant, without picking him up, to see whether he can use the clinician's face and voice to calm herself. This continues for about 10 seconds to see whether it works.

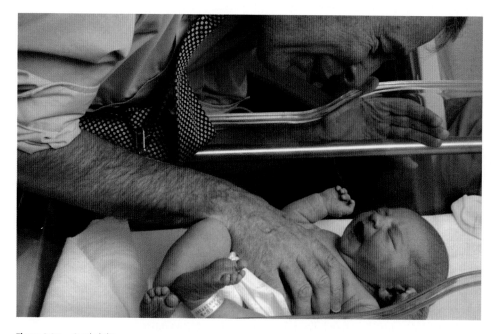

**Figure 3.25.** Soothability.

- If the infant is still crying, the clinician continues talking and then places his or her hand on the infant's stomach to see whether this is successful.

- If this does not succeed, the clinician holds the infant's arms and legs.

- The next step involves picking the infant up and holding him.

- If the infant is still crying, the clinician begins to rock him.

- If that does not succeed, the clinician tries a pacifier.

If, however, the infant shows an inclination to bring his hand or thumb to his mouth, the clinician should give the infant time to see whether she uses this maneuver to organize or calm herself. Some infants also may quiet themselves using their body movements or even by locking onto some visual stimulus in the environment (see Figure 3.26).

## Recording

Soothes easily: Easily soothed and/or consistently self-soothes

Soothes with some difficulty: Can be soothed with clinician support and can settle after rocking or swaddling by the clinician

Soothes with great difficulty: Difficulty responding to clinician's efforts to help infant stop crying or settle; never self-soothes

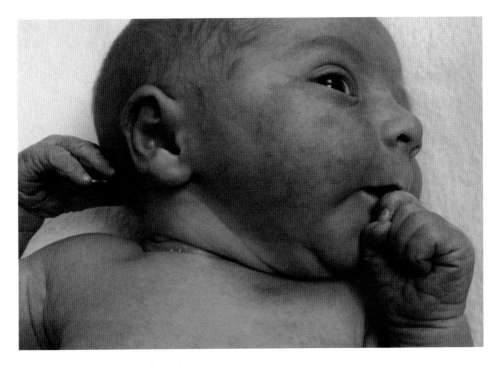

**Figure 3.26.**   Hand to mouth (self-soothing).

The infant who is easily soothed or is able to soothe herself is coded as 3, while the infant who tends to need clinician support and takes time to settle and become calm is coded as 2. The infant who cannot settle and continues to cry despite the support of the clinician is coded as 1.

## Interpretation

Just as there are wide variations in newborn crying behaviors (Sander et al., 1979), so, too, is there a wide range of individual differences in infants' responses to soothability procedures. Some infants quiet when left alone, but most require some kind of soothing stimulation such as cuddling, rocking, vestibular stimulation, or merely face and voice (Korner & Thoman, 1972; Thoman, 1975). Each infant will communicate the level of intervention or calming technique that best serves him or her to quiet and reduce distress.

## Developmental Sequence

Continuous excessive crying can create tension among family members and have a negative effect on family functioning. It can lead to parents' development of negative perceptions of the infant, and this in turn can undermine parents' confidence in their ability to parent. A longitudinal study reported an increased risk for externalizing behaviors (hyperactivity or conduct problems) and more parent-reported negative emotionality in 8- to 10-year-olds with a history of persistent crying in infancy compared with children without such a history (Wolke, Rizzo, & Woods, 2002).

## Implications for Caregiving

Although there are marked cultural differences in beliefs about responding to infants' crying, once parents do respond, they seem to follow similar patterns (Barr, 1990). They say something, touch, pick up, search for sources of discomfort, and then feed. Korner and Thoman (1972) found that when crying infants are picked up and held to the shoulder, they not only quiet but also become alert and begin to scan the environment. Conversely, there are times when prolonged and increasingly varied efforts by caregivers to soothe an intractably crying infant become too much; an exhausted infant at some point may need solitude rather than companionship.

Parents have reported the following strategies to be helpful in their efforts to cope with excessive crying:

- Anticipating the infant's cry throughout the day by learning his early warning signals indicating overload or overstimulation. Learn how the infant reacts to specific situations that are likely to lead to crying (e.g., if the infant usually cries during diaper changing, the caregiver can learn to reduce the level of stimulation or pay attention to the infant's tolerance for various levels of handling).

- Holding the infant and/or swaddling him have proven to be effective. The more hours infants are held, even early in the day when they are not fussy, the less time they will be fussy in the evening.

- Rocking the infant gently can be very calming.

- Talking and singing lullabies to the infant can be soothing. It is no accident that lullabies have developed in almost every culture.

- Holding the infant in an upright position may help.

- Allowing the infant to suck on something may work; some infants are happy only when they are sucking.

Many studies have reported that preterm infants cry more and that their cries are rated as sounding more difficult to interpret and more aversive than the cries of term infants. Excessive crying is one of the most common problems presented to pediatric professionals during the first 3 months of life in Western societies and has been linked to reduced maternal responsiveness (Boukydis & Lester, 1998; Worchel & Allen, 1997).

Although irritable or colicky infants are hard to soothe, it is helpful to discuss the value of age-old soothing techniques such as swaddling, rocking, and sucking. In most non-industrialized cultures, mothers respond to crying by breast-feeding or by providing immediate physical comfort. However, it should be pointed out that the concentration of breast milk changes during a feeding: The *foremilk* at the beginning is plentiful but low in calories and fat, and the *hindmilk* at the end of emptying each breast is far richer and sometimes more soothing. Sometimes colic can be reduced by allowing the infant to finish the first breast before offering the second. If the infant still seems uncomfortable or is eating too much, then offering only one breast (as often as desired) during a 2- to 3-hour period might give the infant more hindmilk.

In the end, the guidance that is offered to parents of infants who cry a lot and seem to be inconsolable will depend on the clinician's assumptions about the nature and origins of crying in the first months of life. Although some infants cry as a result of gastrointestinal disturbances, there is evidence to suggest that such conditions are rare (St. James-Roberts, 2001). Although food intolerance occasionally can lead to gastrointestinal disturbances, organic disturbances account for less than 10% of the cases in which unexplained crying is a concern for parents. More and more, high amounts of crying in infants during the first 3 months of life are considered to be due mainly to developmental processes that are typical for that age. In other words, it is no longer seen as pathological but as developmental.

In summary, the success of discovering the soothing techniques that are effective in calming infants can serve to enhance parents' feeling of self-confidence and efficacy. In the end, the best form of anticipatory guidance may well be to help parents realize that having in place a social support network—whether partner, parents, friends, or neighbors—perhaps is their most important form of preventive intervention at this time.

## State Regulation

State regulation attempts to capture two central aspects of the infant's development—her level of competency in terms of her ability to regulate her states and her individuality or her preferred style of responding, or temperament. This summary item addresses the following questions: Can the infant integrate her behavioral states to maintain her alertness or protect her sleep? How clear or robust are her states? How well can she modulate her transitions from a sleep state to an awake state to a crying state and back to an awake state? Can she do this with ease or with difficulty? What kind of self-organizing strategies does she have? Can she use hand-to-mouth maneuvers to organize her behavior (see Figure 3.26)? How *readable* is her behavior; in other words, how easy is it to read and interpret her behavioral cues? Is the infant's state profile clear and predictable or unpredictable and difficult to describe? By capturing the infant's individual style of responding, the NBO can also reveal what her unique organizing style or temperament might be. What are her primary reaction patterns? What kind of temperament does she seem to have? Will this style be easy or challenging for the parents?

### Recording

Well organized: States are well defined, robust, and easy to read, and/or state transitions are smooth and predictable

Somewhat organized: States are somewhat well defined, and state transitions are fairly smooth, although not predictable

Not organized: Unable to maintain well-defined states; transitions are unpredictable, abrupt, and difficult to read

The infant whose behavior is well organized is coded as 3, while the infant who has little or no self-regulation is coded as 1. Infants who have achieved some level of organization but whose state control is still not well developed merit a score of 2.

### Interpretation

*Behavioral state* perhaps is the single most important concept that has contributed to the current understanding of the newborn because it demonstrates that the newborn is not at the mercy of her environment but that the behavior of the newborn has an inherent organizational structure. State regulation is a summary description of the degree to which the infant is able to integrate her behavioral states, and how well she can maintain alert states or protect her sleep or modulate her transitions from sleep state to awake state to crying state. The developmental challenge for newborns is to regulate or organize their behavior in such a way that they can play an active role in interacting with their new world. Moreover, observing *how* the infant regulates her behavior can provide insight into her behavioral style or temperament.

The NBO describes this process of state differentiation and integration as the newborn infant learns to control and organize her responses to the new environment. State regulation captures the ease or degree of difficulty with which the infant can move from one state to the next and the degree to which there is equilibrium between the states.

## Developmental Sequence

Research has shown that although infants who are born as late as 34 and 37 weeks' gestation have all of the available states, the states are less well organized than those of term infants. These infants need a great deal of support to develop robust, predictable state organization. In preterm low-birth-weight infants, it may be more difficult to differentiate sleep state from waking state. Active sleep and quiet sleep are less well organized, and because the preterm infant expends much energy defending herself from developmentally inappropriate stimuli, the respective periods of each state are of shorter duration. Supporting the development of robust states in these infants requires parents to be especially attuned to their efforts at state regulation. This is discussed in greater detail in Chapters 1 and 6.

## Implications for Caregiving

In the context of the NBO, the clinician and the parents have an opportunity to observe the infant's efforts to regulate her sleep, wake, and crying states during the course of the session to see how well modulated or robust these states are, how easily the infant moves from sleep to wake states, and how easily she can recover from a crying state. Newborns whose states are easily identifiable, who are able to maintain long periods of quiet alertness, and whose state transitions are smooth are referred to as *readable* or *predictable*. and may be perceived by parents as having an "easy" temperament (Worobey, 1997). While the well-regulated newborn is an infant whose state organization is such that the pattern of sleep, wake, and crying states is defined clearly and easily identifiable, self-regulation cannot be achieved without the support of the caregiving environment. Infants whose behavior is easy to read or decipher are more likely to receive the kind of care that will meet their needs. In the case of the so-called "easy" baby, it is simpler for parents and infants to achieve a "goodness of fit" in terms of their interactions with each other, whereas it may be more difficult if the infant's behavior is more unpredictable and difficult to fathom. The less well-organized infant will need a great deal of support to help her develop more predictable, robust states that make it more likely for the parent to decipher her needs and respond accordingly. The NBO therefore attempts to help parents develop a clear appreciation of the status of the infant's self-regulation and also can reveal the unique pattern of the infant's sleep–wake–crying sequences—in other words, the infant's individuality and uniqueness.

## Response to Stress: Color Changes, Tremors, and Startles

Throughout the NBO, signs of physiological stress such as color changes, tremors, and startles are noted.

### *Administration*

Response to stress is a summary observation of the capacity of the neonate to maintain neuromuscular and neurovascular balance in the face of various degrees of stimulation and in various states. The color changes, tremors, and startles that are seen in newborns are the result of the neurological balance of reflexes and muscle or vascular tone, and these have a typical developmental curve that, although influenced somewhat by experience, is strongly under the influence of myelinization and other neural and vascular developments. A wide individual variability in these behaviors is seen in the newborn period. This item describes the ability of the infant to assimilate and accommodate stimulation and the ease or difficulty the infant encounters in doing this. During the course of the session, the clinician observes the infant's response to stimulation. An infant with a robust and well-organized autonomic system will be able to maintain good color, show few if any tremors (especially during alert periods), and have few if any spontaneous startles. If stress cues are observed, the clinician observes when they occur and what triggers them. The infant who is frail or fragile and who is overloaded or stressed easily is deemed to have a low threshold level.

The startle response is described by focusing on the sudden, abrupt quality of the movements of the arms and legs. Unlike the Moro response, in the startle, the elbow is flexed and the hand remains closed. (In the Moro, there are more outward and inward arm movements [Illingworth, 1983].) The clinician also points out the behaviors that may follow the startle, such as color changes and crying.

The clinician describes the tremors when they occur, noting their frequency and amplitude. Tremors are described as signs of the relative immaturity of the CNS in its ability to control muscle activity and often appear in infants who are hypersensitive to environmental inputs.

As the session progresses, the clinician describes changes of color and vascularity using the infant's initial color as a baseline. The clinician describes the degree of the color changes, the examples of acrocyanosis or mottling, and the time it takes the infant to recover his initial color.

### *Recording*

Not stressed: No tremors, no more than one startle, minimal color change; high threshold for stimulation

Moderately stressed: Moderate color change, tremors, and startles; can tolerate moderate levels of stimulation

Very stressed: Very tremulous; startles and extensive color changes present; very low threshold for stimulation

The infant who is physiologically stable and seems to be able to manage stimulation without any compromise to his physiological system is coded as 3, while the infant who manifests some moderate amounts of physiological stress is coded as 2. The infant whose physiological system is easily compromised, who is easily stressed, and who can tolerate little environmental input merits a score of 1.

## Interpretation

As described above, signs of autonomic stress—color changes, tremors, and startles—are signs of how robust or frail the infant's autonomic system is and reveals the capacity of the infant to respond to various levels of stimulation. This is a measure, then, of the newborn's threshold for stimulation and his ability to adapt to and cope with his new, extrauterine environment. Each of these is now described, beginning with color changes.

## Color Changes

Autonomic stress in infants may be observed as paling, acrocyanosis, uneven coloring, or mottling. The healthy term newborn is likely to demonstrate mild color changes during the examination in response to the physiological demands of the various handling maneuvers as the observation progresses. As the handling becomes increasingly more invasive, the infant's color may exhibit mottled, uneven acrocyanosis in the limbs as he attempts to control loss of body heat (see Figure 3.27). The lability of skin color and the amount of time it takes to regain the initial baseline color is an index of the degree of the infant's autonomic stability. Extreme paleness and cyanosis may be a sign of a depressed or overstressed autonomic and vascular system, whereas marked color changes that vary from minute to minute during the NBO can be interpreted as evidence of autonomic stress.

## Tremors

Usually only the arms are involved in tremors, but often they appear in the legs and the feet; occasionally the whole body may show trembling movements. During the first few days of life, high-frequency, low-amplitude tremors often are found in typical, term infants while asleep but especially when infants are crying vigorously and even when they are not crying. However, sustained low-frequency, high-amplitude tremors are associated with a low threshold for startles, the Moro response, high-activity levels, and hypertonicity. Tremors in the newborn period are signs of autonomic stress and may be increased by crying or hunger. Noting the state in which tremors occur is important because they may be

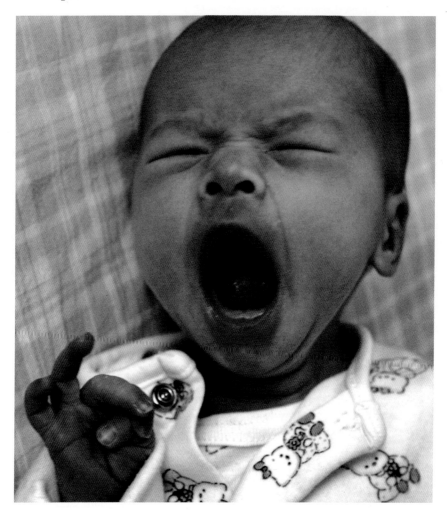

**Figure 3.27.** Response to stress: color change.

significant if they are persistent or present when the infant is in an alert state, especially after the first few days. (*Note:* Less than six times per second is considered low frequency, and more than six times is considered high frequency; less than 3 cm is considered low amplitude, and more than 3 cm is considered high amplitude [Prechtl, 1977]).

## Startles

The clinician notes the context in which the startle was elicited. It may be a response to a sudden loud noise or a response to an abrupt handling movement by the clinician (see Figure 3.28). Whatever the context, it can be interpreted as a sign of autonomic stress. The threshold of the infant's responsiveness to the various levels of stimulation will be reflected in the number of startles that occur during the session. Furthermore, the level of stimulation that tends to elicit a startle can

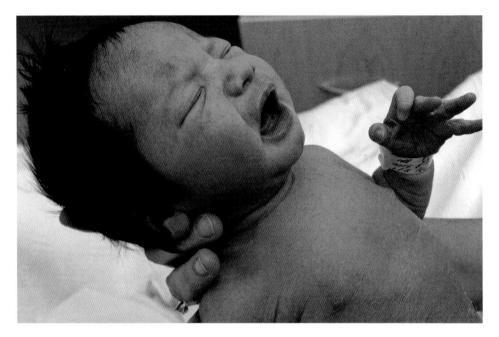

**Figure 3.28.**   Response to stress: startle.

indicate the infant's threshold level to stimulation and the relative fragility of the infant's physiological system.

## Developmental Sequence

In the healthy term infant, startles will decrease during the first month, and tremors tend to disappear after the first few days. They may appear for longer periods during or after vigorous crying in the first weeks of life. In hypersensitive infants with a low threshold for environmental stimulation, they continue to be present during the first month changes. During the first months, the autonomic system of the newborn becomes more integrated and stable as the infant grows and develops.

## Implications for Caregiving

One of the most important conceptual breakthroughs from clinical and empirical work with frail or high-risk neonates has been the concept of a *lowered threshold* for taking in, using, and responding to stimuli (Brazelton & Nugent, 1995). A frail neonate or one whose physiological system still is frail has such a low threshold coupled with an inability to habituate to negative, unpredictable stimuli that he is overwhelmed easily. Such an infant is likely to become disorganized, or become active or start crying to shut out these overwhelming stimuli. The infant's efforts to manage his autonomic system means that he will have little energy to modulate motor behavior or sleep–wake states. When the infant is disorganized, when he is still struggling to organize his motor system, for example, he will be unable to focus on environmental cues. Hence, the opportunity to take in and learn from the environment is seriously endangered. These infants can accept reduced stimuli but with only one modality at a time—touch, visual, auditory, or kinesthetic—but two modalities cannot be dealt with. Respecting this need for reduced input, the infant will learn over time to handle more complex stimuli and organize his CNS to interact with a more and more complex environment. Each of these autonomic signs will be now described in terms of the implications for caregiving.

## Color Changes

Maintaining physiological stability is demanding for the newborn, especially for immature or fragile infants. Parents usually respond spontaneously to marked color changes in their infant by covering or swaddling their infant, which effectively helps him regain his initial color. The changes during the examination also can be explained to parents in terms of the quality and level of stimulation that elicited the change of color. This in turn can sensitize parents to the level of stimulation that stresses their infant and can help them become more aware of the techniques that restore their infant's physiological stability.

## Tremors

Observing tremors and the context of their occurrence can sensitize parents to the level of fragility of their infant's autonomic system functioning. These stress signs can communicate to parents the kinds of touching and handling that may be inappropriate for their infant's autonomic recovery. Parents can be helped to identify the environmental inputs that elicit tremulousness in their infants and then proceed to modulate their inputs to reduce the amount of tremulousness and facilitate the infant's overall autonomic stability. Such interventions may include regulating visual and auditory environmental stimuli and developing handling, swaddling, and soothing techniques that reduce stress. Although the techniques will be individualized for each infant, the goal remains the same: to promote autonomic stabilization.

## Startles

Observing the context of startles and the level of stimulation that produces startles in the infant can sensitize parents to the impact of various levels of stimulation on the infant's physiological system. Identifying the causes of startles can enable parents to recognize startles as signs of an immature CNS and thereby enable them to modulate their handling procedures to reduce the number of startles.

By observing the infant's stress signs and threshold of responsiveness, parents can learn which level of stimulation is appropriate or inappropriate for their infant. This is particularly important in the case of high-risk or preterm infants for whom the impact of various kinds of intervention is critical for the infant's survival. In this case, the infant's behavioral cues provide the caregiver with the feedback necessary to determine the appropriateness or inappropriateness of his or her handling or interactive strategies. This can be presented as an opportunity for parents to facilitate the infant's recovery and smooth functioning. The preterm infant's energy is almost totally involved in shutting out, so there is little energy available for the more affective behaviors such as visual tracking and following, which are of particular significance and meaningful to new parents. Specifically, the NBO can demonstrate to the parents how certain handling techniques or postural adjustments can promote the infant's sleep states and reduce the amount of energy that is spent in shutting out. The parents then will become more confident as they are encouraged to use these techniques and observe how they can help their infant reduce his motor activities, modulate respiration, and ultimately begin to maintain a well-organized sleep state. Much of the involvement of parents of preterm infants will be related to facilitating the infant's sleep–wake cycles, so the NBO can help parents become better observers of their infant's behavior and can serve to develop a sense of competence in their role in promoting their infant's recovery.

## Activity Level

During the NBO, the infant's activity level is observed, particularly when in an alert state.

### Administration

Activity level summarizes the amount of motor activity during the course of the whole session. It is observed best when the infant is supine and in alert states and spontaneous movement can be observed. An infant whose activity level is deemed to be optimal is observed when her movements or activity level does not interfere with her ability to organize herself or to orient to whatever stimulation is offered. If the infant has a difficult time staying still or if her movements are frantic and uncontrolled, then she may get a lower rating. If, for example, the clinician has to swaddle the infant to elicit the orientation items, then it may reflect the infant's high activity level.

### Recording

Optimal: Well-modulated activity level

Moderate: Moderate level of activity

Very high/very low: Either persistently high or extremely low level of activity

The optimal activity level, which merits a 3, is assigned to the infant who displays appropriate levels of activity in supine, shows smooth arm and leg movements, and does not move excessively. The infant's spontaneous activity level does not interfere with her ability to respond to her new environment, and she needs little or no clinician support to settle or remain calm. The infant whose activity level can be described as moderate displays levels of activity that may move from high activity levels to low activity levels during the course of the observation. This raised level of motor activity interferes with the infant's ability to respond to her environment so that she tends to need clinician support to return to a more even level of motor behavior. This level of motor behavior merits a score of 2. Infants who are highly active or hyperexcitable even in alert states, and who always need clinician support to help them inhibit their motor activity level, are coded 1. Similarly, infants who show extremely low levels of spontaneous activity, are extremely lethargic, and who always need clinician support to arouse their motor activity are also coded as 1.

### Interpretation

The well-regulated, healthy newborn is able to maintain a flexed posture with smooth movements and optimal activity levels, which enables her to maintain settled sleep states, on the one hand, and quiet alert states with minimum activity and movement, on the other hand. When the infant is agitated, the level of activity will increase, but the well-organized infant can return easily to a more settled motoric state, either on her own or with environmental support (see Figure 3.29). Infants with high levels of activity tend to have a low sensory threshold and a bias toward a sympathetic nervous system reaction (Williamson et al., 2000). These infants are unable to inhibit random movements and they exhibit high levels of spontaneous activity, even when not agitated or crying. This high level of activity makes it difficult for the infant to organize her responses, whether to settle into a good sleep state or to respond to the caregiver.

Infants who have very low activity levels tend to have a high sensory threshold and require a lot of sensory input to achieve arousal and become active. This is discussed in more detail in Chapter 6.

### Developmental Sequence

Fetal movement begins in the sixth week after conception with the first spontaneous movements of the entire body, which is still one third of an inch long. The number of fetal movements peaks at midgestation and then slows while some movements come under the control of higher brain centers. This level of activity is critical for strengthening muscles and refining the infant's developing motor circuits. Even after birth, most of the newborn's movement is directed by lower brain regions. Activity levels involve a delicate balance between nature and nurture, between a programmed sequence of neuronal maturation and the kind of support or activities that are provided by the infant's environment.

### Implications for Caregiving

Parents tend to respond to highly active infants by swaddling them to inhibit their activity level and to give them a sense of security. For infants who have high-ac-

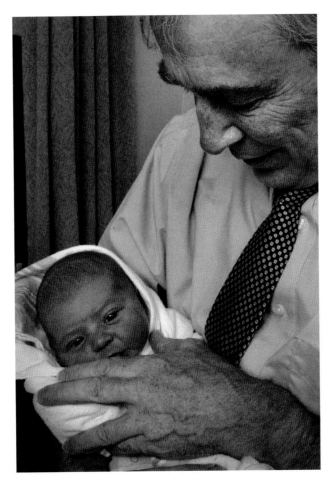

**Figure 3.29.**  Swaddling can help infants contain random motor activity.

tivity levels, it will be important to contain their movements to optimize their motor equilibrium and homeostasis. Some infants may be able to use hand-to-mouth maneuvers to self-soothe and reduce the high-activity level, but most active infants will need to have their limbs contained through holding or swaddling to be able to settle and return to a more optimal state. The sensitive caregiver will tailor his or her responses to the infant's cues and provide the level of support that the infant needs to settle. Covering the infant with a blanket that is tucked into the sides of the bassinet or providing rolled blankets or bumpers can inhibit the infant's motor activity levels and may reduce the kind of distress that is caused by excessive spontaneous activity levels.

Infants who have low levels of activity, conversely, may need support in becoming aroused. Gentle vestibular stimulation, for example, can stimulate their arousal and make them more available for social interaction. However, as Williamson et al. (2000) pointed out, the influence of sensory input is not always observed immediately, so parents need to aware of the possibility that the cumulative effects of sensory input may overload the infant's system, even if the effects are not readily observable at the time.

After the NBO is finished, the clinician and parent fill out the Anticipatory Guidance Checklist and the Summary Profile and Recommendations together.

## ANTICIPATORY GUIDANCE CHECKLIST

The Anticipatory Guidance Checklist is a checklist of themes for discussion with parents and is filled out by the clinician and parents after the NBO session. Anticipatory guidance helps families understand what to expect during their infant's next stage of development and can be used to review specific developmental goals for children based on the NBO observations. The observed behavior or cluster of related behaviors on the same line on the recording form goes hand in glove with the suggested caregiving theme on the checklist and is designed to provide information that can inform the parent's caregiving practices and ensure that their caregiving is responsive to the individual needs of their child. If, for example, the infant has difficulty habituating to light or sound, the "sleep patterns" and "sleep protection" boxes may be checked. Then the checklist can be used as the basis for a discussion of the development of sleep–wake patterns and how the infant's home environment can be organized to best support his or her efforts at mastering the challenge of sleep regulation. The checklist is not exhaustive but merely suggestive, and, in individual cases, a different set of caregiving questions based on the NBO observations or the parents' questions may emerge.

The Anticipatory Guidance Checklist is individualized and flows directly from the NBO observations of the infant's behavior. By checking off the themes that are of concern, the caregivers and parents can identify the infant's strengths and areas that the infant finds challenging and then develop a caregiving follow-up plan.

Although the manual provides a more detailed description of caregiving implications for each behavior, below are brief summaries of each theme of concern in the Anticipatory Guidance Checklist.

### Sleep Patterns and Sleep Protection

On the basis of the infant's response to the initial light and noise stimulus (while the infant is asleep), the clinician checks these boxes if he or she has observed that the infant seems to be aroused easily from sleep and seems to have difficulty shutting out environmental stimulation and maintaining a deep sleep. The clinician can then discuss strategies to support the infant's sleep protection and ways to structure the infant's environment that do not compromise her ability to develop good sleep patterns.

## Muscle Tone

Checking this item gives the clinician an opportunity to discuss the infant's strength and muscle tone and the kind of support, handling, and facilitation the infant may need to organize his motor behavior.

## Feeding Cues

These behaviors provide an opportunity to address any concerns or questions or present guidelines on feeding. The clinician checks here if he or she sees anything in the rooting or sucking suggesting that the infant may have feeding difficulties. If the infant has a weak root or suck, then this can provide an opportunity to initiate a discussion about feeding, and the clinician and mother may decide that the mother needs additional support in this area.

## Touch and Contact

A check here suggests a discussion of the infant's sensitivity to touch and the importance of touch for the newborn infant. It may include a discussion of how the infant prefers to be held. If the infant is not cuddly, for example, this provides an opportunity to reassure the parents of *non-cuddly* infants, who may interpret this behavior as a sign of rejection.

## Sleep Position and Safety

This can be a reminder to discuss the recommendation that an infant be put down to sleep on her back—Back to Sleep—to avoid the risk of SIDS.

## Social Interaction

This gives the clinician an opportunity to discuss the importance of early parent–infant interactions, to review what the NBO revealed about the infant's social capacities, and to help the parents identify the kinds of interactions and stimulation that will best suit the needs of the infant over the first months of life.

## Vision

The clinician checks here if parents wish to discuss the infant's visual capacities or visual preferences.

## Hearing

The clinician checks here if clinician or parent wants to discuss the infant's hearing competencies or preferences, or if there are any concerns about the infant's hearing. The infant's tolerance for various levels of auditory stimulation also may be noted in terms of how parents can use this information when interacting with their infant.

## Communication Cues

This provides an opportunity to discuss the infant's signs of stress or disengagement cues and her signs of availability and social readiness. Here the clinician may wish to discuss how best to interact with the newborn and how to read the infant's social cues and signs of engagement or disengagement or overstimulation.

## Crying and Soothability

This category allows the clinician to discuss with the parents the infant's crying and their perceptions of and reactions to the crying. The recording of whether their infant cried a lot and how sensitive or irritable he is can reveal how easy or how difficult it may be for the parents to help him settle down. Comforting techniques that may work for this infant can be discussed.

## Self-Soothing

This theme allows parents and clinician to identify the infant's self-organizing and self-comforting strategies, such as the use of hand-to-mouth behavior. It can also provide an opportunity to discuss how parents can support these tendencies in their infant.

## State Regulation

The clinician checks here if there is a need to discuss the overall organization of the infant's behavior: Is it well organized, or does this infant need a great deal of support to become organized? What kind of support does this infant need to support her self-regulation? Checking this also presents the clinician with an opportunity to discuss the infant's behavioral style or temperament, her sensory threshold, and whether she is easily engaged, easily upset, or difficult to console. The concept of "goodness of fit" and how parents need to appreciate and adapt to their infant's unique individual temperament can be introduced here.

## Stimulation Threshold

On the basis of the amount of autonomic stress signs such as tremors, startles, and color changes that were observed during the course of the administration, the clinician checks this off. This can provide the clinician with a basis for discussing the kinds of stimulation that may overwhelm the infant and how the parents can best support their infant's efforts to deal with various levels of stimulation in his new environment.

## Needs Support

Infants with very high levels of activity may need a great deal of support to become organized. The clinician and caregiver can use this opportunity to discuss strategies that may help the infant settle, such as holding or swaddling. The observation of the infant's activity level can also be used to address concerns about the baby's cuddliness or her apparent resistance to being held, which is often of great concern to parents. This box should also be checked if the infant has very low activity levels, because she may need a lot of sensory input to stimulate her arousal level and become available for social interaction.

## Summary Profile and Recommendations (Strengths and Challenges)

This section on the NBO recording form gives the clinician and parents the opportunity to compose a summary statement on the infant's strengths as well as the areas in which the infant may need support. The clinician and parents may wish to fill this section out together (direct quotes from parents are especially helpful). On the basis of the infant's behavior observed on the NBO and the clinician's discussions with the parents, the clinician and parents decide together the kinds of caregiving strategies and techniques that are best suited to the individual needs of the infant and that can best promote the infant's optimal development. This section may include additional comments on the parents' strengths and the degree to which the parents may be stressed and may need additional support to care adequately for their infant. The summary profile is used to help make a decision as to whether the infant needs follow-up or support. It does not imply any atypicality or pathology but merely highlights the infant's need for support in certain areas.

## SUMMARY

This manual describes how to conduct the NBO session and how to administer and interpret each of the NBO behavioral items for parents. We presented guidelines on how to elicit and describe the behavior to parents and how each of the observed behaviors should be recorded and coded. Each behavior was described and interpreted in terms of its adaptive and developmental significance—the developmental sequence of the behavior through the first months of life was also described—all of which can serve as resource material for the clinician to help interpret the infant's behavior for the parents. Finally, the possible implications of this behavior for caregiving were presented.

The NBO administration procedures described must be refined and internalized by the clinician so that he or she is able to administer the specific maneuvers in a way that is responsive to the individual infant and at the same time allows the clinician to communicate with the parents. It goes without saying that while all clinicians who use the NBO must be trained in its use, experience is critical to ensure that clinicians can internalize the administration procedures and reach this required level of expertise. (The NBO training program provides clinicians with mentoring in the weeks following the training to ensure that they are competent in the administration of the scale. Only then are they certified in its use.) This level of competence is critical, because it is the smooth administration of the NBO that ensures that the infant is able to reveal the full range of his behavioral repertoire. This level of clinical expertise will also enable the parents to see their infant's behaviors as integrated and cohesive rather than as isolated responses to a series of discrete handling maneuvers. Because the goal of the NBO is to initiate and promote parent–clinician discourse in a relational model of family-centered care, the clinician should not be preoccupied with the proper way to elicit the behaviors or be ill at ease in handling the newborn infant. Well-established, confident handling skills are essential if the NBO is to achieve the relational goals for which it is developed. Only when these administrative skills are well established and the clinician has the flexibility to be able to respond to the infant's state changes will the NBO become second nature to the clinician, and he or she can begin to use the NBO as a relationship-building tool. The next chapter offers guidelines and strategies for clinician–parent communication that can enhance the relationship between them and strengthen the relationship between the parents and their child.

# 4

# RELATIONSHIP BUILDING WITH PARENTS AND THEIR INFANTS IN THE NEWBORN PERIOD

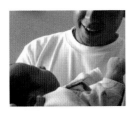

Providing parents with information on their child's development and offering caregiving guidance are best done in the context of relationship-centered care if they are to have a significant effect on child health and development (Feldman, Ploof, & Cohen, 1999; Shelton, 1999; Tresolini, 1996). The Bayer-Fetzer Conference on Physician–Patient Communication in Medical Education emphasized the importance of relationship-centered care and the need for pediatric professionals to communicate with parents and include them as partners in the decision-making process (Makoul, 2001). Karl, Limbo, and Ricker (1998) demonstrated that a close relationship between the family and the primary care provider helped to improve the pattern of health care use by families who lived in disadvantaged areas. Brousseau, Meurer, Isenberg, Kuhn, and Gorelick (2004) found improved continuity of care (indicating strength of the clinician–parent relationship) to be associated significantly with a decrease in emergency department use in the early months of an infant's life.

The Newborn Behavioral Observations (NBO) system provides a structure for parent–clinician discourse about child behavior and development in a relational model of family-centered care. This chapter offers guidelines and strategies for clinician–parent communication that can enhance the relationship between them and strengthen the relationship between the parent and the infant in the newborn period and in the first months of the infant's life.

## SUPPORTING PARENT–INFANT ENGAGEMENT IN THE NEWBORN PERIOD

This chapter begins with consideration of uniquely pediatric ways of helping parents become engaged with their infants and examines aspects of the postpartum experience that make it an unexcelled opportunity to foster relationships between parents and infants and between parents and clinicians. Chapter 2 described the psychobiological characteristics of postpartum parents that allow them to attach so readily to their infant and to caregivers. What follows here are steps that pediatric clinicians can use to take advantage of this tendency to attachment.

This approach begins with attention to the newborn's behavior. As described in Chapter 1, newborn behavior is organized and meaningful. The newborn infant whom parents take home from the hospital, the newborn who will challenge them and guide them, consists, for them, primarily in his or her behavior and interactions. Behavior is the language of the infant and is at the heart of communication between parents and clinicians (Brazelton, 1995). With the NDO, experienced clinicians can read or interpret an infant's behavior and set up a system of communication between the parent and the clinicians, and enhance communication between parent and infant.

Three key relational phenomena heighten the potential for building relationships during critical transitions in an infant's development (Bokhorst et al., 2003; Brazelton, 1992):

The new behavior of the infant may confuse the parents.

The parents' confidence in caring for their infant can be shaken.

The clinician–parent relationship can be a mechanism to guide parents' understanding of their infant's behavior and to enhance parental competence.

In contrast to most other developmental transitions in early childhood, in which a change in the child's behavior may challenge parents, in the newborn transition, the infant's behavior not only is changed but also truly is unknown. During developmental transitions in later months, the parents will have had their experience of understanding and adapting to their infant's previous behavioral changes as a guide for how to approach the new behavior. Parents' previous interactions with their infant and their previous negotiations in those interactions during times of behavioral change exist as a historical reference to be applied to the new behavior. However, the parents of a newborn have no such history for guidance. Fetal movement and ultrasound pictures do provide evidence of behaviors that may shape the parents' images of the child, but their perception and attribution of the whole child still must be constructed. Until the moment of birth, the live infant, who requires active care and responses that are specific to him or her, is an unknown.

For parents, the postpartum condition includes a heightened openness to making attachments and a clarity of awareness that will leave memories for that time strong for life (Klaus et al., 1995; Simkin, 1996). Those who are privileged to enter this *sphere of attachment potential* (i.e., to be present with families at this time) have been given a solid base for developing a strong relationship with the parents. Behind the parents' heightened openness to relational attachments lies the disorganization of the parents' current relationships—to spouse, to parents, to other children. In the reorganization of those attachments, new relationships can grow and old relationships can be strengthened. The disorganization allows the parents to reorganize in a new relationship around their particular newborn, the infant who will elicit their emotional strengths and weaknesses and will call up their "angels and ghosts in the nursery" (Lieberman et al., 2005; see Chapter 2).

## STRATEGIES FOR RELATIONSHIP BUILDING IN AN NBO SESSION

The clinician can take advantage of the opportunity in an NBO session to build toward a positive outcome for the parent–infant and the parent–clinician relationships. An NBO observation session with parents includes the following strategies:

1. Observing the infant in the parents' presence.

2. Narrating to the parents what the clinician is doing and what he or she sees.

3. Involving the parents actively in the session.

Each of these strategies can affect the relational outcome of a pediatric encounter in several ways, as is described next.

### Observing the Infant in the Parents' Presence

Parents' observation of the "unfolding" of their newborn infant during the NBO session places the clinician within the *sphere of their attachment potential;* a relationship with them is ensured. The clinician can lose that attachment, but it will be the clinician's to lose: The clinician is granted it solely by his or her presence at this time.

The clinician's sharing with parents the observation of their infant denotes respect and mutuality. In addition, parents who observe the clinician's examining their infant have an experiential basis for trusting him or her with the care of their infant and themselves. The clinician's reassurances to them, now or later, can be much more effective than if they had only a theoretical basis for trust. They now know that the clinician knows their infant.

## Narrating to the Parents What the Clinician Is Doing and What He or She Sees

Aside from being a simple courtesy, the clinician's telling the parents what he or she is doing to their infant is a way to inform and educate them for their role as parents. Young parents often do not know anything about what newborns can do, so the clinician should tell them, for example, that 1) a newborn infant's movement and posture are based on reflexes (automatic, invariant, patterned movements) but also on complex and volitional patterns, 2) some infants can console themselves and that is why the clinician is letting the infant cry for a moment's observation, and 3) infants can see and hear at birth and the clinician might be able to demonstrate that in their infant.

New parents will see their infant through several lenses. One will be that of the infant of whom they have dreamed, another that of an infant with a much-feared problem, and another that of the actual infant whose behavior they can experience directly. The more the parents understand their infant's behavior through the lens of actual experience, the more appropriate will be their caregiving responses. New parents' minds are sponges for learning, particularly for information and sensory experience regarding their infant. The clinician's narrating the infant's behavior provides confirmation to the parents that they do understand their infant.

The clinician's looking at and stretching and turning the infant are mysterious procedures to parents. The clinician's describing what he or she is doing and what he or she is finding, in understandable terms, not only educates but also empowers parents. They can understand their infant. They will become the clinician's allies; the clinician's trusting them with this information increases their confidence and competence.

## Involving the Parents Actively in the Session

Touch contributes significantly to the biopsychosocial process of attachment of parents to infants and of infants to parents (Ferber et al., 2003; White, 2004). The clinician can support that process by allowing, even encouraging, parental touch during the observation. For example, a mother may stroke the infant's head or let the infant suck her finger to provide some comfort during disturbing maneuvers such as undressing or placing prone. When the infant cries, the father can be invited to gently restrain the infant's hands or arms as part of the consoling sequence. Parents usually are thrilled when their infant grasps their finger. When the grasp reduces generalized or disorganized movements, the parents have first-hand, experiential knowledge of their role as facilitator of the infant's organization of motor behavior. Parents are empowered and their anxiety is lessened when they can share the touch and view of the infant with the clinician. The clinician's acknowledging the importance of their being involved in the behavior observation can increase parental self-worth.

The clinician's fostering relationship in the newborn period refers to two relationships: that of the clinician and the family and that of the parent and the child. The clinician is acknowledging the power of the newborn period to foster attachment relationships. The importance of these relationships cannot be overestimated; neither should the unique value of the newborn period for the development of these relationships be ignored.

## ELEMENTS OF BUILDING RELATIONSHIPS

Relationship is the state of being connected to another through mutually determined and shared goals. This section describes five key elements for the creation of a healthy relationship:

1.  Contingent responsiveness

2.  Respect

3.  Empathy

4.  Time

5.  Tolerance for mistakes

### Contingent Responsiveness

A parent's responsiveness to the needs of his or her infant is the most fundamental of these five elements for development of a healthy relationship. In providing the infant with direct, tangible experience of his or her presence, the parent also introduces an experience of contingency. The infant learns that his or her communication through motion or vocal expression brings reliable and satisfying responses. This, of course, requires the parent's attention to the infant and an ability to recognize the message in the infant's behavior. The use of the NBO with parents is designed to heighten their skill in observing and responding to the infant's signals.

### Respect

Parents show their respect for their infant by allowing the infant's expression of his or her individuality. The parents' acceptance of the range of an individual infant's behavioral style helps the infant to build toward a sense of self and self-esteem.

### Empathy

Empathy includes recognition and understanding of the state of mind and emotion of the partner in the relationship (Jordan, 1989). One of the major gifts of a relationship is the experience of being known, even as much as being understood. With empathy, the parent reflects the infant's emotion and provides scaffolding for the infant's regulation of state, as in the following example of a 4-week-old infant and his mother at home:

✳

The infant, Asa, was sitting upright in the infant seat in a calm, alert state. Suddenly, a door slammed shut, making a loud noise, and Asa startled and began to cry. His mother approached him with a look of concern and empathy, saying, "Ooh, Asa dear, that was a loud sound and it frightened you," as she gently picked him up and cuddled him to her chest. He continued to whimper for a moment, during which his mother stroked his head, rubbed her cheek to his, and made soothing sounds. Asa then stopped crying and resumed his alert state.

✳

Through experiences such as this, an infant grows into a sense of being known, through being mirrored. This and the contingent responsiveness in this experience create the basis for the infant's sense of security and trust.

## Time

Creation of a relationship between people of any age requires a minimal amount of time in contact with another to begin to know that person as an individual. Many of the important details that one knows about friends, spouses, or children are learned unconsciously, during the course of many physical and social interactions, from the mundane knowledge of how many sugars one's spouse likes in his or her coffee to the relevant knowledge that most mothers have, within a few days of giving birth, about their infant's preferred position or way of signaling hunger versus wet diaper. The time in contact during those interactions allows accurate and detailed knowledge to inform the relationship.

## Tolerance for Mistakes

Last and most important, although it may be somewhat counterintuitive, a relationship tolerates mistakes and offers avenues for repair. Examples of this are examined from clinician–parent relationships and parent–infant relationships.

In an established relationship, the five elements at work will have led to

1. A sense of security and trust that the other partner will be there when needed

2. An understanding that the responses of the partner will be appropriate and timely

3. An understanding that one's personal style, both its endearing features and its irritating features, will be accepted

4. An expectation that one's feelings will be understood

5. An expectation that one will be given the time necessary for working together

Many well-functioning clinician–parent relationships have these characteristics, enabling those relationships to survive relational mistakes. The following is an example of such a relationship:

---

Dr. Miller misread anger in Mr. Smith's anxiety about his 4-day-old infant's failing the hearing screening. Fortunately, they had begun to form a relationship during the time that Dr. Miller spent assisting Mrs. Smith with some difficulty in breast feeding in the first 3 days of life. Mr. Smith felt self-confident enough to correct Dr. Miller's attribution of anger, and Dr. Miller was able to apologize. The experience of that mistake, on Dr. Miller's part, and its repair, as Mr. Smith and Dr. Miller confronted and apologized to each other, would serve to strengthen their relationship in the future, when the infant's hearing problem required diagnosis and treatment.

Similarly and with the same family, as the Smiths were growing in their relationship with their infant, at approximately 6 weeks of age, Mrs. Smith abruptly turned away from the infant while he was smiling at her, and he reacted by crying and falling slightly forward in his infant seat. She quickly responded by stroking his arms and using his grasp to help him help himself return to an upright position. With that, their gaze met, and the infant quickly smiled in response to Mrs. Smith's activating her face and smiling at him.

---

Research on face-to-face interactions between mothers and their infants shows that typical, healthy pairs spend up to 30% of interaction time misreading each others' signals and violating rules (Tronick & Cohn, 1989). In the process of discovering what happened and returning to a balanced and satisfying interaction, the pair learn to repair potential breaks in the relationship and, in fact, weave an even stronger connection.

## THE IMPORTANCE OF THE PARENT–INFANT RELATIONSHIP IN DEVELOPMENT

In a positive relationship, both partners experience clarity of self, a sense of competence, a sense of self-worth, and a desire for more relationships. A special energy often accompanies these relational experiences of mind and emotion. Referred to as *zest*, it fuels development and change (Jordan & Dooley, 2000; Miller, 1986). Relational processes fuel development and healthy change in infants and in parents.

The parent–infant relationship is the main effective agent for development in infants. The quality of the relationship between parents and infants is critical to

**Table 4.1.**  Link from parent–clinician relationships to child development outcome

Skilled, caring communication between clinician and parent →

Relationship between parent and clinician →

Parental self-worth* →

Positive parent–infant interactions →

Optimal child development: physical, intellectual, emotional, and social

*Also empowerment, clarity of self, energy or zest, and desire for more relationship

the socioemotional, cognitive, and physical development of their children (National Scientific Council on the Developing Child, 2004). In pediatrics, a positive relationship between the clinician and the parent is an essential component of care that leads to better health outcomes in infants (American Academy of Pediatrics Committee on Hospital Care, 2003; Nobile & Drotar, 2003). A positive relationship between a child's health care clinician and his or her mother promotes sound outcomes for the infant's mental and emotional development (Owen et al., 2000; see Table 4.1).

The NBO clearly represents a model for parent–infant–clinician discourse about child development and behavior in relationship-centered care. Pediatric care such as the NBO, which is focused on the infant's behavior while centered on the family, can be practiced with families of young children of any age. Development and use of the NBO, however, acknowledges the unique power of the newborn period to foster attachment relationships.

## THE ROLE OF COMMUNICATION IN DEVELOPING A RELATIONSHIP: GUIDELINES AND STRATEGIES FOR COMMUNICATION THROUGH THE NBO

Evidence-based studies show that clinicians' interpersonal and communication skills have a significant impact on patient care and correlate with improved health outcomes and health care quality (Nobile & Drotar, 2003; Stewart, 1995; Stewart et al., 1995). This section offers guidelines and strategies to help NBO trainees communicate with parents in a way that can enhance the parent–provider relationship. This includes a description of basic techniques of skilled communication and guidance on attitude and expression of intent and caring. Communication is a core clinical skill, with defining actions that can be taught and learned. Use of these skills in communication with parents promotes positive relationships. Although many variations of these descriptions and guidelines are available in the literature of psychology, nursing, and medicine, the basic skills and attitudes are similar across the variations, with self-reflection at the heart of the process (Hafler, 2005; Schon, 1983).

The basic communication skills are presented, and guidance on applying those skills to express a caring attitude in interaction with parents is offered. The effective use of these communication skills for building relationships depends on

1.  Self-reflection and awareness of one's own biases

2.  Respect for individual differences in parents' styles of communication

3.  Careful observation of the environment and the flow of the NBO interaction

In addition, the clinician offers a commitment to the parents to work from their strengths.

The description of communication skills is organized in a temporal framework that includes three phases in a typical NBO encounter:

1.  Pre-NBO encounter: mental preparation before the interaction

2.  Within-NBO encounter: three levels of focus

3.  Post-NBO encounter: preparation for seamlessness of care

In the central *within-NBO encounter* phase are three levels of focus: 1) an immediate mental "snapshot" of the scene followed by 2) a "narrowing focus" to the parent–infant interaction and 3) a "widening focus" on the breadth of contextual factors for the family.

## Pre-NBO Encounter: Mental Preparation Before the Interaction

Clinicians should attend to every aspect of their behavior and attitude, beginning before initiating the face-to-face encounter with the parents. Before approaching the family space, be it in a hospital room, home, or clinic, clinicians should reflect, as follows, on two of their own inner states: attention and attitude.

Where is my attention directed? The clinician should note especially distracting thoughts about professional or personal issues that would prevent full attention to the task at hand, which is to get to know this infant and family through the infant's behavior and in a way that supports the parent–infant relationship and that prepares the way for an effective relationship between the parents and the clinician.

What is my attitude toward this family? Great care should be taken to be alert to attitudes toward the family that are based on little information, particularly secondhand information. Knowledge of everything about the family, even others' opinions, can be helpful, but all should be suspended for an attitude that is free of assumptions or at least aware of potential inaccuracies that could interfere with the development of a relationship with the parents. With this approach, the clinician is left in a position to view the parents as people with whom a relationship is possible. Progress and support are possible only in the context of a relationship.

## Within-NBO Encounter: Three Levels of Focus

Aspects of each of the three levels of focus may overlap in time or may occur simultaneously or sequentially. For example, while "mental snapshot" will likely occur first, throughout the encounter the clinician may very well have his or her attention redrawn to the way participants have situated themselves (in relation to one another, to the clinician, or to the infant). On the other hand, even before completion of a mental snapshot of the scene, the clinician may be drawn to a question or comment by a parent, and, in this way, be called upon to use communication techniques from the level of "narrowing of focus." Similarly, the clinician may be offered information on the context of the family's life anywhere in the encounter, although we have listed it third among these levels of focus of the "within-encounter phase."

### Immediate Mental "Snapshot" of the Scene

An NBO session may occur in various places: in a general setting (e.g., a hospital room or nursery, a clinic, a home), in a specific space (e.g., the infant in a bassinet, on the father's lap), or with a particular audience (e.g., from only one parent to the extended family). The clinician should make careful observation and a mental note of the spatial relations in the room and the emotional tone. These findings may become useful in understanding the family and in application of the NBO with them.

The clinician should pay attention to the environment. Is his or her back to one of the parents? Is the infant between him or her and the parents and close enough for the parent to touch the infant? Must the parents face a bright window light, or can that be used to reflect on the clinician and the infant from behind them? If others are present, then do the parents want them to stay? The clinician's attention to these situational characteristics can affect positively the result of the encounter.

### "Narrowing Focus" to the Parent–Infant Interaction

Communication techniques for the level of *narrowing the focus to the parent–infant interaction* tell one what to say and how to say it while doing the NBO. Communication with parents and the infant stands at the heart of an NBO session, and the following basic strategies are designed and suggested to allow that communication to achieve its intended goals of creating a relationship between the parents and the clinician and enhancing the relationship between the parents and the infant. The strategies fall into three categories: active listening (Hafler, 2005; Mishler, 1985), clear speaking, and mutuality of action (see Table 4.2).

#### Active Listening

The clinician should use open-ended questions because they leave the parents in charge of the order in which topics are raised, in itself an important piece of information. The clinician will learn about what he or she did not know to ask. The most important nonverbal listening strategy is to pause for at least 3 seconds before speaking after asking a question; it will seem like a very long time, but many studies show that, even for people who have something to say, they may need at

**Table 4.2.**  Communication techniques for narrowing the focus to the parent–infant interaction

Active listening (OPERA)

    O  Use <u>O</u>pen-ended questions

    P  <u>P</u>ause

    E  Make <u>E</u>ye contact

    R  <u>R</u>epeat

    A  <u>A</u>void judgment

        <u>A</u>sk opinion

        <u>A</u>dvise last

Speak clearly (be a SUPER speaker)

    S  <u>S</u>peak slowly

    U  <u>U</u>se simple sentences and lay terms

    P  <u>P</u>ace yourself to the parents' attention

    E  <u>E</u>mphasize important words and transitions

    R  <u>R</u>eview parents' understanding

Act mutually (you CAN)

    C  <u>C</u>ollaborate: respect/recognize

    A  Be <u>A</u>uthentic: present/real

    N  <u>N</u>egotiate: respond/repair

least 2½ seconds to find it or phrase it (Napell, 1976). The clinician must learn to maintain eye contact that is appropriate to the parents' tolerance and use other nonverbal behaviors to signal understanding. Some brief eye contact virtually always is necessary, but the frequency and the intensity of it, after an initial checking in, should be modulated in accordance with the parents' signals. The clinician's repeating the last few words of what a parent has just said or repeating what he or she believes to be what the parent intends to say confirms to them that he or she is listening and hearing and allows for clarification in the event that the clinician's repetition was not accurate. The clinician also should check in for clarification of the parents' emotional experience.

Throughout the NBO session, the clinicians should avoid judgment of what the parents say and of the parents' actions or emotions and assume that they want the best for their child. Any possible knowledge of their past successes, failures, or inadequacies must be held outside this moment with them. The clinician must accept them as they are, for that is the only place from which to begin support and work with them.

During the NBO session, the clinician should ask the parents' opinion on an issue before offering his or her own opinion or standard advice. When clinicians allow parents to express all of their concerns and ask questions, many important characteristics of health improve; for example, satisfaction with care, compliance with treatment, effectiveness of intervention, and maternal adaptation to the child (Percy, Stadtler, & Sands, 2002).

Engaging in this type of interview may be threatening to a novice's sense of or need for control; with experience, clinicians can learn to recognize the change in a parent's discourse style that indicates that he or she has expressed him- or herself sufficiently. Although many clinicians fear that allowing the parent to lead will consume too much time, in fact, most parents will finish to their satisfaction with in 1 minute and virtually all within 3 minutes. By giving the parents time to express their issues and opinions first, the clinician will learn what advice they are seeking, and the clinician's advice can be tailored specifically to their individual needs (Mishler, 1985). Giving parents time at the beginning of the NBO often shortens, not lengthens, the time that is necessary for the session.

## Clear Speaking

The clinician should communicate clearly, speaking slowly and pacing his or her speech to the parents' attention. In the postpartum period, mothers may be slow to process information, because they are distracted by pain or by the effect of narcotic medication. They also are being presented with an enormous amount of information from at least a dozen different people. The clinician should use simple sentences and lay terms and avoid medical jargon. The clinician should test him- or herself by phrasing as if he or she were speaking with a nonprofessional member of his or her family. In that mode, he or she is likely to be clear without being condescending. The clinician should not only use simpler words but also fewer words, rather than more. After speaking three sentences, the clinician should pause and review the parents' understanding.

The clinician should emphasize important words and announce transitions (Mishler, 1985). For example, "*Now* [announces a transition; emphasize it and pause] watch how her *hands move* [alerts the parents to the activity of interest] when she focuses on the red ball," or, as the clinician says, "*Now*, I want to ask about the *jitteriness* that you noticed," the parents have time to realize that the topic has changed and bring to mind what they noticed in the infant's hand movements, rather than wonder how what the clinician is doing (uncovering the infant's hands) relates to the infant's turning to the parent's voice, which has delighted her, and the parent may not be thinking about her earlier worries.

Then, periodically or when the parents' attention seems to wane, the clinician should review the parents' understanding of what has been said, eliciting the parents' confirmation and questions about the issue or the findings. Although listening is the most important feature of discourse for relationship building and the message and the information must be well founded and accurate, the manner of the clinician's speech is crucial for the parents' full understanding and mutual collaboration.

## Mutuality of Action

Mutuality of action is the key process to which the clinician brings the listening and communication strategies described in the previous two subsections (Jordan,

1986). For example, collaboration requires listening actively and speaking clearly but also includes agreeing to ask the opinion of the other and agreeing to take no action without the understanding of the other. The strategies of listening and speaking are important, but a relational encounter consists of more than strategies alone. The collaboration itself recognizes the parents as competent partners with the clinician in understanding and caring for their infant. That recognition shows the clinician's respect for the parents and supports their own feelings of self-worth.

Relational care is authentic, caring, and emotional (Miller et al., 1999; Suchman, 2006). Being fully present with the parents allows the clinician to be his or her authentic self; the clinician's caring and emotion become apparent but not forced. This state of presence is what the clinician aims for when he or she does pre-encounter reflection. It leads not only to effective care but also to compassionate care that supports the development of effective and even therapeutic relationships.

Striving for authenticity may lead to mistakes and misunderstandings, but mistakes are part of the process of coming to know the other, which is an intermittent but ongoing task in a relationship. Distraction and lack of full attention (i.e., inauthenticity to the parents) more likely will lead to mistakes. Mistakes create a dissonance and tension; we must pause and reflect on the situation. They require mutual exploration and negotiation, which can lead to repair, and often leave the relationship even stronger for the new knowledge gained about the other and the demonstrated caring and commitment to the relationship.

These basic principles of respectful and effective communication are outlined with acronyms in Table 4.2. These are relational processes of listening, speaking, and acting. In summary, in active listening, the clinician asks the parents' opinion, pauses for a reflective answer, avoids judgment, and holds back on advice. In clearly communicating, the clinician paces him- or herself to the parents' attention and reviews the parents' understanding. In mutuality of action, the clinician collaborates with and respects the parents and recognizes his or her strengths.

## "Widening Focus" to the Breadth of Contextual Factors

For the level of *widening the focus to the breadth of contextual factors*, techniques are those that may tell the clinician what to think about while doing an NBO. Simultaneous with communication with the parents and the infant, the clinician's focus must widen beyond the infant and parent–infant relationship to include the following four perspectives:

1. Story of the pregnancy and birth

2. Emotional tone in the family

3. Values, beliefs, and techniques of child-rearing practices

4. Context and history of the family's life

The clinician need not question the family on every one of the four elements. Primarily, he or she should listen for evidence of them in the parents' narration and discussion. Throughout the encounter with the parents, some elements may reveal themselves to be more pertinent to this family and may warrant further exploration.

## Story of the Pregnancy and Birth

A family's narrative of the birth of a child holds more meaning than a simple report of the facts. In relating the facts in a story mode, the parents are arranging the facts in a meaningful way, informing the clinician and themselves about the relationships, expectations, and worries about their new life as a family with this particular child. The story will hold meaning that a report of the experience cannot convey, giving it power to affect the relationship with the clinician (Bruner, 1990). Studies of outcomes in occupational therapy demonstrated that the relationship between therapist and patient, particularly through the co-creation of a narrative of the patient's illness, was the significantly effective element, more so than the specific exercises, in shortening the period of disability and need for therapy (Mattingly & Garro, 2000). At the time of a birth, any previous pregnancy loss, particularly the demise of a term or near-term infant, will be re-experienced. This infant may very well continue to be a member of the family, psychologically, and acknowledgment of the infant or the loss may uncover that infant's role in the family and the status of the family's mourning that loss.

## Emotional Tone in the Family

The narrative provides the cognitive facts and structures about which and from which a range of intense emotions may arise. Expressing the feelings alone can be therapeutic for parents—especially feelings of fear and anger. Sharing the expression of those feelings with a caring, nonjudgmental clinician can be therapeutic and potentially healing into the future.

The relationship between the new parents and their parents may hold keys to how these young parents will perform in their child-rearing roles. Certainly, the clinician is privileged to observe the other siblings as they greet the new infant. Even more so, the parents' responses to and concerns about the reaction of the other children to the new infant are important information for clinicians who are beginning a relationship with the family through the NBO. For example, with questions such as, "Was the first-born, now 2 years old, similar in her ability to self-console as we see in this new infant?" "How does the 2-year-old behave now when frustrated?" the clinician demonstrates his or her availability to the parents should they want to discuss their other children.

The clinician's observations of the newborn's behavior with the parents during an NBO provide a shared platform for discussing sibling reactions to the new infant and parents' plans for how to manage those reactions. This is an example of how clinicians can join in collaborative problem solving even before they and the family know each other well.

## Values, Beliefs, and Techniques of Child-Rearing Practices

The explanations that parents give for their child-rearing practices, their explanatory models, are cognitive, mental constructs that often are unconscious yet can have a strong effect on a family's behavior as parents (Harkness, Super, & Keefer, 1992). They guide most families to culturally appropriate ways of being with their infants so that the outcome of a healthy adult of that culture is ensured. In other words, parents choose child-rearing practices (techniques) on the basis of beliefs about how children grow and develop and about what makes a good parent. Those techniques then tend to shape children's behavior toward valued characteristics (LeVine et al., 1994; Whiting, Fischer, Longabaugh, & Whiting, 1975).

For example, traditional Japanese families view the newborn infant as detached from the family, requiring close and continuous contact to ensure a strong attachment to the family and to give the infant the sense of being connected to the family (Doi, 1991; Shimizu & Levine, 2001). This belief supports the parental practice of sleeping with their infants in the same bed. Underlying this system of belief and explanation and concomitant practice is the Japanese cultural value of a highly connected society, one in which the group could be more important than the individual.

In contrast, many American families see the newborn infant as dependent, requiring practices that would support a separation and less contact; therefore, they place their newborns in a separate crib and often from an early age even place the infant in a separate room. Underlying these American practices and beliefs are the cultural values of independence and the primacy of the individual (Harkness, Super, Keefer, Rahgavan, & Kipp, 1995).

The clinician should know as much as he or she can about the public information on any particular culture, but knowing how they play out in the function of a particular family is essential for relational care. In some instances or regarding certain issues, a system of techniques, beliefs, and values is unique to a family. Functionally, understanding a family as a microculture can be helpful when a clinician is involved in helping to solve problems with the family. For example, some parents want their newborn to use his or her hand to suck and comfort, whereas others will not tolerate that activity. The clinician will find a range of explanations and beliefs about why the parents subscribe to one or the other of these attitudes. Some come from the health/medical model ("Teeth will not come in straight") or an economic model ("I don't want to pay for a lot of dental work"). Others will rely on aspersions to character ("That's for sissies, and I don't want him going to school with his thumb in his mouth"). Along the lines of character, some parents value an independent, self-regulating infant who can contribute to his or her own learning of state regulation.

The task for clinicians, who may subscribe to one or another of these beliefs themselves, is to allow the parents' expression of opinion and their exploration of underlying values that the belief supports. Perhaps, if the parents express ambivalence over their practice or their exercise of the practice leads to struggle with the infant or other caregivers, then the clinician may help the parents to explore other options. Great care should be taken, however, to avoid simply replacing the parents' belief and practice with that of the clinician.

### Context and History of the Family's Life

Knowledge of the current social, economic, and physical conditions of a family also is essential to a clinician's giving optimal care and facilitating a healthy relationship between the family and the clinician. The history of the family as a unit and its members individually certainly will affect how they use a clinician's help and may explain much of the family's narrative, emotions, values, and beliefs.

## Post-NBO Encounter: Preparation for Seamlessness of Care

The clinician should make him- or herself known clearly throughout the session, beginning by using the name that he or she wants the parents to use. The clinician again should make clear the purpose of the NBO session. Trust will be built by projections into the future: The parents will wonder when they will see the clinician again and whether they will be able to reach him or her. Even if the NBO encounter is a singular event between the clinician and the parents, the clinician can support the maintenance of trust by knowing who the next clinicians will be and using their names, making reference to his or her knowing them (whether they are in the same discipline or another), and demonstrating his or her willingness to communicate to them about the NBO. A moment of reflection on the relational aspects experienced in the session, while documenting the event, could be part of the clinician's self-improvement of communication skills. In addition, if the NBO session is the beginning of a long-term caregiving role for the clinician, even brief notes about these aspects of the session, especially a direct quote from the parent, can be bridges for powerful reconnection and deepening of the relationship in the next encounter. Parents will feel held by the clinician and the system; the clinician is scaffolding their transition to the next encounter with a health care professional and into the future.

## SUMMARY

This chapter has defined *relationship* and reviewed the importance of relationships in child and family development and in effective interventions by pediatric professionals in a variety of disciplines. Although the task of establishing a helping relationship with parents is a challenging one, this chapter has pointed out how certain postpartum conditions make the newborn period highly opportune for parents to establish relationships. The openness of parents to attachment at this time provides the pediatric professional with a remarkable opportunity to enter into a supportive relationship with the family.

At the same time, parents' current relationships become disorganized so that they can reorganize around their newborn infant. This creates a critical developmental challenge for the parent–infant interactions. With the NBO, clinicians can offer a reflection on the child's individuality, strengths, and challenges, bringing the shared observations of actual behaviors to the parents' construction of the meaningful infant. Highlighting the newborn's competencies and individual appeal with the NBO facilitates the mutual affective regulation process between the parents and the infant and may reduce the risk for abuse or neglect of the infant.

This chapter also reviewed a variety of communication skills and organized them as strategies for use at all phases of an NBO encounter, from pre-encounter reflection, through the collaborative heart of the encounter, to a model for scaffolding parents into the future. Relationships that are formed at this time are likely to be resilient to a variety of communication errors, but the new relationships may flourish better with careful attention to modes and manners of skilled interpersonal communication.

# 5

# INCORPORATING THE NEWBORN BEHAVIORAL OBSERVATIONS SYSTEM INTO THE NEWBORN NURSERY ENVIRONMENT

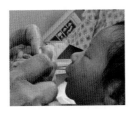
The birth of a child is a major life event and as such presents a unique opportunity for clinicians who work with and support families at this critical life transition. The arrival of this new person stimulates significant changes for parents and reshuffles roles within the family system (Belsky, 1985; Brazelton, 1992; Klaus et al., 1995; Lerner et al., 2002; Minuchin, 1985; & Stern, 1995). The clinician who has the privilege of caring for families during this life-changing time can join with parents as they discover their strengths and work through their vulnerabilities.

Traditionally, the goals of newborn care in the postpartum environment are to identify and treat potential medical complications in the newborn infant and to give parents necessary anticipatory guidance before hospital discharge. As critical as these goals are, the postpartum hospital stay also is an opportunity to accomplish much more with families. Clinicians can support families in their developing relationship with their newborn, helping them to build self-confidence in their ability to understand and appreciate the uniqueness and individuality of their newborn. These first encounters with newborns and their families are also wonderful opportunities for clinicians to model and begin a healthy, family-focused relationship with the parents. The Newborn Behavioral Observations (NBO) system helps clinicians accomplish these goals. It offers a tool to observe behavior and to describe the unique individuality of each newborn. As such, it provides a framework within which to characterize the newborn's developmental strengths and vulnerabilities beyond the labels *typical* or *not typical*. Most important, it does so in a collaborative manner with parents. The clinician brings expertise with respect to newborns in general; the parents bring expertise with respect to their particular infant. This collaboration has powerful relationship-building potential not only for the parents and the infant (Das Eiden & Reifman, 1996) but also for the parents and the clinician. The strength of these relationships has the potential to contribute subsequently to the family's caregiving abilities (e.g., Rutter et al., 1990).

## THE NBO AS A TOOL FOR DEVELOPING RELATIONSHIP-BUILDING SKILLS IN THE NURSERY ENVIRONMENT

The NBO is a practical tool that can be used to guide clinicians who value the importance of relationship in their work. Through the use of the NBO, the clinician has an opportunity to practice several core principles of good relational medical care:

1. Being a keen observer

2. Being flexible; in this case, adapting the encounter to the infant's state—the sleeping, bright-eyed, crying, or hungry infant—and always keeping the newborn at the center of the interaction

3. Taking a sincere interest in the family and respecting their knowledge about their own newborn

4. Valuing the concept of continuity and demonstrating a sense of personal commitment to families

### Keen Observation

Keen observation of newborn behavior is central to the NBO. This point must be emphasized. The clinician also must understand the core concepts of newborn and infant development as they apply to the various systems of the young infant: the autonomic, motor, state, and social/interactive behavioral systems. The clinician must learn to use the NBO to carefully observe the infant's level of organization in each of these realms and generate a behavioral profile of the infant, thereby providing meaningful observations to share with parents.

### Flexibility

By its nature, the clinician must carry out the NBO with the participation of the family. The infant must be at the center of the interaction so that observations can be shared. Such shared observations can relieve anxiety and give parents the ability to refer to the shared observations in future conversations about their child's development with each other and with their clinician. The clinician also must learn to use the NBO flexibly on the basis of the infant's state and the particularities of the situation. If the infant is crying, the discussion is about the healthiness of infant cry and the different kinds of cry and about soothing. If the infant is sleeping, the clinician can talk about habituation and the ability to shut out unwanted noises and light and give suggestions for helping the infant protect his or her sleep. As the infant moves from state to state during an encounter, the conversation turns to regulation, the importance of organization, and the infant's cues for decompensation and need for support. The parents then have an opportunity to see how the clinician manages these various aspects of typical newborn behavior. When these shared, flexible, newborn-centered observations are woven into physical examinations and other aspects of clinical care, they provide a rich context for clinicians and families to discuss many aspects of the infant's health and upbringing. In contrast to this model, clinicians often examine and care for newborns in the hospital nursery, away from parents. This likely occurs for a variety of reasons: convenience and time constraints, better lighting, force of habit, or discomfort with the possibility that an atypical finding will need to be thought through in the presence of family members. What is lost is a powerful opportunity to allow the family to see all the ways in which the clinician has examined and cared for their newborn instead of merely hearing, "I looked at her in the nursery and she looks fine." Also lost are opportunities to remind the family of questions they had and to share their infant with a caring professional: in short, to build a relationship. As an exercise, some pediatric residents (physicians in a post-graduate residency training program) in the authors' nurseries are asked to compare consciously the quality of experience with two families: one whose infant they examined alone in the nursery and one whose infant they examined in an interactive manner with the family. The differences between the two encounters are clear not only for the families but also for the clinician.

## Respect for the Newborn and Family

Beyond its use for sharing observations, the NBO provides a powerful tool for the clinician to establish a collaborative relationship with new parents and to demonstrate his or her sincere interest in and respect for the newborn and the newborn's family. It is worth emphasizing the importance of *language* here. Given the power of the moment, it perhaps is not surprising that pediatric encounters in the newborn period are ones that can be remembered for a lifetime. Most parents can recount the story of their child's birth as though it occurred only yesterday, recalling experiences and exact words and phrases used by their doctor, especially comments that were significantly positive or negative (Simkin, 1991, 1992). One can well conjecture that words such as *strengths, talents, skills, challenges,* and *opportunities* convey an empowering message of confidence to new parents. Words such as *abnormal, weakness, deficit,* and *problem* may exacerbate parents' vulnerabilities or discourage or alienate them, with possible long-lasting effects. A health issue as common as neonatal jaundice in the first few days can lead to persistent parental perceptions of a child's ongoing vulnerability, with sequelae as diverse as disruptions in the parent–infant relationship, early termination of breast-feeding, and increased medical visits (Hannon, Willis, & Scrimshaw, 2001; Kemper, Forsyth, & McCarthy, 1989). In short, whether the infant is term and healthy or faces multiple medical concerns, clinicians must choose their language carefully, understanding both the vulnerability and the sense of possibility in each newborn family. Using words such as *sharing* instead of *teaching* helps to put the relationship on the level of partnership rather than paternalism. Carefully and thoughtfully chosen words can reinforce the parents' position as the primary caregivers. For example, asking the parents how they think their infant prefers to be held affirms their authority and capability as parents. Observing the infant with his or her parents, the clinician asks the parents what *they* have seen. Rather than expect that the parents do not know their infant and do not understand newborn care, the clinician adopts an attitude that parents *do* know their infant and, in most cases, know him or her better than anyone else does. Not uncommonly, when asked about what they have noticed in their infant, mothers will laugh and describe the infant as though she has been with him or her for years, even though the infant is less than 24 hours old. The mother may even say something like, "Oh, he has always been like that!"

## Commitment to Continuity of Care

Finally, continuity of care is of fundamental importance to families (Mainous, Goodwin, & Slange, 2004). The NBO can provide a common language—the language of infant behavior—that can be transferred easily from one clinical environment to the next. As the clinician notices key aspects of the infant's behavior during the NBO in the hospital, he or she may remark, "Won't it be interesting to see what he is doing when I see you next!" At the next visit, referring to the past shared observation (e.g., head lifting when in prone position), the clinician notes, "Remember how he could only briefly hold his head up in the nursery? Look how much longer he is able to hold up his head now!" This seamless thread that the clinician has created between one encounter and the next serves to establish a trust in the parents' minds that the clinician cares about their infant and does *remember* the infant. As this trust is established, the relationship between the parents and the clinician can grow. In the realities of current pediatric care, of course, different clinicians are often seeing families from one pediatric encounter to the next. In these situations, the common language of the NBO can be a powerful tool that can be shared by various providers to help create a sense of a continuity of caring for families. For example, at an initial office visit with a healthy 4-day-old infant, Dr. Smith, a covering physician, observes the baby's ability to briefly hold her head up when in a prone position. He notes this milestone aloud to the baby's mother and documents his observation in the medical record. When Dr. Jones sees the infant at her 1-month check-up, he is able to refer back to the baby's neck tone and observe aloud with the mother what gains the infant has made in only 3 weeks: "Remember when you were here at your last visit? She could only hold her head up briefly. Look what she is able to do now!"

## The NBO as an Educational Tool for Clinicians in Training

The NBO is a useful educational tool for even the newest clinicians as they learn about newborn care. In the authors' nurseries, for example, the pediatric physicians-in-training (residents and medical students) are introduced to the principles of newborn neurodevelopment and the NBO and are given an opportunity to practice at least parts of the NBO in a variety of situations. Trainees in other disciplines caring for newborns can also be introduced similarly to the NBO. For example, during a newborn examination, the trainee may focus more on the behavioral cues of the infant that are most relevant to breast feeding (hand-to-mouth activity, rooting and suck, state organization). In another encounter, he or she may spend time with parents as they observe the social aspects of the infant's behavior. Most important, the trainee is taught to *notice aloud* what he or she sees in the infant. If the infant is observed self-soothing with hand-to-mouth activity, then the trainee shares with the parents what he or she has seen. In this way, the parents become partners with the trainee, and they gain as much from the process as the trainee does. Trainees should have an opportunity to use the NBO in a variety of situations. For example, a mother with postpartum depression, adolescent parents, and parents of a preterm infant each may benefit from different aspects of the NBO. As a result, trainees learn to use the NBO to develop an understanding of the neurodevelopment of newborns and to hone their communication skills with new families, each with its unique needs.

Trainees also should be encouraged to discover and adopt their own style of administering the NBO with parents, because the NBO is not meant to be rote or mechanical. The authenticity that is required to carry out relational care with the NBO (see Chapter 4) necessitates that clinicians bring their own character and temperament to the interaction. Individual styles of clinicians could make an NBO on virtually the same family look quite different in someone else's hands. Some clinicians, for example, are quiet and watchful, some are energetic and enthusiastic, and some are measured and serious. Some may be more likely to listen for information about siblings, whereas others will focus more on parental adjustment. A clinician's effectiveness in using the NBO to form relationships with parents and to support parent–infant relationships stems specifically from the combination of a particular and shared set of skills and attitudes with the clinician's individual style of caring practice.

Beyond the knowledge and skills learned by clinicians in training, the NBO is a model for teaching these young adult learners. Just as the administration of the NBO with parents and infants requires a collaborative and respectful attitude on the part of the clinician, teaching it requires a similar degree of collaboration and respect for the learner. Following guidelines from current research on medical education, trainees are expected to articulate their goals, skill level, and mode and pace of learning (Hafler, 2005). In this collaborative teaching model, trainees can be observed through their time in the nursery and given an opportunity to demonstrate the skills they have achieved (Hafler, 2005). They can then be helped to recognize where their skills, attitude, or knowledge breaks down, not to grade or demonstrate failure but rather to allow them to identify openly those areas as a place from which to work toward improving their skills and abilities. Using a collaborative and respectful teaching approach will help ensure that the trainee will assume the same attitude when caring for their own patients.

## SCENARIOS USING THE NBO IN THE NURSERY ENVIRONMENT

This section describes ways in which the NBO can be used by a variety of clinicians in the newborn period. We begin by outlining the use of the NBO during the most common types of visits that clinicians encounter during the well-newborn hospitalization. Following that is a broader discussion of the concept of the developmentally rich newborn nursery and how the NBO can be used in a multidisciplinary way.

In the United States, newborns are hospitalized with their mother for approximately 2 to 4 days, depending on whether they are born vaginally or by cesarean section. This then becomes a time of intense interaction between parents and many clinicians: physicians, nurses, nurse practitioners, lactation consultants, and health aides. After hospital discharge, mothers typically bring their new infant to the primary clinician's office for follow-up, at least once or twice within the first weeks, and they also may be getting home-visiting support from registered nurses, lactation consultants, or other family support services, depending on the need. The use of the NBO in the early newborn period is discussed with this care structure as the reference, but it is hoped that the concepts discussed can be adapted beyond the North American model.

### Use of the NBO During Common Pediatric Encounters in the Early Newborn Period

For convenience, the role of the NBO for clinicians in the early newborn period is outlined somewhat chronologically. Although every interaction differs, common themes do emerge from one family to the next, providing a framework for discussion. Although this is to some extent an artificial organization of concepts, the following themes are discussed as a "rounding" pediatrician or nurse practitioner might encounter them:

Day 1: The first encounter—strengths and needs within the family system

Day 1/Day 2: Feeding support and easing transition

Day 2/Day 3: Crying and soothability

Day 2 and beyond: Individualized caregiving guidelines

The reader will see how concepts from one theme weave throughout other themes and how the NBO adapts itself to a variety of professionals. As is discussed in the latter part of this chapter, the NBO is most powerful when it is used by all of the clinicians the family encounters; it helps if everyone is using the same language.

## Day 1: First Encounter—Strengths and Needs within the Family System

The first pediatric physical assessment often is the first meeting between the clinician and the family. The pretext of the visit is to complete the physical examination of the infant and discuss newborn health maintenance issues. Its richness, however, comes from clinician and parents looking together at the new infant as a person. Therefore, as discussed earlier, this examination should be done, whenever possible, in the presence of the family. Although each provider builds relationships in his or her own style and there are cultural differences in the ways in which such an introduction may be presented, a useful first question is, "How did you choose his name?" Most parents care deeply about the name they have chosen for their infant; usually much thought has gone into their decision. There often are stories that spring from the parents as they begin to recount their story of the infant's name. Listening carefully to the answer, the clinician can elicit important social and family history without asking uncomfortable or intrusive questions (e.g., the father's involvement, key support people who participated in choosing the name, religious and cultural traditions, hopes and dreams for the new infant). Using the infant's name throughout the subsequent examination gives parents one of their first opportunities to hear their infant addressed by his or her name—an intimate joy to share.

Early in this first encounter, the clinician can invite the parents to bring their concerns to the fore: "What questions do you have about your infant so far?" Typical concerns may revolve around unresolved worries or fears from the pregnancy, prenatal testing findings, medication exposure, effects of maternal illness on the infant, delivery room events, transitional difficulties that the infant may have experienced, or physical findings that were noticed by a parent or other family member. Many of these issues, of course, may not be raised at first. Nevertheless, the question should be posed at the start of the visit as a standing invitation for parents to raise concerns when they feel comfortable doing so. Indeed, in a study by Wolke, Dave, Hayes, Townsend, & Tomlin (2002), the opportunity to discuss health care issues during a newborn's routine physical examination was found to be related significantly to mothers' satisfaction with the clinician who was performing the examination.

The only question on the minds of many parents at first is, "Is my infant healthy?" Even if the clinician narrates every item of the examination for families—"Her heart sounds normal, her belly feels fine . . ."—if he or she forgets to end it with a summary pronouncement of health, someone in the room is likely to ask for it. The importance of this opportunity presented by the simple physical examination of a typical child must not be underestimated. "This looks like a healthy infant to me," is just what each parent has hoped to hear after the many months of pregnancy. Even when the clinician finds a medical problem, such as a clavicle fracture or a dislocated hip, he or she has the opportunity to frame these findings more easily when sharing the examination with the family at each step.

Conducting the physical examination in the presence of the parents can be both a way of communicating with them and a means of gathering important information about the family (Kennell & Rolnick, 1960). The examination, when infused with the principles and spirit of the NBO, offers an opportunity to draw in those who are present in the room. Siblings may be invited to stand beside the bassinet. A perhaps reticent father can be invited to feel the fontanels or, if culturally appropriate, to calm his infant during the examination by helping the child to suck on his or her hand or even on the father's finger. Commenting on the infant's tone or level of activity may prompt a question about what he or she was like in utero, thereby honoring some of the mother's already developed intimate expertise on her infant. Noticing aloud how the infant calms in response to the familiar voice of the mother or father acknowledges the uniqueness of the parents' roles in this particular newborn's life. In so many ways, the clinician's openness to the family while looking together at the newborn provides opportunities to support and recognize the parents' competence and expertise, often even before they are aware of these things themselves. Furthermore, observing the family's responses to the examination—indifference, joy, anxiety, surprise, conflict—can begin to help the clinician understand where some of the strengths and vulnerabilities in this family system may be. Moreover, the very experience of focusing on the infant together provides an environment of trust and often will prompt families to offer unsolicited information about their strengths and needs. Of course, this is not the time to draw firm conclusions but rather to begin to gather information that will help guide future interactions. Finally, honestly enjoying the infant—tiny fingers, searching eyes, even a cry—signals to this family that the clinician truly cares, really does see how special this individual is, and sincerely wants to help them succeed in their parenting.

### Day 1/Day 2: Feeding Support and Easing Transition

In the first 24 to 48 hours of their newborn's life, many parents observe an array of state changes in their infant as he or she makes the transition to a new, extrauterine environment. They experience their infant's erratic early feeding behaviors and may have trouble making any sense of it all. The NBO is ideally suited to helping guide families through this early, confusing time. Here, the critical concept is that of *state and organization of state.* The pediatric care clinician can share aloud observations of the newborn's states and how he or she moves through them. Many parents can identify easily the common quiet alert state in the first few hours of life, often followed by a prolonged sleepier period, and are comforted to know that this is a normal pattern. Sometimes, transient medical complications that require separation of mother and infant occur in the first few hours after birth. These families, having missed that initial alert period, may need more reassurance about the subsequent sleepiness. All infants are individuals, of course, and may have a variety of behavioral patterns. Some parents may report that their infant has been very wakeful, wishing to be held constantly. Perhaps the clinician notices that an infant has difficulty habituating to light or sound and/or moves jaggedly from crying to sleeping. The skilled clinician will share his or her observations with parents in a way that helps them make sense of their experience and guides caregiving choices while avoiding labeling and prediction. There is a world of difference between being told, "I notice that she is disturbed quite easily when asleep. Protecting sleep is a skill that each infant learns at his or her own pace. We'll have to keep an eye on this with her," and, "You sure have a fussy infant on your hands!" Observations should be made in the spirit of "what is being seen together on this day, at this time." Parents then are given the tools to make their own observations, confirmatory or otherwise, as they move forward. The critical goal is not to hand the family a complete understanding of who this infant is and what his or her individual personality is like, but to look together and help to identify what to look for and a developmental context in which to place it.

For example, the NBO is used frequently as a way to help parents of near-term newborns understand their infant's less mature state organization.

✳

One mother was working very hard in the first days to help her infant of 36 weeks' gestation learn to breast-feed. Although the infant had a mature suck and swallow, her feeding was inconsistent. While observing the mother attempt breast feeding, the postpartum nurse noticed that the infant alternated between crying and sleepy staring. The nurse talked to the mother about feeding cues and infant states and reinforced the idea that breast feeding typically takes some time to be established. This made sense to the mother and alleviated her anxiety. Although initially perplexing to the mother, when it was explained that the infant's ability to regulate her state still was immature, that it was still developing, the infant's behavior—and what to do about it—made sense to her. The next day, the mother reported, "She did that same crying-staring thing again last night, so I just let her rest on my chest for a while and she was able to feed better a little later." This mother understood the concept of state regulation in the context of her infant and was using it to adapt her caregiving; the result was successful breast feeding.

✳

*Behavioral state* also is a central concept when helping parents make sense of early feeding behaviors of mature, term newborns (Hughes, Townsend, & Branvin, 1988; Kennell & McGrath, 2003). Before meeting their infant, crying may be the only feeding cue that many parents recognize or know. Crying is a *late* feeding cue and often results in an infant who is too disorganized to calm and latch onto the breast, a situation that will be frustrating for all involved. Observing rooting, sucking, and hand-to-mouth behaviors and distinguishing between deep and light sleep all serve to help teach parents the "sign language" of feeding readiness (Gill, White, & Anderson, 1984). Although each infant may differ in feeding skills at birth, helping parents to identify their infant's states and sense of his or her state organization as well as early feeding cues will go a long way toward making the most of each unique situation (Karl, 2004).

## Day 2/Day 3: Crying and Soothability

Listening to their infant cry presents a challenge for many parents, especially when the reasons for the cry are unexplainable (Barr, St. James-Roberts, Keefe, 2001; Brazelton, 1962; Donovan, Perlstein, Atherton, & Kotagal, 2000; St. James-Roberts, 2001). Told that they would recognize their infant's different cries—hunger, dirty diaper, pain—they more often stare with panic, wondering which one is which and why they do not seem to know the language. They fear that the crying is unpredictable, that they are incompetent to stop it, and that they will be unable to help their infant in need. Although some newborns may cry even the first day, crying periods may lengthen after the infant emerges from the postbirth sleepy period. Crying may be related to feeding cues or it may be unrelated to hunger. A common scenario is to arrive at the hospital room on the second, third, or fourth day and be greeted by a tired mother who says, "I think something is wrong with him. He kept me up all night crying." Most typical, the infant now, of course, is asleep either next to the mother or in the bassinet. Concepts from the NBO can be very helpful in these situations. For example, in an earlier encounter, the clinician may have heard the infant's cry and commented on its strength and vigor, what seemed to trigger it, and what seemed to calm him or her. In other words, the clinician can value crying, not that the infant should not be consoled, but that it is a typical thing that infants do.

By expressing interest in the infant's crying, the clinician can talk with the mother about variations in crying and response to consoling measures. The parent and the clinician then can look together at this infant to examine these issues. In these encounters, the clinician hopes to see the infant cry. This can be stated explicitly to the parent, "Maybe we will have a chance to see Sarah crying together now while I am examining her. What have you noticed that sets her off? What have you noticed so far that works to calm her?" Most often, even if they had not yet realized this themselves, parents will be able to describe patterns that they have already noticed: "Well, she really likes it if Hakim [father] holds and sings to her. It's just that we can't put her down!" The clinician watches how and when the infant cries in his or her own hands as well as the stepwise series of consoling maneuvers, which the clinician can narrate as he or she moves through them, remembering also to notice the infant's attempts at self-consoling. This may be an opportunity, for example, to affirm the parents' awareness of their infant's preferences. Parents also may have the validating experience of seeing their infant crying and being difficult to console in a professional's arms ("She's really crying all out. What a strong cry she has, although I can see what a challenge it is for her to calm down!"). Many times, once the clinician hands the inconsolably crying infant back to mother, everyone will have the opportunity to see the infant calm promptly in those familiar arms, with that familiar voice and scent. In summary, the goals are 1) to focus on the crying, placing it the context of the infant's individual pattern of state regulation and soothability; 2) to help parents identify and extend their own emerging expertise in reading their infant's behavior; 3) to empathize with the difficulty of coping with a crying infant; 4) to identify efforts at the infant's self-consoling, even if not yet fully successful; and 5) to normalize the sometimes surprising amount of external support that some infants may need and to place it in a developmental context.

## Day 2 and Beyond: Caregiving Guidelines and Anticipatory Guidance

As the time for discharge from the hospital approaches and during the first days and weeks at home, parents are able to turn their attention from the issues of early transition to the concerns of caring for their infant at home. Pediatric clinicians often have laundry lists of topics to discuss with new parents before discharge. Meanwhile, parents, exhausted and overwhelmed, have their own sets of questions that may or may not overlap with a clinician's agenda. Providing guidance in the context of the NBO allows clinicians to give advice that is individualized and presented in a collaborative style. For a clinician who is conducting a discharge examination, for example, the NBO may take the form of a combined physical and behavioral examination, similar to that outlined as an adaptation of the Neonatal Behavioral Assessment Scale (NBAS; Keefer, 1995). What follows is a template for such an encounter, based on a discharge pediatric hospital visit. Ideally, this visit will be at least the second or third time the clinician and family have met so that the clinician can refer to and build on earlier discussions.

As already discussed, parents must be invited genuinely to share their concerns and to influence the agenda. Therefore, many an encounter will not "fit the mold." It is not necessary to have every topic on the clinician's mental list addressed if the encounter was informative and meaningful from the parents' point of view. In fact, a thorough discussion of every topic outlined next probably would exhaust everyone!

✳

As the clinician approaches the infant, he or she may begin with skin inspection. This is an ideal time to look for jaundice and to discuss this topic and any necessary follow-up with families. The heart and lungs can be auscultated at this point. If the infant is still sleeping and has not been disturbed, then habituation items may be administered, prompting discussions such as where the infant will sleep at home, maturity of state regulation, or sibling adjustment (because it may be the sibling who disrupts the infant's sleep). As the infant is unwrapped a bit and placed on his or her back, a good opportunity is presented to discuss sudden infant death syndrome prevention while demonstrating proper sleep conditions and positioning (American Academy of Pediatrics Task Force on Sudden Infant Death Syndrome, 2005; Hauck et al., 2003).

The clinician may take this moment to inspect and show the parents the healing cord and guidelines for its care and surveillance; to examine and show the healing circumcision site, if applicable, and review circumcision care or notice the umbilical cord; to check for robust femoral pulses; and to perform a hip examination. The undiapered, supine infant also provides an opportune time to talk about temperature taking as well as infection prevention at home. Often, the infant will have cried by this point in the examination, prompting discussion about the parents' experience thus far with the infant's crying, soothability, and predictability. The clinician may have noted some rooting or sucking or may have found urine or stool in the diaper, all of which make for good opportunities to talk about feeding guidelines. The clinician then may look together with the parents at the infant's muscle tone and pull him or her to sit, allowing for a conversation about robustness as well as the level of head support that the infant seems to need at this point. Putting the newborn in the prone position naturally prompts a discussion of "tummy time" for encouraging extensor muscle development.

Many parents are surprised and delighted by their infant's neck strength or mention having seen this neck strength themselves while holding their infant on their chest. If the infant comes to a reasonably quiet alert state during this time, the clinician may take the opportunity to observe the infant's ability to respond to visual and/or auditory stimulation, inanimate and animate. This is an ideal time to discuss issues around social readiness, stress cues or signs of possible over stimulation, and decision making around exposure of the new infant to the family's social world. Finally, if the opportunity presents, there can be no nicer way to end the encounter than by asking one of the parents to call the infant's name and watching the infant turn to his or her mom or dad and then returning the infant to their arms.

✳

Sometimes patient encounters are not so straightforward and not at all what the clinician is expecting. A mother's hidden fears may express themselves in seemingly surprising worries or concerns. On such occasions, the relationship-building power of the NBO can be invaluable. The following vignette describes such an encounter, showing how newborn behavioral observation also can be used to great advantage as a way of discovering, prioritizing, and addressing parent concerns. Here, the Lopes twins, born at 38 weeks and 7 pounds each, have been thriving in their first days and are ready to be discharged. Their mother is recovering well from her cesarean section and has multiple family members supporting her. Nurses have found her to be coping well with her infants, although a bit nervous.

※

Upon entering the room, Dr. Zhu sees that Ms. Lopes is anxious about taking her newborn twins home. Dr. Zhu puts aside her discharge teaching "agenda" to explore Ms. Lopes's anxieties. Ms. Lopes expresses her concern that maybe her twins are not ready to go home. Dr. Zhu is perplexed because, looking at the medical record, the infants are healthy, term infants who have transitioned well and are medically stable for hospital discharge after 4 days of life. Rather than explain the medical reasons for why the infants are ready to go home, Dr. Zhu listens. She proposes to Ms. Lopes that they unwrap the infants and look at them together. Immediately, Dr. Zhu senses Ms. Lopes's anxiety decrease as she perceives that her concerns are being heard. Dr. Zhu uses the language and structure of the NBO to share with Ms. Lopes, with her own infants, the aspects of their examinations that are healthy and typical. The two also look at those important areas of the infants' physical and developmental stage that will require extra care, such as attention to head control and careful bundling of small newborns. At the end of this brief encounter of shared observation, Ms. Lopes is visibly more open to Dr. Zhu's opinion regarding safety for discharge. Recognizing Dr. Zhu's genuine interest in her and her infants, Ms. Lopes volunteers her fear: She describes a friend whose infant died at home. Dr. Zhu acknowledges the mother's fear and does not meet it with superficial assurances that these infants are typical. Instead, she proposes another option: a visiting nurse to check on mother and infants after discharge. Having been reassured, Ms. Lopes now is mentally available to take in important anticipatory guidance. Having been shown through her own infants aspects of their health, she is less likely to be anxious at home and to convey that anxiety to her infants. Moreover, in the brief minutes that Dr. Zhu spent during this encounter, her relationship with this mother has been strengthened and a key trust has been established.

※

## The Developmentally Rich Newborn Nursery

The NBO has much to offer to the entire multidisciplinary team that cares for newborns and their families in the first days of life. Concepts of newborn neurobehavior can be incorporated into many aspects of newborn care, such as routine nursing tasks (vital sign assessment, immunization administration, diapering, and infant care instruction [White, Simon, & Bryan, 2002]), infant bathing classes

(Amy, 2001; Karl, 1999), breast-feeding support (Hughes, Townsend, & Branvin, 1988; Karl, 2004), care of fathers and other family members (Myers, 1982), and infant massage (Field et al., 1996). As the various members of the nursery staff learn the same infant developmental language, parents who are exposed to important concepts in various environments during their nursery stay will remember what they have learned because of its repetition and consistency. For example, the lactation consultant talks about feeding cues (hand-to-mouth behavior, eye fluttering upon awakening, and rooting) during her breast-feeding instruction. The pediatrician emphasizes the same feeding cues during her discharge examination, and the nurse reiterates the same newborn behavior as she observes rooting behavior while she is in the room checking on mother and infant. In this way, a very important concept about infant feeding, one that may have serious negative consequences if not understood at home, is communicated effectively without undue time or effort on the part of the staff. These important items can easily be documented and added to the infant's record for communication.

Following are five vignettes that focus on the work of clinicians in the postpartum environment. These illustrate how the NBO can contribute to creating a developmentally rich newborn nursery environment. In each case, the clinician uses core concepts of the NBO to share keen observations of newborn behavior and keep the newborn at the center of the interaction. The clinician attends to the family's concerns, seeks and values parents' expertise regarding their own child, and maintains an openhearted approach to building relationships with families to help make the most of the first days of family life. The NBO serves as a concrete tool to provide structure for behavioral observation.

## Nursing Tasks

Mother–infant nurses must complete multiple tasks with many different patients during the course of an 8- to 12-hour shift. The following vignette illustrates how a skilled nurse with training in understanding newborn behavior can turn tasks into learning opportunities for her work with a newborn family:

❋

Joy, a registered nurse, is caring for four mother–infant pairs, among them Mrs. Gupta and her infant, Raj. Joy needs to take Raj's vital signs, administer his hepatitis B vaccine, and begin preparing Mrs. Gupta for discharge the next morning. As Joy greets Mrs. Gupta at the beginning of her shift, she notices Raj stirring gently in his sleep in the bassinet, occasionally rooting. "Oh, look at him, he's sleeping lightly now. Have you noticed how he's sometimes in a deep sleep and sometimes in this lighter sleep? Have you seen those rooting movements?" "Yes, I was just getting ready to feed him," replies Mrs. Gupta. Joy gently unwraps Raj's blankets. She checks his heart rate and respiratory rate. His arms begin to wave, so she calms him by letting him grasp her finger. As she puts the thermometer under his arm, he begins to cry. "So sorry to disturb you, Raj," Joy coos. She soothes him with her voice and softly but firmly gathers his arms toward his chest. Joy speaks directly to Raj, "Hey, hey, hey, little Raj, I see you like when I talk to you and cuddle your arms for you. That helped you stop crying, didn't it?" As Joy finishes taking Raj's temperature, she asks Mrs. Gupta what she has noticed about Raj so far. Has he cried much? How has she calmed him? How are things going in general? Joy notes that Raj easily recovers from being disturbed and now is wide-eyed and alert. She compliments him on his ability to wake up so smoothly. "Not every infant can do that in the first days, you know," she informs Mrs. Gupta, who smiles proudly.

Raj is Mrs. Gupta's second infant, and breast feeding is going smoothly so far, so Joy suggests that Mrs. Gupta get Raj settled on the breast in preparation for his hepatitis B vaccine. She explains that breast feeding is analgesic in painful procedures (Carbajal, Veerapen, Couderc, Jugie, & Ville, 2003; Gray, Miller, Philipp, & Blass, 2002), something that may be helpful for the many immunizations that he will need in the coming months. After Raj latches and begins feeding (an opportunity for Joy to confirm firsthand that breast feeding is progressing well), Joy administers the vaccine in his thigh. Raj yelps once, unlatches, shakes his head back and forth for a few seconds, then relatches and continues feeding contentedly. "Wow, you're good at that, Joy," Mrs. Gupta marvels. "And you're good at *that*," replies Joy, noticing aloud how Raj is sucking and swallowing rhythmically. A brief few minutes have allowed for a rich discussion. Joy has accomplished her vital signs on the infant for this shift, assessed breast feeding, and given the necessary vaccine. Her warm and respectful approach allows Mrs. Gupta to trust her in a deeper way. Mrs. Gupta now is able to volunteer how she misses her 2-year-old at home and how she hopes this time around she is not as anxious and depressed as last time. She and Joy talk a bit about typical "baby blues" versus postpartum depression. Mrs. Gupta is surprised to hear how commonly postpartum depression occurs. Joy offers her the opportunity to speak with a social worker for referral numbers in case she needs them. "You know your infant so well and take such good care of him. Let's be sure you're getting cared for as well." All this has taken up only 15 minutes of Joy's shift.

✳

## Father Care

It often is the case that mothers are given special attention in the nursery and fathers unwittingly are marginalized. Furthermore, the adjustment to fatherhood comes with its own unique set of challenges and changing role definitions (Barclay & Lupton, 1999; Pruett, 1983). The NBO can be used as a tool to include fathers in the nursery environment.

✳

Joy leaves the Guptas' room and moves on to check on Ms. Jackson, a 17-year-old first-time mother, and her infant. Ms. Jackson gave birth vaginally the day before. Mr. Davis, 18, the infant's father, is lying on the pull-out bed in the corner of the room, engrossed in a music video, seemingly oblivious to the infant's stirring and fussing whenever he loses his pacifier. Joy introduces herself to Ms. Jackson and Mr. Davis (Mr. Davis does not respond) and explains that she needs to check the infant's vital signs. Joy uses the opportunity of the infant examination to bring the father to the center of the experience. "Hey, Mr. Davis, would you mind giving me a hand here for a moment?" asks Joy. Joy instructs Mr. Davis on how he can calm the infant by offering a clean finger to suck on. The father laughs with surprise and pride over his son's strong suck. Joy asks Mr. Davis what the infant's name is. When Mr. Davis tells her his name is Clarence, Joy asks how the name was chosen. Mr. Davis tells her that the infant is named after Clarence, his older brother who was killed last year. Joy expresses her sympathy on the loss and remarks on his thoughtfulness in naming his son. She is finished with vital signs now, so she shows Mr. Davis how to swaddle Clarence. Clarence is bright-eyed and awake now. Asking Mr. Davis to stand near Clarence and gently say his name gives Joy an opportunity to comment on Clarence's behavior and on the relationship between father and infant. "Yeah, my father was never there for me. I want to show my son something different," remarks Mr. Davis. Clarence turns and searches his father's face. Joy uses the opportunity to discuss infants' amazing abilities to see and hear right from birth, their preference for familiar people, and their need to interact with those around them. She hands Clarence over to Mr. Davis, who now is conversing with his newborn son. As Clarence responds to his father, Joy has taken the opportunity to validate the father in a very brief but powerful encounter.

✳

## Breast-Feeding Support

Although natural, breast feeding can feel anything but natural to a new mother who is tired, overwhelmed, and insecure about her ability to provide adequate sustenance for her newborn infant. Sometimes, hospital staff attempt to counter these fears with a barrage of information about human lactation combined with a variety of rules for mothers to follow when feeding their infants. Alternatively, nursery staff can take a partnering approach with mothers, specifically recognizing their stress and helping them to understand the importance of the newborn's contribution to successful breast feeding (Hughes, Townsend, & Branvin, 1988; Karl, 2004; Lothian, 1995). The following vignette demonstrates the latter approach:

✳

Claire, a lactation consultant, visits Mrs. Miller and her 36-hour-old infant Kate in her room. She finds Mrs. Miller sitting awkwardly in bed, struggling to breast-feed a wailing Kate. She observes the infant's flailing arms and legs and sees the mother's angst. Rather than immediately point out the positioning problems, Claire sensitively begins by encouraging the mother and asking her what she thinks: "You're working very hard! How is it going?" The mother replies in frustration, "He's hungry and I don't have enough milk!" Instead of refuting the mother's opinion with a host of medical knowledge about colostrum and sufficiency of breast milk, Claire gently observes Kate's behavior. She notes her flailing feet and suggests swaddling to help her get organized. She notes her strong cry and suggests that a little break may help calm the infant. Claire and Mrs. Miller talk about typical infant states and hunger cues. With infant and mother a little calmer, Claire is able to make a few more recommendations: She encourages Mrs. Miller to move to a chair, swaddles Kate, and begins to help Mrs. Miller position Kate at the breast. She is affirmed as Claire recognizes her hard work, and she is empowered as Claire describes Kate's cues and proposes possible solutions. Helping the infant latch, Claire now can talk about the first week and how Kate will learn, assuring Mrs. Miller that it will not always be this difficult. Mrs. Miller now is open to hearing Claire talk about colostrum and the sufficiency of the mother's milk. As the infant latches, the mother is more likely to be open to the possibility of her breast-feeding success and is more likely to persevere. After a brief encounter, a trust is established between Claire and Mrs. Miller. The next day, Claire returns to Mrs. Miller's bedside. She makes sure to mention the previous day and asks Mrs. Miller how the past 24 hours have been. She affirms the mother's hard work and offers support when needed. In this way, Claire serves as a partner, and her skills and expertise can be welcomed rather than unintentionally discouraging and overwhelming for the mother.

✳

## Bath Class

All nurseries provide instruction to parents in the bathing and physical care of the newborn. This routine task provides a wonderful opportunity for nursing staff to share information about newborn neurobehavior and to do so in a collaborative, rather than didactic, and an individualized, rather than a generic, manner (Amy, 2001; Karl, 1999).

✳

A nervous Mrs. Haddad watches as Barbara, the nurse, prepares the warm bath water for Mrs. Haddad's new infant, Ibrahim. As Barbara gently unwraps Ibrahim, she shares with Mrs. Haddad what she notices about the infant. "Look how he startles a little as I undress him. Look at his strong arms and legs, just a sign of how well you took care of him inside of you! You fed him well!" Mrs. Haddad giggles a little and sighs with relief. Barbara continues as she places the infant in the water, quietly speaking and assuring the mother that "there are no rules. You can bathe your infant every day if you like. It may be especially soothing in the early evening if he becomes colicky." If Ibrahim settles into the bath easily, then Barbara can comment on his relaxed tone, even skin color, and comfortable breathing. If he is in a quiet alert state, then Barbara can notice how he is alert to voices and faces, particularly his own mother's voice. If Ibrahim becomes distressed and cries as he is placed in the bath, then Barbara can comment on the signs of his distress: cry, color change, and increased tone. As she gently shifts him to make him comfortable, her calm demeanor will give his mother a signal that all is well. This state is typical for an infant. Barbara, through her behavior, gives permission to Mrs. Haddad to respond as calmly at home. The nurse talks about crying—its importance for newborns—and about the infant's preferences: Does he like the warm water? How does he adjust, and how much time does he need to transition? This will change over the next few weeks, and that is expected too. Barbara reminds herself to observe Ibrahim's state and his cues and to plan the next steps accordingly. If he is in a quiet alert state, then the mother and the nurse can proceed with confidence and provide the infant with re-assurance vocally and visually. If he begins to fuss and tremor, then Barbara can let Mrs. Haddad know that he is signaling to move more slowly. The mother's anxiety diminishes as the three proceed with the bath. Slowly, Barbara steps back and gives Mrs. Haddad the lead. Now Barbara has done the most important thing; in stepping back, she affirms the mother's capability. The nurse serves as an important professional witness to a mem-orable moment: This mother is the new mother of this brand-new infant, and she now feels competent to meet her infant's needs.

*

## Infant Massage Class

Ideally, members of different disciplines of the nursery staff—nurses, doctors, lac-tation consultants—understand newborn behavior and development and use the principles and structure of the NBO. Families then benefit from the common and consistent language and approach among the members of their care team. Here, infant massage classes can reinforce families' understanding of their new infant during their postpartum hospital stay. There is evidence that massage therapy contributes to more organized sleep patterns, weight gain, and more positive in-teraction patterns thought much of this research has been done with preterm neonates (e.g., Diego, Field, & Hernandez-Reif, 2005; Dieter et al., 2003; Ferber et al., 2002; Field, 1998; Onozawa et al., 2001; Wheeden et al., 1993).

*

As she begins to massage one of the infants in a massage class, Alicia, the therapist, de-scribes aloud the infant's responses to touch. She notices any color changes, startles, and hiccoughs and names them with parents as the infant's signs that he needs less stim-ulation. Alicia talks about the kinds of stimulation to which infants are exposed: light, sound, touch, smell, and taste. She talks about the preferences of the infant, some pre-ferring auditory over visual stimulation, and reflects with parents what this infant's pref-erences may be. Noticing this infant relax with a soft, predictable, and rhythmic touch, Alicia shares with the parents that the baby appears calmer with predictable, rhythmic strokes and deep touch rather than light strokes. He prefers simple strokes to compli-cated strokes, which could easily overwhelm him. At the end of the brief session, the therapist has an opportunity to affirm how much the parents already know about their infant, how natural they seem, and how much they provide for him (with their faces, voices, touch, and smell) without having to purchase any extravagant equipment. In this simple session, in yet another way, the parents have had an opportunity to learn about their infant's behavior.

*

## SUMMARY

The NBO is a set of observations to be shared with families. However, to be effective as a relationship-building tool, the NBO must be approached with a set of qualities and attitudes on the part of the clinician to meet its goal of fostering the parent–infant relationship. First, the clinician must be a sophisticated observer of newborn behavior. He or she also must have a deep understanding of infant development to notice and interpret behaviors and, in so doing, share observations with families, taking great care to watch his or her chosen language. Next, the clinician must be able to place the newborn at the center of each conversation and respond flexibly to each situation, welcoming the unique opportunities presented—for instance, by an encounter that begins with a crying infant and anxious parent as well as a sleeping infant and relaxed parent. Clinicians who use the NBO in their work also must sincerely respect the parents' expertise regarding their own child, beginning on the first day of his or her life. Language that is used with families should be chosen carefully to reflect this respect and to recognize both the vulnerability and the sense of possibility of the newborn period. Finally, the clinician must be nonjudgmental in his or her approach to families, valuing the clinician–family relationship and demonstrating how he or she remembers them from one encounter to the next. Undoubtedly, many readers will recognize rightly that these are merely some of the qualities that characterize a good clinician. Therefore, respecting the wisdom, experience, and expertise that clinicians already possess, the NBO can be thought of as a practical tool that can be used to build on and extend what they already know about observing infants and caring for families.

The newborn period represents a major stage in the infant's behavioral adaptation to his or her new environment. It also marks a unique transition for parents and presents a significant window of opportunity for their growth as family roles shift with a new infant's arrival. The clinician who enters into a partnership with parents at this vulnerable time can use the NBO to facilitate the development of positive parent–infant and clinican–family relationships. Incorporating the NBO into routine nursery care can help create a developmentally rich nursery environment and contribute to a meaningful and memorable birth experience for families.

# 6

# Using the Newborn Behavioral Observations System with Preterm or Medically Fragile Infants

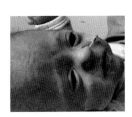

At term age, all infants, regardless of their prenatal or perinatal histories, have a wide range of behavioral competencies. However, although high-risk infants can see and visually track objects, hear and locate sounds, and show their preferences toward auditory or visual stimulation, they may do so at increased cost to their physiological, motoric, and state systems and with increased need for support and facilitation. They tire more easily and show their limits through changes in their skin color, in their breathing patterns and muscle tone, and in becoming fussy or drowsy. They may not be as capable as healthy infants to signal their needs clearly and may not be as successful in maintaining self-regulation during interaction. The behaviors that they have available to disengage from social interaction, such as gaze aversion, can be subtle and not always perceived by the parent as a clear signal for a break in the intensity of the interaction, so although high-risk infants may demonstrate voice preference and auditory orientation to a stimulus, they can only do so if the input is carefully timed and is matched to their individual sensory thresholds for stimulation.

The main purpose of this chapter is to describe the behaviors that high-risk infants use to communicate with the outside world and to describe how the Newborn Behavioral Observations (NBO) system provides a model of behavioral observations that is well suited to the needs of preterm or medically fragile infants and their families. It should be pointed out that although the NBO is an observational tool, it is not an assessment tool per se. It is a relationship-building tool that is designed to promote the parent–infant relationship and the relationship between the clinician and the family. (For a formal assessment of preterm behavior, the Neonatal Behavioral Assessment Scale [NBAS] has been used, whereas the Assessment of Preterm Infant Behavior [Als et al., 2003; Als, Lester, Tronick, & Brazelton, 1982] was designed specifically to assess preterm and at-risk infants, and the NICU [neonatal intensive care unit] Network Neurobehavioral Scale was developed to assess drug-exposed and other high-risk infants [Lester & Tronick, 2004].) The NBO is appropriate for use with preterm infants and for medically fragile infants who are close to discharge or already have been discharged from the hospital and is designed specifically to refine the parents' ability to recognize their infant's thresholds of and preferences to stimulation.

The first section of this chapter discusses the impact of preterm birth on the parents to help clinicians recognize some of the special considerations to be given to parents who are taking home an infant who was born early. The second section provides a framework for understanding high-risk infant behaviors. Als's (1982, 1986) model for neurobehavioral functioning of the preterm infant is the best theoretical model available to understand the behaviors of young infants and is adapted for use with the NBO in this chapter.

In the second section, Als's traditional regulatory and stress behaviors are categorized further using the "traffic light metaphor," which was adapted from the authors' work with the NBAS (Higley, Cole, Howland, Ranuga, & Nugent, 1999). The traffic light metaphor's observational system will assist the clinician in two ways. First, it will refine the clinician's ability to understand infant behaviors in terms of degrees of self-regulation, and it will provide the clinician with a system to communicate these observations to parents. Second, it will guide both the clinician and the parents during the immediate decision-making process that takes place when having to decide on the modifications that are necessary to best support the infant's efforts at self-regulation.

The third section of this chapter focuses on the NBO model of intervention with high-risk infants and describes how it can help parents better understand their infant's behavior, threshold for responsiveness, and cues of readiness for interaction, thereby supporting the "goodness of fit" between the infant and his or her parents and new home environment. The last section of the chapter provides a detailed discussion of anticipatory guidance on specific caregiving themes and developmental issues for the high-risk infant. Although this chapter is written with the preterm infant as its main focus, the proposed model is judged to be appropriate for use with infants who present with a wide range of developmental disabilities, whether preterm or term (e.g., Down syndrome, small for gestational age, failure to thrive, genetic syndromes).

# IMPACT OF PRETERM BIRTH ON THE PARENTS

The preterm delivery of an infant often is a very traumatic event for parents, but the experience may vary depending on the nature of the delivery. For some parents, the pregnancy may have been diagnosed as high risk, which often results in hospitalization before delivery. This may lead to discussions with medical professionals over the possibility of a preterm delivery, a visit to the NICU, and time to educate and prepare the parents on the medical issues that face their infant at birth (Vergara & Bigsby, 2004). For other parents, the precipitous delivery of their infant after sudden premature rupture of membranes or rapidly progressing preterm labor leaves them with no time to prepare for this event. Although previous knowledge of the possibility of preterm birth may soften the intensity of the experience at first, all parents of preterm infants are particularly vulnerable throughout their infant's neonatal period. First and foremost are issues of survival followed by concerns over the quality of the infant's developmental outcome once survival is ensured. In general, mothers of preterm infants are at risk for feelings of depression and failure and generally experience significantly greater psychological stress than mothers of term infants (Eisengart, Singer, Fulton, & Baley, 2003). Their feelings of anxiety and depression may be rooted in the mother's viewing the preterm birth as a personal failure, because she believes that she was unable to bring her infant to term. The mother's own expectations and the dream of having a perfect "fantasy baby" have been shattered (Bruschweiler-Stern, 1997).

Most preterm infants will require a hospital stay in the NICU. Although efforts are made to include the parents in the decision making and caregiving of the infant while in the hospital, Redshaw (1997) demonstrated that the experience of separation for mothers of preterm infants in the NICU can be associated with the temporary loss of a sense of parental role and identity. Nursing and medical staff, on whom the infant depends for lifesaving care, spend more time with the infant than the parents and inadvertently may erode further the parents' role in the NICU. The stress that is experienced during the newborn period extends far beyond the first few weeks of life for the preterm infant and may flare up all over again when the infant is discharged home at an age close to his due date. Indeed, mothers of infants who require ventilation may feel overwhelmed, worried, and even panicked when told that their infant is well enough to go home and may feel less confident about taking their infant home than do mothers of healthy infants. The phase immediately after discharge from the hospital is one of anxious adjustment during which mothers express their lack of confidence and insecurity in caring for their preterm infant (McHaffie, 1990). Eventually, most mothers accommodate and become confident, but this initial phase after discharge is a great source of stress and anxiety for these mothers.

Several investigators have noted interactional difficulties between mothers and their low-birth-weight children (e.g., Melnyk, Feinstein, & Fairbanks, 2002). It may be that the difficulty that parents of a preterm infant experience in responding to their preterm infant is due, in large part, to the fact that these infants tend to be less responsive, are more fretful, smile less, and give less readable communication signals than do term infants (Spiker, Ferguson, & Brooks-Gunn, 1993). Because their communication cues are more difficult to decipher, this may result in interactive disturbances—"parental misattunements"—between parent and child. Significant efforts by health care professionals have to be made to alleviate such parental stress and anxiety. Costello and Chapman (1998) attempted to alleviate maternal anxiety through a care-by-parent program in the hospital before discharge. Interviews with the mothers after this type of intervention suggested that the experience helped them learn about their infant's patterns of behavior and their own responses to their cues so that they could meet their needs better. Because the ability to read and attend to their infant's cues both consistently and contingently is important in the development of a secure attachment relationship, the degree to which parents can develop this ability becomes an important clinical issue (Fish & Stifter, 1995).

A number of studies have demonstrated that during the difficult hospital stay, assisting parents in understanding their infant's behavior seems to be critical in helping them maintain their role as parents and mitigate levels of stress and depression (Browne & Talmi, 2005; Lawhon, 2002; Loo, Espinosa, Tyler, & Howard, 2003; Parker, Zahr, Cole, & Brecht, 1992; Redshaw, 1997). Helping parents read their infant's cues and providing them with feedback on how their infant responds to them can help to mobilize confidence in their efforts to develop a relationship with their young infants. Als et al. (1994) demonstrated that individualized, developmentally based intensive care can reduce the stress that is caused by the NICU environment and can improve outcomes, both medically and developmentally, for the preterm infant. These studies show that developmentally appropriate interventions, which are characterized by helping parents read their infant's cues and are designed to enhance parent–child interactions and support the parent–child relationship, can improve outcome and can promote the child's cognitive and socioemotional development (Als et al., 1994; Kleberg, Westrup, & Stjernqvist, 2000; Nugent & Brazelton, 2000; Sameroff, 1997). Therefore, it is proposed that developmentally appropriate interventions that are designed to enhance parent–child interactions and support the parent–child relationship can improve outcome and can promote the child's cognitive and socioemotional development.

## BEHAVIORAL COMPETENCY OF THE PRETERM INFANT

In Chapter 1, the developmental task of the newborn was described as the unfolding of sequential achievements in the four behavioral dimensions:

*A* The infant first must organize his or her **autonomic,** or physiologic, behavior.

*M* The infant must regulate or control his or her **motor** behavior.

*O* The infant must **organize** his or her behavioral states.

*R* The infant must regulate his or her **responsivity,** or affective interactive or social behavior, through interaction with his or her social and physical environment and orientation to animate and inanimate objects.

These sequential achievements allow the infant to organize his or her behavior so
that he or she is actively able to influence and guide caregivers in the choices they
make to provide the best care needed for the infant's optimal development (Als,
1982; Brazelton, 1962). It is through the meticulous observation of behaviors
within each of these dimensions that the infant's level of maturity to this first developmental task can be determined. An infant who is capable of organizing, regulating, and modulating his or her behaviors displays competent self-regulation
and therefore is better equipped to deal with the demands of everyday life than
the infant who has not yet fully accomplished this first developmental task with
full integrity. Self-regulation, defined as the successful integration of the four behavioral dimensions, is the optimal goal of this first developmental challenge and
is the construct being measured during behavioral observations. Therefore, the
behaviors that the infant displays in each of the four behavioral dimensions form
the lens through which caregivers can determine the current degree of self-regulation that the infant has mastered.

To assist clinicians and parents to understand the "quality" of self-regulation
of a given infant, Als (1982) categorized behaviors within each of the dimensions
as either *approach/regulatory* or *avoidance/stress* behaviors. Regulatory behaviors indicate a state of well-being and are observed when an infant's self-regulatory abilities are able to support the social and environmental demands that are placed on
him or her. The infant then is described as *organized.* Stress behaviors indicate a
state of exhaustion and are observed when the infant's threshold for self-regulation is exceeded by the demands that are placed on him or her. The infant then is
described as *disorganized* (D'Apolito, 1991). Table 6.1 provides a list of specific behaviors that are categorized as approach or avoidance behaviors for each of the
behavioral dimensions.

A regular respiratory rate, good color, and stable digestion are noted in physiologically organized infants, whereas infants who are showing signs of disorganization in this behavioral dimension may have irregular breathing and poor color
and be gagging and straining. Within the motor subsystem, smooth movements
and balanced flexor-extensor tone are considered organized behaviors, whereas
jerky movement quality and overuse of extensor movements are considered disorganized behaviors. An infant with a well-organized state system has a broad

**Table 6.1.** Behavioral dimensions (AMOR) and their individual regulatory and stress behaviors

|  | Autonomic | Motor | Organization of state | Responsivity |
|---|---|---|---|---|
| What to observe | skin color, breathing patterns, visceral functioning | muscle tone, posture, movements | range of state, robustness and clarity, transition pattern | ability to maintain alertness, responds and interacts with animate (people) and inanimate (ball or rattle) objects |
| Regulatory behaviors | pink, stable color; regular respiratory rate; stable digestion | smooth, balanced flexor-extensor tone; tucking, hand to face or mouth, foot bracing, hand clasping, grasping, facial frown, soft cheeks, sucking | deep sleep, light sleep, drowsy, alert, active, crying; bright eyes, robust sleep and cry; smooth transition from state to state; easily soothed | able to achieve and maintain shiny-eyed alertness and able to maintain interactive periods at least briefly |
| Stress behaviors | pale, red, mottled, dusky, or cyanotic color; irregular breathing; pauses, apnea, tachypnea, sighs, yawns, regurgitation, grunting, straining bowel movement, twitching or startles | jerky, overuse of extensor movements and postures observed in the face, neck, trunk, fingers, hands, arms, legs | not all states may be available or observed; states may be difficult to identify; gaze aversion, floating eye movements, closed eyes, rapid state changes, difficult to soothe | strained, low level alertness; hyperalert and unable to break away from interaction |

*Source:* Als, H. (1986). A synactive model of neonatal behavioral organization: Framework for the assessment of neurobehavioral development in the premature infant and for support of infants and parents in the neonatal intensive care unit. In J.K. Sweeney (Ed.), *The high-risk neonate: Developmental therapy perspectives* (pp. 3–53). New York: Haworth Press; adapted by permission.

range of well-defined states available with smooth transitions from one state to the next. A less well-organized infant may have a narrower range of states, states may be more diffuse, and the infant may have rapid state changes. Infants with well-organized attention-interaction can achieve and maintain shiny-eyed alertness and well-modulated interactive periods at least briefly. A less well-organized infant may have strained, low-level alertness or, conversely, may be hyperalert and unable to break away from interaction that may be too intense. It is especially important to share this type of information with parents to help them understand that they are not causing their infant's sensory overload but rather that their preterm infant's ability to self-regulate in varied situations and conditions still is limited in duration and quality. By adjusting their approach on the basis of the behavioral cues of the infant, parents can provide better matched opportunities for interactions with their child.

Because self-regulation is fluid and affected greatly by the changing interactions and demands of the moment, the traffic light metaphor is useful in detailing ongoing degrees of self-regulation and can guide the clinician's and parents' choices of responses to support the infant during the NBO (see Table 6.2). The *green light* behaviors communicate readiness, organization, and stable neurobehavioral functioning with little evidence of stress; they are the regulatory behaviors as proposed by Als (1986). These behaviors indicate to both the clinician and the parents that it is appropriate to continue the NBO with little or no adjustments. Breaking down stress behaviors into two categories (*yellow light* and *red light*) helps the observers pay more attention to the thresholds to stimulations and emergence of loss of self-regulation (yellow light) and separate those events from the moment when complete loss of self-regulation is attained (red light; see Table 6.2). The yellow light behaviors indicate some level of stress and that a sensory threshold may have been being reached. The yellow light behaviors suggest pausing and observing the infant's behavior to see whether he or she recovers or gets worse before deciding which action to take next. The parent can be guided to change the way the infant is handled, spoken to, or held or even to change the lighting in the room. The clinician's sharing of his or her observations with the parents is always important but is particularly important during the observation of yellow light behaviors. This possibly is the ideal time for parents to observe the efforts that their infant makes and strategies that he or she uses to reach and maintain self-regulation. The red light behaviors indicate primarily a state of stress, exhaustion, and loss of self-regulation. The stress level indicates that the demands that are placed on the infant during the NBO are too stressful for and overwhelming to the infant's regulatory capacities. These behaviors signal the need for the parents and the clinician to stop handling the infant and give the infant a prolonged break while offering support and facilitation.

Often, clinicians and parents have difficulties in identifying and understanding the meaning of infant behaviors that are in the yellow light category. The two extremes in self-regulation—its presence or its total loss—are more easily identified and understood by observers of infant behaviors, but it is the path, or the infant's behavioral story, between those two conditions and its meaning in the spectrum of self-regulation that often are misunderstood and lost. Clinicians are urged to devote the most time and attention to learning the yellow light behaviors and to develop the complementary clinical skills that will support the infant's at-

**Table 6.2.**  Traffic light metaphor for observing regulatory and stress behaviors and its applications during the NBO

| Behaviors | Degree of self-regulation | Traffic light metaphor | NBO decision making |
|---|---|---|---|
| Regulatory | Indicate well-being, self-regulation | "Green light" | Continue while observing infant |
| Stress | Indicate threshold to stimulation | "Yellow light" | Pause, time-out before continuing |
|  | Need for support, loss of self-regulation | "Red light" | Prolonged break, discontinue NBO |

tempts to avoid loss of self-regulation. Although recognizing behaviors in all dimensions and categories is required, parents will benefit the most from strategies that will assist them in helping their infant achieve or maintain self-regulation. This is accomplished best through the use of the yellow light behaviors.

When compared with the healthy, term infant, the preterm infant's ability to self-regulate seems compromised and limited in duration. Sensory thresholds to stimulation that lead to loss of self-regulation are reached more easily as compared with the typical, term infant. For example, a young infant with chronic lung disease may demonstrate the ability to turn to the sound of a voice and may be able to track his mother's face with his eyes but only with carefully timed stimulation matched to his sensory thresholds. When the mother speaks to her infant, the infant may pause his breathing when he first hears her voice and after a brief pause shift his eyes toward her. These initial behavioral responses (pause in breathing and delayed eye shift toward voice) let the mother know of the infant's initial efforts to respond. The mother, in turn, comes to realize that she needs to adapt her voice to the infant's level of response before they can begin to interact. In this case, if the mother responds by giving the infant a brief time-out by not talking for a few seconds, then the infant may be able to regulate his breathing and orientation responses and turn toward the sound of her voice. Conversely, if the mother does not read the initial infant behaviors as indicating a need for support or a need for a break in the intensity of the stimulation and continues to ask the infant to respond to her voice, then the infant may respond by closing his eyes and turning away from her voice.

An infant with poorly organized self-regulation therefore will require more assistance from his or her caregivers and the environment to achieve and maintain integration of the behavioral dimensions. The need for assistance in the quest for self-regulation forms the basis of an intervention approach that is highly individualized to the needs of the infant. These individualized intervention strategies are accomplished best when environmental and social demands support the infant's self-regulatory limits and when they take into account the infant's sensory thresholds (Blanchard & Mouradian, 2000). Within this perspective, intervention is aimed at facilitating prolonged periods of organization, thereby decreasing the manifestation of disorganized behaviors while reinforcing the infant's individual self-regulatory style. For example, well-organized, term newborns and infants may be observed bringing themselves into a sleep state by placing one hand against the back of the head or behind the ear with the other hand close to the mouth. Less well-organized, preterm infants may attempt to do the same but may not be as successful at maintaining these comfort postures. Building on these observations, the clinician or the parent can assist the infant by swaddling him or her, by bringing the hand close to the mouth, by offering a finger to hold, or by tucking the legs and allowing the infant to brace his or her feet against the caregiver's hand until he or she settles down and is able to maintain a state of organized functioning. Meeting an infant's needs with such individualized and well-timed support leads parents to develop a deeper understanding of their infant's developmental status, strengths, and challenges. Detailed intervention strategies toward specific developmental issues of the high-risk infant are included in the last section of this chapter.

## THE NBO SESSION WITH HIGH-RISK INFANTS

The individualized nature of the NBO renders it responsive to the particular needs of individual infants and families (Nugent & Blanchard, 2006). By eliciting, describing, and interpreting the newborn's behavior, the clinician has the opportunity to engage the parents in identifying the kinds of responses that the infant will make to the environmental demands and the kinds of caregiving techniques that can best promote his or her organization and development. The NBO thereby offers the clinician and the parents a forum to observe the infant's level of functioning during the first 3 months and together arrive at a behavioral profile that captures the infant's individuality. Although the immediate goal of the NBO is to help reveal to parents the infant's unique adaptive and coping capacities, the long-term clinical goal is to influence positively the infant–parent relationship by developing a supportive therapeutic alliance with the family at what could be called the formative moment in the development of the family. The NBO thus is seen as the first stage in the development of a supportive relationship between the clinician and the parents that should continue beyond the newborn period.

Before the NBO begins, the clinician notes the infant's behaviors across the behavioral dimensions and aspects of the physical environment and social surroundings. For example, the clinician would note the state of the infant and his or her color, breathing pattern, posture of arms and legs, and quality of movement and also note aspects of the social and physical environment. After this initial observation, the NBO maneuvers become the event through which the infant's neurobehavioral functioning is challenged and measured. The behavioral observation continues throughout the duration of the NBO with concurrent observation of specific environmental or social events and maneuvers of the NBO itself that challenge self-regulatory control. Once the NBO is completed, the observation is continued for some time to document the infant's recovery from the demands of the interaction.

The recommended sequence of maneuvers in the NBO manual may not always be followed as suggested and will vary in response to the infant's behavioral state. For example, if the infant is sleeping, then habituation can be observed. A crying infant needs to be consoled, whereas an alert infant can be observed for either the motor items or the orientation items. During the course of the NBO, infants may become fussy or drowsy, start crying, or become disengaged. When this happens, the clinician's sensitivity to the infant's behavioral manifestations of disorganization (yellow light) and his or her ability to capture the moment at which the first signs of disorganization occur and to respond contingently to facilitate the infant's return to an organized state become critical to a successful NBO experience (Blanchard & Mouradian, 2000). These clinical skills, combined with the ability to identify key events during the NBO such as handling or social demands that trigger such loss of self-regulation and, therefore, loss of organization, help the clinician identify the infant's sensory thresholds and developmental challenges and subsequently make recommendations to parents for individualized intervention strategies (Blanchard & Mouradian, 2000).

The following section provides a detailed example of an NBO with Eric, who is a preterm infant born at 24 weeks of gestation, weighing 590 g. Soon after his birth, Eric was intubated and remained dependent on the ventilator for 2½ months, after which he received oxygen through nasal cannula until close to discharge home. While he was in the hospital, he suffered a grade III intraventricular hemorrhage, which since has resolved as his last cranial ultrasound before discharge showed no residual signs of the hemorrhage. He developed stage 3 retinopathy of prematurity, for which he required laser surgery to both eyes before his discharge home. His hearing was tested in the NICU and found to be normal. He was discharged home from the hospital 1 week before his due date and was referred to his local early intervention program, home-visiting nurse agency, and community pediatrician. Cheryl, Eric's mother, is 22 years old and has two other children: Aaron, who is 8, and Maggie, who is 4. Cheryl has had a difficult life, having been raised in foster care and having her first child at 14. She is a drug user and lives alone with Eric; her two other children are in foster care with family members. Eric's father is in jail.

The vignette's medical and social contexts for this young infant are based on the true story of a young, poor mother living with her infant in an urban environment and show the complexity in the lives of many families in the community. The mother wishes that her infant could develop as other children do and wants to do everything she can to nurture him properly, but she soon may be drawn back to the streets and to the life that she knows. Her social isolation soon will weigh on her and increase her stress to a breaking point. The home visitor has to meet her agency and administrative responsibilities, provide services that are within the scope of her professional knowledge and expertise, and hopefully make a connection with this family. Both the mother's and the clinician's agendas have to be met for this collaboration to be successful. The relationship-based NBO offers a context that is nonjudgmental and open to the mutual discovery of this infant through shared observation of his behaviors. The following description of an NBO session will help the reader to see how the NBO can make a positive difference in a young mother's life and help to lay the foundation for a successful collaboration between the mother and her home visitor. The NBO session was conducted at the first home visit by the family's home visitor, Theresa, a physical therapist from early intervention.

＊

During this visit, Theresa and Cheryl were in Cheryl's bedroom with Eric on the bed. Cheryl seemed to have difficulty relaxing and moved around a lot, folding laundry, going to the bathroom, and finding "busy work" to do in the room, but she answered Theresa's questions about Eric's medical history and was somewhat attentive. After paperwork was completed, Theresa decided that the NBO would be useful in getting to know Eric and to engage Cheryl in a conversation about her infant and about her goals for her son. Cheryl had warned Theresa that Eric would be getting hungry soon, so Theresa decided to stroke the corner of his mouth and elicited a strong rooting reflex. He turned his head and opened his mouth as if searching for a nipple. Theresa commented to Cheryl on how strong he was and that he was searching for his bottle. With gloves on, Theresa felt his suck on her finger, which was very strong as well. Cheryl remained on the periphery, never sitting down on the bed but watching from where she stood. Theresa placed her index fingers near Eric's palms, and he immediately grasped them with both hands. Theresa pulled him to sit. Eric held his head up throughout the pull to sit and kept it up while Theresa called his name and counted out loud to see how long he could hold it up. Cheryl's face brightened, and she smiled while watching. Theresa commented again on how strong and robust Cheryl's son was. Cheryl smiled but did not say anything. Theresa picked Eric up and placed him on his stomach on the bed. Eric immediately lifted his head up and started crawling on the bed. He actually moved forward and kept his head up for some time. He then found his hand, relaxed, and started sucking his fist. Theresa was impressed with his abilities and shared her delight with Cheryl. Theresa and Cheryl talked about his sleeping position, which was in the supine position.

Theresa picked up Eric and held him in her arms and asked Cheryl whether she had noticed his listening to her voice or looking at her. Cheryl said that she had not seen him do any of this. She laughed and said he was too young for that. Theresa invited Cheryl to sit down next to her and asked her to call Eric's name. As soon as Eric heard Cheryl's voice, he turned his head toward her and looked at her. Cheryl was stunned and said that she thought it was just coincidence, that she did not think he could do that. Theresa turned Eric around so that his other ear now was near his mother and asked her to call his name again. Sure enough, Eric turned his head toward his mother as soon as she called his name. Theresa then brought his head back to midline and asked Cheryl to call him while Theresa called his name on the other side. Eric again turned to his mother immediately. By then, Cheryl was beaming. She said over and over again how she could not believe that he was already able to do this. She clearly was more interested in what Theresa was doing at that time and remained seated on the bed with her. Theresa took out a red ball, and Eric tracked the ball to his left and right and a little bit in the vertical. Theresa shook a soft rattle to each side of his head, but by this time, Eric was getting tired and started fussing. He became fussy and more active and needed a break. Cheryl decided that it was his time to eat, so she went to get him a bottle. Theresa followed her into the kitchen while holding Eric and asked her what she does to quiet him when he gets fussy like this. Cheryl said that Eric loves to be held up on her shoulder. When Theresa positioned Eric on her shoulder, he quieted immediately and started looking around. Theresa commented on how well Cheryl knew what Eric liked and on how alert and aware he was of his surroundings. He loved to watch his mother prepare his bottle.

The telephone rang, so Cheryl handed Theresa the bottle so that she could start feeding Eric. To Theresa's delight, she heard Cheryl recount the visit to Eric's grandfather in great detail. She was so excited and was laughing as she described Eric's crawling skills on the bed and how he was able to hold his head up and look around. When she told him about Eric's turning his head to her voice, it sounded as if he did not believe her, because she kept saying, "I tell you, he did it, he turns to me when I call his name and even likes my voice better than the physical therapist's, who is here right now from early intervention." Theresa was so pleased to hear Cheryl say these wonderful things about her son. And so, their relationship began. Cheryl kept her next appointments and looked forward to Theresa's visits. The NBO did not erase the complexity of Cheryl's life, but it gave her the opportunity to witness her son's potential in a way that she had never seen it before.

*

Every NBO session presents the observer with unexpected decision-making challenges when the infant's behavior, at times obvious and at times subtle, demands that the observer pause and consider the next step in the item administration sequence. At times, these pauses can be momentary and barely noticeable but still play a critical role in assisting the infant in reaching and maintaining a state of self-regulation (Higley et al., 1999). The following vignette with Eric illustrates what an NBO session may look like given different types of responses of the infant. Using the traffic light metaphor ( ), the infant's response to handling and item administration is followed by a description of the clinician's response and adjustments made to match the infant's level of self-regulation. For further assisting the reader, behaviors and characteristics within each traffic light category are in boldface type. For the purposes of this exercise, it is assumed that the NBO is administered item by item as presented in Chapter 3. The behavioral scenario that is provided next is but one of many possible scenarios, and infants in other NBO sessions may display other types of behaviors than those portrayed here. Each item of the NBO creates an opportunity to talk about many different developmental topics, which are detailed in Chapter 3.

## Habituation to Light

Eric first responds to the light with a **mild squirm** and **facial twitch.** His response decreases after each light presentation; after the fifth presentation, his only response is a slight blink of the eyes.

Theresa shares Eric's success with habituation with the parent and continues with the NBO while observing Eric.

Eric first responds to the light with a **full body squirm,** and he **extends** his arms and legs away from his body. His fingers remain extended. He remains in that position and has 2- to 3-second **respiratory pauses** after each light presentation.

Theresa shares Eric's efforts at self-regulation and habituation with Cheryl and continues observation of skin color and length of respiratory pauses. If either increases in severity, then Theresa will discontinue habituation and allow recovery of color and breathing pattern before continuing with habituation to the rattle.

After the third light presentation, Eric is very **pale** and shows **duskiness** around the mouth and bridge of the nose. He is lying with a **limp** posture and starts **gagging.**

Theresa discontinues habituation and guides Cheryl to place Eric on his side and tuck his arms and legs close to his body by swaddling him with his blanket or with her hands; when gagging ceases, Theresa waits until Eric regains color and regular breathing pattern. Theresa talks to Cheryl about Eric's sensitivities to this type of stimulation, his efforts to maintain self-regulation and achieve habituation, and his recovery after his signs of exhaustion. Theresa explains to Cheryl that this item requires Eric to be in an undisturbed sleep state and that because Eric's sleep has been interrupted, it is no longer possible to continue with habituation. Theresa continues with the next NBO item while observing Eric.

## Habituation to Sound

Eric responds to the first rattle presentation with a **mild startle,** causing him to adjust his position in the blanket. He regains **regular breathing** within seconds and remains **pink.** By the fourth rattle, Eric is in **deep sleep** and does not respond any longer.

Theresa shares Eric's success with habituation with Cheryl and continues with the NBO while observing Eric.

Eric first responds to the rattle with a **full body startle.** His response decreases over the next three rattle presentations but comes back in full force at the fifth presentation. He is now **breathing rapidly.**

Theresa points out to Cheryl Eric's breathing rate and pattern, and they observe jointly how it changes with each rattle presentations. If his breathing rate slows down and becomes regular, then Theresa will continue with another rattle presentation. If his breathing rate continues to increase and color changes are noted, then Theresa will explain to Cheryl that he is showing ongoing signs of stress and that it is best to discontinue habituation to the rattle.

 Eric responds to the first rattle presentation with a **full body startle** and becomes quite **frantic,** unable to stop his movements. He becomes increasingly active and starts **crying.**

Seeing Eric cry may be distressing to Cheryl and difficult to watch without attempting to calm him right away. Theresa engages Cheryl in a joint observation of Eric's efforts to self-quiet at this time and describes how his behaviors reveal whether he needs consoling immediately or is showing signs of self-quieting. When crying persists, Theresa discontinues habituation to rattle and proceeds to the consolability maneuvers. Because Eric is no longer sleeping, Theresa explains to Cheryl that the habituation item cannot be completed.

## Supine, Uncovered, Rooting, and Sucking

 Eric stretches his arms and legs but is able to **tuck** them back in close to his body. He rubs his face with his hands and **braces** one foot against the other leg. He **opens his eyes** slightly and seems to be waking up. He shows a strong response to both rooting and sucking.

Theresa points out to Cheryl Eric's display of robustness in his motor system and transition to an awake state during this item and continues with the NBO while observing Eric.

 Eric becomes **active** by moving his arms and legs and starts **fussing.** He tries to tuck himself in but is unable to maintain the position on his own for more than 1 to 2 seconds. He shows a very strong response to both rooting and sucking.

Theresa encourages Cheryl to support Eric's efforts to tuck himself in by showing her how she can hold Eric's arms and legs close to his body with her hands. She also can be encouraged to bring one of Eric's hands close to his mouth and observe his efforts to suck. He also could be placed on his side if he remains active and swaddled softly with a blanket as needed.

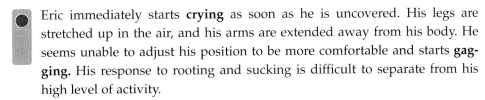

Eric immediately starts **crying** as soon as he is uncovered. His legs are stretched up in the air, and his arms are extended away from his body. He seems unable to adjust his position to be more comfortable and starts **gagging**. His response to rooting and sucking is difficult to separate from his high level of activity.

Theresa follows the same procedure as for habituation to the rattle and proceeds with consolability maneuvers when appropriate.

## Consolability

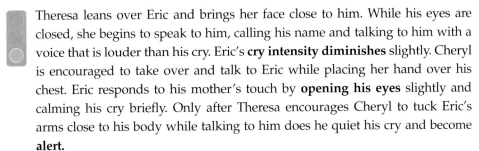

Theresa leans over Eric and brings her face close to him. While his eyes are closed, she begins to speak to him, calling his name and talking to him with a voice that is louder than his cry. Eric's **cry intensity diminishes** slightly. Cheryl is encouraged to take over and talk to Eric while placing her hand over his chest. Eric responds to his mother's touch by **opening his eyes** slightly and calming his cry briefly. Only after Theresa encourages Cheryl to tuck Eric's arms close to his body while talking to him does he quiet his cry and become **alert.**

Theresa continues to the next NBO item while observing Eric.

At first, Eric seems to respond to Theresa's voice by decreasing the intensity of his cry for a brief moment. His crying then intensifies again during the holding of his hands close to his body and even when picked up by Theresa. He attempts to bring his hand to his mouth but is unable to maintain it there. He is very red, and a dusky color shows around the mouth and bridge of the nose.

Theresa continues with observation of skin color, breathing pattern, and crying state. Theresa always asks Cheryl what works best to calm Eric when he is this upset. If he remains upset but stable in color, then Theresa will proceed rapidly to rocking, swaddling, and pacifier (if permitted by Cheryl), giving each maneuver a few seconds before introducing the next.

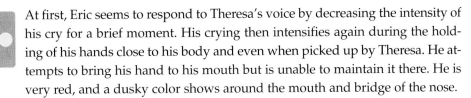

As soon as Eric begins to cry, his color changes to red and dusky. He begins to gag and suddenly loses tone in his body.

Theresa swaddles and picks Eric up immediately while asking Cheryl what works best when Eric gets this upset. Theresa uses the pacifier, after getting Cheryl's permission, and lets Cheryl take over. Theresa observes and comments on Eric's ability to quiet when held by Cheryl. Theresa gives Eric a prolonged rest before proceeding to the next item.

## Orientation Animate

Eric is **alert,** and his gaze is **oriented toward** Theresa; he has **soft cheeks** with **pink** color, and his hands are **tucked** near his face with his body resting comfortably in the blanket. He follows Theresa's face with or without voice with

**slow, smooth movements of his eyes and head**. He **turns his head** to each side when called and finds his caregiver.

Theresa shares with Cheryl how focused and attentive Eric is to the human face and continues with the next NBO item while observing Eric.

 Eric **pauses** in his breathing, **looks away,** moves his fingers, and **squirms** slightly in the blanket. He stills when he hears Theresa's voice and shifts his eyes but is **unable to turn his eyes or head** toward the source of the voice. His **fingers are splayed,** and his arms are pushing out of the blanket.

Theresa slightly distances her face and softens her voice. She gives Eric a time-out, rocks him gently in a vertical motion, and tucks him in a blanket. When Eric looks at Theresa, she moves slowly and stops when Eric's gaze shifts away from her. She waits for him to come back before continuing. Theresa stops when Eric repeats the sequence of shifting his gaze again and proceeds to the next item. When calling his name on each side, Theresa softens her voice, observes his response, and keeps encouraging him to turn with a soft voice. She stops after Eric shows consistency in the level of response twice. Theresa shares the richness of Eric's behavioral response with Cheryl.

 Eric **looks away** from Theresa, his gaze is **dull, his mouth is open,** his fingers are **stretched** out, and he lies with a **limp** posture in the blanket. He is **breathing fast** and is becoming **very pale.**

Theresa stops and gives Eric a break from the intensity of the interaction. She swaddles him and offers a pacifier after getting permission from Cheryl. Theresa tries the intervention strategies that were described in the yellow light section and adds breaks, swaddling, and rocking to her facilitation efforts. Theresa dims lights in the room and proceeds slowly and very gently and does not keep insisting on a higher level of response from Eric. Theresa tries each stimulus twice and notes Eric's best response. Again, she shares with Cheryl the range of behaviors that Eric displayed and highlights his efforts at communicating his needs for breaks from the intensity of the interaction.

## Orientation Inanimate

 Eric is **bright-eyed** and looks at the red ball with **intent** and a slight **frown** of his eyebrows; his entire body seems to follow the ball, with fingers from both hands **clasping** to one another. He shows **robust tone** and **even color.**

Theresa continues with the next NBO item while observing Eric.

 Eric's **eyes are moving as if floating** without clear focus and ability to follow. His eyes **overshoot** to the side as the red ball is moved; he is becoming **active** and is **not responding to the sound of the rattle.**

Theresa slightly distances the ball. She gives Eric a time-out, rocks him gently in a vertical motion, and tucks him in his blanket. She tries to get his attention on the red ball by shaking it gently. Once Eric's eyes are on the ball, Theresa moves it slightly to one side and waits for Eric to catch up should he look away. Theresa gets Eric's attention again by moving the ball; she makes sure that he is following the ball and not the other way around. Theresa engages Cheryl in a discussion of Eric's efforts to maintain his attention on the ball while pointing out his difficulty in doing so for prolonged periods of time.

 Eric is **breathing faster,** and the color around his mouth has turned **dusky.** His eyes are wide open as if **hyperalert,** and he is **grimacing** and **grunting.** He suddenly becomes frantic; his arms and legs move and stretch, and he starts **crying** loudly.

Theresa stops and observes with Cheryl whether Eric will self-quiet. If he is unable to quiet, then Theresa will begin consolability maneuvers but will move quickly if she is unsuccessful in consoling Eric. If Eric settles and quiets again, then Theresa will try intervention maneuvers that were described in yellow light section and pay close attention to Eric's responses. Theresa proceeds slowly and very gently and does not keep insisting on a higher level of response from Eric. She tries each stimulus twice and notes Eric's best response. It is important to capture with Cheryl the events that led to Eric's loss of attention and self-regulation and to talk about the modifications that may help Eric to achieve a higher level of performance for this item.

### Hand Grasp, Pull-to-Sit, and Crawl

 Eric responds with a **strong grasp and tone** in his neck and shoulders when pulled to sit. He is able to **pick his head up** and hold it steady for a few seconds. When placed on his stomach, he lifts his head and **makes crawling movements** with his legs. He is **robust** and **alert** while looking around. He seems to enjoy the handling and stimulation.

Theresa engages Cheryl in the observation of Eric's developmental competencies during this item and his motoric robustness while maintaining himself in a nice, awake state. Theresa continues with the next NBO item while observing Eric.

 Eric **curls his fingers** around Theresa's finger and maintains a **moderate grasp** while he is pulled to sit. He **fusses** and has a **head lag,** and it is difficult for him to bring his head forward on his chest, but he eventually succeeds in doing so. He is **unable to keep his head to midline.** He **fusses** again when placed on his stomach. At first, he **lies with his face down** and **does not move his legs.** He eventually turns his head to one side and makes weak crawling movements with his legs while **fussing.**

Theresa places her finger in Eric's hands, making sure that her other fingers are not touching the back of his hand. She stimulates his grasp by pushing gently inside his palm with her finger. Once he is grasping, she holds his hands and gently tugs at his arms as if lifting him. If the head lag persists, then Theresa will place her fingers gently behind his neck to offer him more support when pulling him to sit. Once in a sitting position, Theresa calls his name to encourage him to lift his head. She gives Eric a break before placing him prone by holding him or cradling him with her hands on the mattress. She gently turns him around onto his stomach and places her hands on his feet while pushing on them gently to trigger his crawling movements. If he keeps his face down on the mattress, then she will turn him onto his side.

 Eric is very **floppy** and shows **little grasping** response and **no ability to hold his head** while pulled to sit. He is **drowsy** and is **fussing** as Theresa attempts to pull him to sit. Once in sitting, he keeps his **head flexed on his chest** and makes no attempts to lift it. On his stomach, he makes **no attempts to free his face** and seems to be falling asleep.

Another possibility is for Eric to be **extremely active and upset.** He **cries** as soon as he is pulled to sit and seems to have great tone in his neck and shoulder muscles. He is able to keep his head straight in sitting, but he **arches** his back and his cry increases in intensity. On his stomach, he continues to cry and **arches** his back while making **exaggerated crawling movements** with his legs.

If Eric is very floppy and drowsy, then Theresa will pick him up and rock him gently in a vertical motion in an attempt to arouse him.

If Eric is very active or crying, then Theresa will need to console him and bring his behavioral state down to an alert state. Theresa can attempt the consolability maneuvers by holding, swaddling, and rocking him or using the pacifier.

Theresa uses the intervention strategies that were described in the yellow light section but observes carefully and decides to proceed or not on the basis of Eric's response. Theresa will not insist on a response if Eric repeatedly returns to a drowsy or crying state.

## ANTICIPATORY GUIDANCE: SPECIFIC CAREGIVING THEMES FOR THE PRETERM INFANT

During the course of a home visit, many questions that concern the overall development of preterm or medically fragile infants arise. Although the questions may vary, most relate to the following themes: sleep issues, touch and handling, feeding difficulties, crying, chronological versus corrected age, stimulation, and interaction. The following section provides background information that clinicians may find useful when answering these questions (Nugent et al., 2007).

## Sleep Issues

Many preterm infants are discharged home with a history of apnea and still may have ongoing respiratory issues with chronic lung disease, whereas some still may be on oxygen therapy or home cardiorespiratory monitoring equipment. This equipment is known to sound its alarm when the infant moves even slightly, causing numerous interruptions during sleep and preventing parents from enjoying uninterrupted rest at night. Research also shows that preterm infants have immaturity of their sleep organization when assessed by electroencephalogram. These infants also often are noisy breathers, with snuffling, snoring, and grunting, so parents tend to be worried about breathing difficulties and are more likely to be disturbed by their infant at night.

Infants who have been in a busy NICU that does not have normal night and daylight cycles may have their night and day mixed up once at home. Parents of preterm infants often report that their infant is most alert in the middle of the night. The calm environment in terms of noise and levels of lighting that is typical of the home night environment may well be the reason for that increased level of alertness. Infants who come home after a NICU stay have become accustomed to the continuous background noise and light that are typical of those environments. These infants learn to habituate to noise and light and may even find that these disturbances help them sleep (Vergara & Bigsby, 2004). Changing the intensity of the lighting in the room in which the infant is placed during the day, pulling the shades, or dimming the lights may support the infant's efforts to reach and maintain an alert state. Swaddling the infant and providing grasping opportunities through finger holding helps the infant maintain a relaxed posture for longer periods and can assist the infant in efforts to respond to his or her parents' voices. In general, a calm daily routine of low-key events will nurture and support appropriately the development of the preterm infant's competence (Mouradian, Als, & Coster, 2000). During the day, infants should be in a quiet and calm home environment with opportunities to sleep in a room that is free of television or conversation noises. They can be swaddled or "nested" in blanket rolls, which provide opportunities for bracing their feet against the boundaries of the nest. Limiting the number of visitors and caregivers will help to establish a predictable routine that is planned around the infant's developing sleep–wake cycles and feeding schedule. Supportive reassurance regarding the common occurrence of these problems in preterm infants and an acknowledgment that their sleeping problems are more complicated and most likely will take longer to resolve than in term infants also are helpful for anxious parents. The following vignette tells the story of Amanda, a little girl who was born preterm at 24 weeks' gestation and now is home after a prolonged stay in a big urban NICU.

✳

During the NBO at the first home visit, Amanda showed difficulty in habituating to the rattle. Although she did not wake up, her level of response to repeated presentations of the rattle kept alternating between low and high with no shutdown. Her mother Ellen mentioned that she had her day and night reversed: She would sleep soundly during the day, and it seemed that nighttime was playtime. Ellen was visibly exhausted and asked whether there was anything she could do to change this. The home visitor, Connie, had noticed that Amanda's bassinet was placed next to a big-screen television in the living room and asked Ellen where Amanda slept during the day and night. She said that she slept in the bassinet during the day and in a crib that was placed in the parents' bedroom at night. Ellen did not feel comfortable letting Amanda sleep in her crib during the day because she felt the need to have her within eyesight. Connie suggested that Ellen gradually move the bassinet away from the television by placing it in the adjoining dining room, for example, until she felt comfortable letting Amanda sleep in her crib in a quiet room during the day. At the next home visit, the bassinet was near the living room but removed from the television. Ellen mentioned that she was trying to keep the volume as low as possible while Amanda's brother watched television during Amanda's daytime naps. By the third visit, Amanda's mother proudly announced that the bassinet was now in Amanda's room and that she was able to take all of her naps in that room. Nighttime waking now was limited to feeding times and was of much shorter duration. Ellen clearly was proud of being able to solve on her own an issue that was affecting the whole family.

✳

## Touch and Handling

In the course of the NBO, the infant's response to touch and handling can be observed during the administration of the motor items or when the infant is held. Many preterm infants respond to being handled with extension and stretching movements of their arms and legs. This response can be brief and followed by tucking and flexion of the extremities toward the body. For other infants, this response is more difficult to inhibit and may lead to disorganization. The NBO offers the opportunity to observe the kind of support that the infant needs when handled. For example, some infants prefer to be picked up with their arms and legs kept tucked in. They also respond better to being placed on their back or side while tucked in. The tucking support can be provided by the parent's hands or through the use of a blanket that is wrapped loosely around the infant.

The importance of touch now is understood better, and parents are encouraged to hold their preterm infants with skin-to-skin contact, practicing *kangaroo care*. Research has demonstrated the positive effects of extended skin-to-skin contact, or kangaroo care, for preterm infants and parents alike (Anderson, 1991; Ohgi et al., 2002). A meta-analysis of the effects of extended skin-to-skin contact revealed slightly improved Neonatal Behavioral Assessment Scale scores for habituation, motor maturity, and range of state and reduced stress (Vickers, Ohlsson, Lacy, & Horsley, 2002). Likewise, in older infants, massage therapy has been used, and results suggest that it may improve weight gain in preterm/low-birth-weight infants and may have an effect on decreasing length of hospital stay (Dieter et al., 2003; Ferber, Kuint et al., 2002). After discharge home, massage therapy, taught by a trained professional, also may provide a positive experience for parents and infants. Because deep touch such as that provided through swaddling or contained holding is organizing for most infants (Browne, 2000), these infants may be calmer when held during the day. Although this may be comforting for the infants, many mothers find it difficult to go about their daily routine when an infant prefers to be held a lot. Therefore, the use of infant carriers when the infant reaches the appropriate size may be another way to continue this close contact. Responses to light touch may vary among infants (Vergara & Bigsby, 2004). Some infants will enjoy it and turn toward the source of light touch, whereas others quickly become disorganized. Observing the individual response of an infant to touch is important and will help the caregiver adjust his or her approach to meet the needs of the infant better.

## Feeding Problems

Feeding problems are common in high-risk infants during the first year of life, particularly in infants who have had prolonged mechanical ventilation and nasogastric tube feedings (Dodrill et al., 2004; Rommel, De Meyer, Feenstra, & Veereman-Wauters, 2003; Thoyre, 2003), and can be categorized as resulting from medical, oral, and behavioral sources (Rommel et al., 2003). These problems commonly are multifactorial, with medical problems such as gastroesophageal reflux, which results in feeding-associated pain and triggers oral sensitivity with oral defensive behavior. Most preterm infants will have been fed through a nasogastric tube while in the hospital, and for many of these infants, the full transition to breast or bottle feeding was achieved just days before discharge home from the hospital. While in the NICU, preterm infants also are fed according to a strict schedule, which varies between every 3 and 4 hours. Feeding success often is reported to the parent in terms of volume ingested and grams of weight gained daily. The reality that parents face at home will be different. Most infants soon will ask to be fed on demand and therefore will not follow the schedule that was established in the NICU. Sleep issues may interfere with the feeding schedule, because many infants may sleep most during the day and feed more often at night. Parents become increasingly worried about weight gain, because the daily feedback on weight gain no longer is available to them.

The observation of the rooting and sucking reflex during the NBO creates the opportunity to ask the parents about feeding. Many parents will have much to say and offer a detailed rendition of the feeding history of their infant. When asked how the infant is feeding, many parents may respond with the volume ingested and ounces gained, which was how feeding was reported to them while the infant was in the NICU. The clinician should ask parents appropriate open-ended questions regarding feeding, which will allow discovery of more information on "how" feeding is really going. Information on the duration of the feeding, state of arousal of the infant during feeding, reflux, postfeeding recovery time, and schedule of feeding for a 24-hour period can help the parents to identify potential sources of problems during feeding. If a feeding problem is identified, then a thorough evaluation needs to be completed by a competent and highly trained therapist. Vergara and Bigsby (2004) provided a comprehensive list of common feeding problems as belonging to 1 of 10 categories:

1.  Low arousal

2.  Fatigue/increased work of breathing

3.  Poor coordination of swallowing and sucking

4.  Poor coordination of breathing with suck–swallow

5.  Weak suck and/or hypotonicity

6.  Limited tongue and jaw mobility and/or hypertonicity

7.  Oral hypersensitivity

8.  Irritability

9.  Poor lip closure

10. Inadequate intra-oral suction

Because feeding problems can be very complex, only highly trained therapists should provide feeding intervention. An experienced therapist can assist the parents in the selection of appropriate nipples for the infant, in proper positioning during feeding, and in the awareness of how levels of stimulation affect arousal and feeding (Vergara & Bigsby, 2004). The NBO is useful in identifying infants and parents who may benefit from such specialized feeding support and intervention.

## Crying

Before the NBO session begins, the clinician should describe briefly the events that will take place, one of which is the possibility that the infant will cry. The clinician then can ask the parents' permission to let the infant cry briefly so that they both can observe what makes the infant cry and his or her self-consoling attempts and response to being consoled by either the clinician or the parent. This preparation is critical for a successful NBO, because parents may not understand why the clinician would choose to observe an infant cry rather than console immediately. Once permission has been granted to observe the infant cry, a comfortable setting for discussing crying issues has been put in place. Irritability and excessive crying are among the most common problems reported by parents during the first 3 months of life, and research shows that this is truer of preterm infants than of term infants (Barr, Rotman, Yaremko, Leduc, & Francoeur, 1992; Sobotkova, Dittrichova, & Mandys, 1996). There is no doubt that caring for a child who cries a lot is extremely stressful for parents. Many parents of a preterm infant may feel depressed or overwhelmed by the continuous and sometimes inconsolable crying of their infant. It is especially important, therefore, for the clinician to recognize that parents need to talk about their feelings of frustration and their feelings of inadequacy in the face of their infant's excessive crying. The best form of anticipatory guidance may well be to help parents realize that having in place a social support network—whether partner, parents, friends, or neighbors—is perhaps their most important form of preventive intervention at this time.

In the past 10 years, much research has been done to understand crying. Although this knowledge may not by itself offer solutions to everyday crying issues in the home, it offers the clinician some insight to share with parents during a home visit. The following is what is known about crying, with a focus on the preterm infant:

- First described by Brazelton (1962), crying shows an increase in duration up to approximately 6 weeks of life, followed by a gradual decrease at approximately 4 months (Hopkins, 2000).

- Barr et al. (1996) compared the crying patterns of healthy, term infants with those of healthy preterm infants from 40 weeks' gestational age through 24 weeks' corrected age and found that preterm infants still cried significantly more than term infants after 40 weeks' gestational age, with a peak and evening clustering at 6 weeks' corrected age.

- At both 6 weeks and 3 months of age, mothers of preterm infants, as compared with mothers of term infants, reported that their infants cried more and were more irritable than term infants (Sobotkova et al., 1996).

- Not only do preterm infants cry more, but also their cries are rated as sounding more difficult to interpret and more aversive than the cries of term infants; excessive crying, in turn, has been linked to reduced maternal responsiveness (Boukydis & Lester, 1998; Worchel & Allen, 1997).

How, then, does the clinician help parents respond positively to a preterm infant who they believe cries excessively, has a piercing cry, and is difficult to console?

First, it is important to remind parents that over time, their infant's cry will become more robust and will sound more like the cry of a term infant (Robb & Goberman, 1997). It becomes critical to let parents of preterm infants know that this lower threshold for crying may reflect the preterm infant's lack of ability to regulate behavioral states and not a response to inadequate care and response by the parent. This may present the clinician with an opportunity to help parents listen closely to the acoustics and harmonics of the cry to "befriend" their infant's cry and to recognize that the strength and robustness of the cry is a reliable index of the infant's well-being and development (Nugent et al., 2007). Second, the clinician can help parents realize that the cry is their infant's communication system par excellence. The clinician can help them anticipate the infant's cry throughout the day by teaching them early warning signals that indicate overload or overstimulation. By learning how the infant reacts to specific situations that are more likely to lead to crying (e.g., if the infant usually cries during diaper changing), the parents can learn to reduce the level of stimulation or pay attention to the infant's tolerance for various levels of handling (Nugent et al., 2007).

## Stimulation and Interaction: Promoting the "Goodness of Fit" Between Parent and Infant

The hypersensitivity of the high-risk infant to handling and to social and environmental stimulation has been well documented. Parents and clinicians need to recognize that many infants who were discharged home recently from the hospital will remain sensitive to stimulation for some months after discharge. Therefore, anticipatory guidance that is given to parents should include information on the prevention of overstimulation and the support of self-regulation for the sensitive infant. The AMOR observational structure of the NBO provides an organized way to understand neurobehavioral functioning and to observe the interdependence among the four behavioral dimensions. It helps clinicians to identify the types of stimulations and interactions that lead to loss of self-regulation, the strategies that the infant uses to maintain self-regulation, and the type of support that is most helpful to the infant's recovery.

Preterm infants, even at term age, have limited abilities for multisensory processing (Vergara & Bigsby, 2004). For example, it often is very difficult for a young preterm infant to look at his or her caregiver while being held and talked to at the same time. It is recommended that caregivers take into account the number of modalities that they use when interacting with their infant. The pediatrician can suggest that caregivers limit the number of modalities presented all at once by holding (not rocking) and smiling at the infant but not talking to him or her at the same time. If the infant establishes eye contact and looks relaxed, then the caregiver can greet the infant with a soft voice while watching his or her behavioral signals of regulation to decide whether voice is appropriate at the moment.

For assisting the preterm infant's emerging abilities to maintain self-regulation in a variety of environments, taking the infant on outside errands to the grocery story or the shopping mall should be limited for the first few weeks after discharge home from the hospital. Parents often ask about what are appropriate toys for their young infant. In the first 2 to 3 months of life, the parents themselves are the best "toys" available to their infant. Infants at this age are most interested in faces, especially their parents' faces, and will prefer looking at them than at any given toy. Parents should avoid battery-powered toys that offer continuous stimulation (light or sound) without pause and should limit exposure to television. Early intervention clinicians typically are well versed on which toys are appropriate for very young infants and can assist the pediatrician in making recommendations.

## Chronological Age or Corrected Age: A Dilemma for Parents

In home-based early intervention, parents are asked to identify developmental goals that will guide the delivery of services to their child at home. Very often, parents will say that the desired goal for their child is that "she does what she is supposed to do for her age." Throughout the NBO session, the parent often may ask, "Is my infant okay?" or, "Is my infant doing what she should for her age?" One of the major sources of concerns for parents is the question of how to estimate the infant's age, whether to use the concept of *corrected age* or simply use the infant's actual *chronological age* (Nugent et al., 2007). Most preterm infants are discharged from the hospital within weeks of their due date, and although they match on their corrected age for prematurity, some will be 4 weeks' chronological age, whereas others may be 3 months' chronological age. Parents are unsure which age classification, corrected or chronological, to use an index of the infant's progress or development. When using popular books on early child development as resources, parents also often believe that their infant's development does not fit either age profile and are not sure what to expect in terms of the infant's development. Most parents have been told that their infant will "catch up" within the next 2 years, but at the present moment, they need reassurance that the catching up is taking place. Parents of infants with significant brain injury have been told that their infant most likely will have developmental delays or cerebral palsy, and those parents are very anxious and in need of knowing when those signs become apparent. There is no simple solution to this dilemma, and a good clinician will use the infant as the best index of prediction available. The motor items of the NBO create an opportunity to observe motor robustness, tone, and general motor activity and provide a context to discuss those parental concerns.

It is very important for health care professionals to remind the parents of their infant's corrected age and to point out some basic differences between the preterm and the term infant of similar postconceptual ages. For most healthy, preterm infants who were born at gestational ages of more than 26 weeks, the corrected age quickly becomes appropriate to determine their developmental status, and popular books can be good resources for those parents. For infants who were born earlier or who were medically fragile, however, using the corrected age to verify the developmental status of an infant may not be appropriate for some time. During the first year of life, many preterm infants present *soft neurological signs,* such as lower extremity hypertonicity, truncal hypo- or hypertonicity, scapular retraction, and jitteriness (Drillien, 1972; Georgieff & Bernbaum, 1986; Georgieff, Bernbaum, Hoffman-Williamson, & Daft, 1986). For many years, these signs have been classified under the term *transient dystonia,* and for most preterm infants, they resolve by 18 months of age. For infants with neurological compromise, these signs will persist and increase in severity, with the presence of obligatory and persistent primitive reflexes becoming more evident at an age when integration of those reflexes is expected. For these infants and parents, the use of corrected age is inappropriate, and long-term support and guidance are needed to help the family adjust to the reality of their child's emerging disability.

Early intervention clinicians can be very helpful in assisting the pediatrician, neurologist, or nurse address developmental issues with parents. A simple guideline would be to monitor progress in development over time as seen in the acquisition of early skills and to comment on the quality of the observed skills rather than on the quantity. For example, although a preterm child may be delayed in sitting, he or she may display excellent quality of movement in his or her ability to turn, reach, transfer objects, or play with his or her feet. The comments on the quality of movement can reassure the parents that the infant is showing healthy signs of development. The same principle can be applied to other domains of development. With steady progress and good quality of performance, parents can witness that the progress that their child is making is indicative of catching up and can be reassured somewhat of the absence of major developmental disabilities.

## SUMMARY

This chapter provided a framework for understanding behavioral competence in the high-risk infant with a focus on the preterm infant. Many of these infants are referred to home-based early intervention services after discharge from the hospital. Clinicians have a responsibility to individualize their approach and intervention strategies to meet the unique needs of the infant and his or her family. The NBO is proposed as an effective relationship-building tool to be used in the early weeks and months after coming home from the hospital. The NBO can meet two main goals of early intervention: 1) to support families to provide the best care for their infant and 2) to provide highly individualized intervention strategies that can help them best meet that goal. It offers a positive-adaptive model within which the infant's strengths can be showcased and vulnerabilities can be identified but also can be used as a practical tool for demonstrating developmental progress over time. The NBO is appropriate for use with a wide range of infants who have developmental disabilities and are referred for early intervention services, so its use should not be limited to the preterm infant.

# 7

# Using the Newborn Behavioral Observations System in Postpartum Clinic and Home Visits

Kristie Brandt

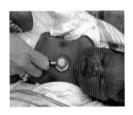

This chapter describes how the Newborn Behavioral Observations (NBO) system can be used by nurses and other health care clinicians in a variety of postpartum environments, particularly during maternal postpartum health care appointments and in parent–infant home-visiting programs, to form a more meaningful relationship with the parents and to support the health and well-being of the family. The first 2 days after birth are a potent and dramatic phase for the parents and infant that sets the attachment process in motion (Bowlby, 1982). The parents come to this moment ready to receive the newborn whom they have longed for, imagined, dreamed of, and feared for during the months of pregnancy (Brazelton & Cramer, 1990). This process has been fueled not only by the knowledge that the infant is coming but also by the first barely perceptible movements and then the clearly apparent presence and activity of the child behind the thin veil of the abdominal wall.

The time immediately after birth affords nurses a rich opportunity to use the NBO in supporting the parents and infant as they encounter and experience one another face to face for the first time, but this period is brief and can be stressful and hectic for parents, who may still be exhausted from the labor and birth, occupied with visitors, continuing to undergo intense medical management, or, for other reasons, unable to receive and process information well. As the new family is organizing during the first 8 weeks postpartum, meeting the challenges and experiencing the fears and joys of parenting the young infant, the NBO continues to provide a systematic and powerful intervention strategy for strengthening the parent–infant relationship and fostering the process of the parents and infant "falling in love."

## THE TRANSITION HOME

For perinatal clinicians, the goals of late pregnancy, labor, birth, and the initial postpartum period primarily focus on ensuring safe passage and optimal health for the mother and infant. After birth, in ideal environments, the focus shifts to supporting the parents and infant through the immediate and potent phase of engagement and dawning acquaintance, although this often is overshadowed by continuing surveillance of the infant's and mother's health and well-being in the first 2 days after delivery (Rooks, 1999; Vareny, Kriebs, & Gegor, 2003). In many countries, including the United States, where mothers typically have frequent prenatal care visits and their infants are born in hospitals or birthing centers, the transition to home that occurs 1 to 3 days after giving birth is highly symbolic of many things, including

- The completion of the birthing and immediate postnatal phase with its accompanying close surveillance and virtually constant presence of health care personnel

- The assumption that both the mother and child are in good health

- The transition to the parents of full responsibility for the infant's continuing health, safety, and nurturance, as well as full accountability for problems in these areas

- The societal belief that at least one parent possesses sufficient skills and enough of a loving connection, or attachment, to the infant to ensure that the infant survives and thrives

- The loss of the intense and vigilant support matrix of the maternally focused prenatal and intrapartum health care system, and transition to infant-focused contacts with the health care system

- The loss of the "known family" and construction of a new family system

This transition home occurs within the context of—or perhaps even exacerbates—intense parental vulnerability (George, 2005). Four factors make this passage a critical time for prenatal and intrapartum clinicians to maintain their connection with the family and their vigilance of the infant–parent relationship or to ensure that a referral is made and the *trust bond* is transferred to another reliable and competent clinician who can accomplish these tasks:

1. Many mothers are emotionally and physically ready for this transition, but others may not be sufficiently recovered from labor and birth and may still be in the postpartum "taking-in" phase (Rubin, 1967), experiencing "baby blues," or exhibiting early signs of postpartum dysphoric disorders (George, 2005).

2. For the team of health care clinicians, the prenatal and intrapartum periods of extreme vigilance and being poised to respond to maternal, fetal, and infant emergencies subside at this time, and the resulting relaxation and distancing of the health care team may be perplexing and disturbing for the mother as the transition to home occurs; she may even experience a sense of abandonment. When birth occurs in the woman's home, she may have a similar experience as birth attendants reduce their vigilance, complete their intrapartum and immediate postpartum care activities, and are no longer a presence in the woman's home.

3. The presence or absence of a supportive circle of family and friends will have an impact on parents, who may vacillate between (and be unable to reconcile) their desire for and fear of being alone with the infant and their wanting proximity to the trusted people in their lives for reassurance and assistance. In this period of vulnerability, adult attachment issues may be activated, and one or both parents may experience an intense yearning for their own childhood attachment figure. The availability or absence of this person and the history of that relationship may be quite meaningful for the new parents, and they may find themselves occupied with memories of their childhood, coupled with concerns about their own ability to parent the new infant. This, in turn, may influence the parents' responsiveness to the infant (Main, Kaplan, & Cassidy, 1985).

4. Patterns of interactions with the infant are being established, and the internal working models, or ways of being together, that are formed in this important period will have a lasting impact on the parents, the infant, the parent–infant relationship, and the lifelong health and well-being of the infant (Carlson & Sroufe, 1995).

This phase will be influenced by many things, including the family's culture and the woman's experience of caring for infants, level of support, temperament, and experience of being parented herself (Britton, 2005), but sooner or later, it dawns on the mother that she alone is viewed by society as being solely responsible for the health and well-being of her infant and for any problems or difficulties her infant may experience (Stern & Bruschweiler-Stern, 1998). This moment typically is a pivotal point in the first postpartum weeks and may be emblematic of the so-called fourth trimester of pregnancy.

For most parents, this phase will have an impact on the budding relationship with the infant as the joy and relief of birth followed by the wonder and awe of experiencing the newborn temporarily shift to apprehension and anxiety about caring independently for the unfamiliar infant (Brazelton, 1981). From a biological perspective, this alarm response can produce tremendous anxiety that parents may attempt to mitigate by turning their attention to scheduled routines of physical caregiving and heightened attention to the infant's physical well-being and safety (Brazelton, 1992). The skilled clinician will find this time to be an opportunity unlike any other to support the parents in identifying and understanding the infant's behavioral language. This complex transitional phase, described by Rubin (1967, 1984) as the "taking hold" and "taking charge" progression, is an opportunity to allay parental anxiety by supporting parents in building their parental mastery and getting to know and understand their unique infant (Brazelton, 1992; Brazelton & Cramer, 1990). It also is an opportunity to use parental anxiety as a potent motivator for developing these parenting skills.

Prenatal and intrapartum clinicians often make referrals to nurse home-visiting programs to ensure that families receive the support and observation of a skilled maternal–child and family nurse (MCFN) during this important transitional period. The benefits of nurses who provide home visits to families with infants and young children, particularly in high-risk households, are some of the best documented in the health literature, and nurse home visiting is considered to be a truly "evidence-based" intervention (Olds & Kitzman, 1993; U.S. Public Health Service, 2000). Olds (2002) posited that the success of home-visiting programs is based partially on the nurse's ability to promote parental understanding of the newborn's behaviors and temperament, foster responsivity to the infant, support development of infant care skills, and validate the mother as she adapts to her changing role.

In the MCFN's hands, the NBO is a multidimensional tool for effectively achieving these goals. Used with newborns from birth to 8 weeks of age, it is a systematic and organized method for the nurse to elicit, observe, and showcase the newborn's individuality as expressed in his or her mastery and clarity of cues and other behavioral repertoire. It also provides nurses with an effective lens for gaining insight into the parents' awareness and understanding of their infant and learning about the parents' experience of the infant and what meaning the parents have made of the infant's behaviors and characteristics.

When used by a highly skilled clinician, the NBO becomes an even more sophisticated and useful tool with the potential to open the clinician–parent relationship to new levels of intimacy and alliance as they explore together the parents' ghosts and angels in the nursery (Fraiberg, 1980; Lieberman et al., 2005), projections, attributions, dreams, fears, and successes and the parents' own model of attachment. The NBO can become the catalyst for establishing sensitive and responsive patterns of parental caregiving that are guided by the infant's behavioral initiation and feedback while providing the clinician with the opportunity to support parental mastery (Brazelton, 1995) as parents meet their own developmental milestones. Finally, the NBO can be a screening tool for identification of concerning behaviors and neurological responses that were not identified in the early newborn period and that may require additional evaluation.

Use of the NBO can be tailored to virtually any environment in which the nurse encounters the family (e.g., hospital, pediatric office visit, home visit) and can be used as easily in an infant-focused pediatric visit as it can in a maternal postpartum examination or a home visit with the family. The flexibility and the applicability of the NBO across this range of environments and clinicians speak to its usefulness and ease of administration in the postpartum period.

In addition, the NBO can be tailored to highlight specific concerns or questions that parents may have. For instance, if a mother has noticed that her infant awakens easily, then there may be greater focus on the habituation, or sleep protection, items. Elements of the NBO can be used on the basis of the state that the infant is in when the examination commences. With a sleeping infant, the observation starts with the habituation items; the motor tone or activity level items can be assessed first when the observation starts with the infant in an active alert state. If the infant is crying, then the NBO can start with the consolability items. Infants who are in the quiet alert state are ready to engage in the visual (tracking) and auditory or social-interactive items. For preparation, the nurse need only carry the small NBO kit.

The benefit of performing the NBO in the presence of the parents cannot be overstated. It is by its very nature an interactive tool wherein the clinician and the parents learn about the infant's repertoire, style, and capacities, with the added entrée into the parents' and clinician's learning more about parental meaning, concerns, and responses. Following is a clinical vignette illustrating the use of the NBO in a postpartum home visit by a public health nurse (PHN).

## Clinical Vignette: The NBO in the Home Visit

❋

The PHN knocked on Maria's front door and could hear an infant crying somewhere in the house. The crying got closer, and Maria opened the door, gently bouncing against her shoulder 4-week-old Adrian, dressed in a diaper and undershirt, crying full force and flailing his arms. Maria: "Sorry. He's just been doing this all day and most of the night." Maria looked tired and frustrated. "Nothing seems to help him, and I've been holding him for hours."

Together on the couch, the PHN and Maria talk about Adrian and Maria's attempts to soothe and calm him. When the PHN asks what Maria has tried and what has worked, she lists a series of things that she has done to help sooth Adrian.

Maria: "I'm just done. I think it must be breast feeding. Everyone tells me to give him formula or cereal and that will help. Maybe that will do it."

The PHN offers to do an NBO, and they place Adrian on the couch between them. For a few seconds, they watch him as he cries and moves his arms and legs actively in the air.

✳

Clinical Comment: This strategy by the PHN models a way for Maria to be with Adrian when he is crying and allows her to watch and learn more about his distress, the behavioral messages that he is giving, his ability to manage his distress, and what he may need from his mother. By not rushing in immediately to alleviate his distress, Maria can both learn more about her son and support him in providing a wider repertoire of cues.

✳

PHN: "Let's see how much support he might need from you to calm himself down or whether he can even do it yet by himself." She leans over and presents her face to Adrian, who continues to cry, and then she says softly, "Hey, what you doing? Adrian, your mommy is right here beside you. Can you calm yourself down? How you doing?"

✳

Clinical Comment: The PHN's carefully chosen language in administering the NBO has established implicitly that learning to calm himself is a developmental task for Adrian. She has also implied that she, the professional nurse, does not know what Adrian wants and that together, mother and nurse will explore what he can do to calm himself. This is a critical strategy that places mother and nurse in an equal partnership as they think together about Adrian and work to understand his abilities. It also has established that Adrian may not be able to do it all alone yet and may need his mother to intervene to support him as he develops this capacity. The parallel process of nurse and mother is evident.

✳

Adrian slows his crying pattern, pauses for a moment, and looks at the PHN. Within seconds, he starts crying again. Maria says that she has seen that her voice sometimes calms him, but "just like now, he starts back up." The PHN asks Maria to place her hand on Adrian's belly; again, he briefly slows his crying, and then resumes. After a few seconds, the PHN asks Maria to gently bring Adrian's hands together and let them rest in the middle of his belly. Adrian stops crying, takes several longs breaths, and then starts fussing.

✳

Clinical Comment: This expert PHN used a very strategic approach in electing to have Maria carry out most of the elements of the consolability steps under her guidance. Being aware of Maria's vulnerability and frustration in understanding the kind of support that Adrian needed to soothe himself, the PHN considered that if she were successful in helping Adrian sooth himself, this may undermine

Maria's sense of competence in her mothering role. During this encounter, the PHN guided Maria through the steps that resulted in effective soothing, and Adrian's progress became a shared success for mother and son, and the PHN could witness and affirm their achievement. This also provided Maria with multi-sensory information about Adrian as she felt his response with her hands, heard the quality and the nuance of his cry, and saw his behaviors while she learned implicitly about strategies for consoling him. The PHN is developing a working alliance with Maria, and she is careful not to violate the infant–parent relationship by performing the activities that might calm Adrian when his mother has been struggling with this issue.

※

Maria: "See, he just cannot stop. I think he cries half the day, eats a little, sleeps, then cries more. Adrian, my little man, what can I do?" The PHN notices that Maria's affect remains warm and concerned toward Adrian and that her body movements are smooth, and she notices the amount of talking and the tone as Maria attends to Adrian. She observes the gentleness of Maria's touch as she gathers and holds Adrian's hands. Adrian looks briefly at Maria, and his face momentarily softens, his eyes widen, and his lips pull forward. As she and Adrian make eye contact for a moment, Maria's face softens, too. "I love you, mijo," she says in a noticeably gentler and more intimate tone.

※

Clinical Comment: Maria's reaction to the infant during the NBO provided vital data for the nurse in her understanding of Maria's parenting skills, responsivity to her newborn, self-regulation, and ability to engage in mutual regulation with her son. The nurse gained insight into Maria's affect as she attended to her fussing child, and the nurse was able to see how Maria used her voice and tone in communicating to him her presence and concern. The nurse also observed Adrian's response to his mother and Maria's ability to notice and respond to extremely subtle cues from her young son.

※

PHN: "You have such a nice way with him. You just seem to know how he likes to be touched and talked to. How did you figure that out?" Maria talks about how much she loves Adrian and the little signals from him that tell her what he likes. Adrian begins crying again. Finally she says, "I figured out everything but this crying." Her eyes fill up with tears.

※

Clinical Comment: In a parallel process, the skilled PHN has observed subtle and sophisticated cues that the mother exhibits, and she comments on these to

Maria in a general statement about her "way" with her son. Then, the PHN carefully positions Maria as the expert on Adrian with a question about how she accomplished this level of skill. Supported in this alliance, Maria now can share her love for and understanding of her son and her vulnerability and concern about consoling him, which is representational of all of her concerns about becoming Adrian's mother.

❋

The next step in the NBO consolability scale would be to pick up the infant and rock him, but the PHN believes that she observed this when she arrived, so she moves to swaddling. She asks Maria to swaddle Adrian but notices that Maria hesitates.

PHN: "What do you think about swaddling him?"

❋

Clinical Comment: The PHN's focus and skills allowed her to observe a very slight shift in Maria's affect when the issue of swaddling was introduced. Rather than making an assumption about Maria's hesitation, the PHN slows the interaction and asks what the mother thinks. Not knowing whether the hesitation meant anything at all and wondering whether there may be a cultural marker associated with this, the PHN brings respectful curiosity into their discussion and positions Maria as the expert on her experience.

❋

Maria: "The nurse at the hospital told me to keep his hands uncovered so that he could get them to his mouth to calm himself. He hasn't been able to do that yet, but I keep hoping."

PHN: "Oh, that's a good idea." Then she suggests that they try swaddling Adrian leaving one hand out so that he can get it to his mouth and asks whether Maria has noticed which hand he tries to bring to his mouth most often. Maria has noticed this, and she swaddles Adrian leaving his right hand free, and then picks him up.

❋

Clinical Comment: Maria's answer to the PHN's swaddling question has provided the nurse with great insight into Maria's understanding of infants' self-soothing strategies and her awareness that learning to self-soothe is an important developmental skill for Adrian. The PHN and Maria have moved into a deeper therapeutic alliance as they mutually problem-solve and develop a strategy for moving forward together. The PHN has asked another pivotal question, positioning Maria as the expert on her son, and finds that Maria has noticed which hand Adrian has tried most often to get to his mouth. The PHN now has more data about Maria's remarkable observation skills.

✳

Adrian takes a deep breath; his chin quivers, and he looks at his mother. She smiles: "Hey there, little man. How are you? Is that what you wanted?" He turns his head slightly and stares at his mother's face. She cradles him and relaxes back against the couch. Mother and son look in one another's eyes for more than a minute without saying anything. She turns to the PHN and smiles: "Look at him. Peace! His body feels so relaxed."

PHN: "I can see how much you know about Adrian. You seemed to know that more talking or movement right now might be too much for him." Together they talk about the kind of support that Adrian needed to calm himself and Maria's style with him and her comfort with swaddling him in this way. The PHN talks about Adrian's ability to learn more about himself in the coming weeks and getting better at telling his mom what he likes.

PHN: "Next time I come, I'd love to hear more about how he tells you what he wants from you."

✳

Clinical Comment: The PHN narrates Maria's and Adrian's experience and validates Maria's skills and competence. The PHN closes the home visit with a comment about anticipating and expecting to learn more from Maria about Adrian at the next home visit. This, again, positions Maria as the expert on Adrian and the PHN as a supportive professional coming alongside the mother to support her.

✳

In this vignette, the impact of the visit was not accidental or a prescriptive formula for a home-visit encounter. The administration of the NBO was expanded by the skill and the experience of the PHN, who used careful observation, pacing, infant-focused questions, and thoughtful, strategic decision making to enhance the effectiveness of the NBO and the efficacy and the impact of the home visit. The PHN did not arrive at Maria's home intending to administer the NBO but rather used this tool to follow the lead of the mother and expand both her own and the mother's understanding of Adrian's capacities and style of communication. In a triadic session such as this, the infant became the focus from which the PHN–parent relationship gained new dimensions of respect, trust, and understanding, and what is known as the *affirming matrix* was expanded as the mother experienced acceptance of her infant and acknowledgment of herself in the mothering role (Rubin, 1967; Stern & Bruschweiler-Stern, 1998).

## THE AFFIRMING MATRIX

In *Neurons to Neighborhoods*, Shonkoff and Phillips (2000) concluded that the most successful primary prevention and therapeutic interventions on behalf of the infant's lifelong health and well-being focus on facilitating the infant–parent relationship and assisting the dyad as they learn to adapt to one another. Fortunately, the postpartum period is particularly potent for achieving this goal because during this time, mothers are seeking to create an *affirming matrix* and have an extraordinary desire to seek out and affiliate with caregivers who affirm their experiences, make them feel secure and trustworthy, and encourage them to explore their parental capacities (Stern & Bruschweiler-Stern, 1998). This need also was identified in Rubin's (1967) four maternal tasks that include ensuring safe passage, seeking acceptance of the infant by others, seeking acceptance of herself in the role of mother, and learning to give of herself in the role of mother.

In this time, mothers have a great need to be accepted and affirmed in their new role, to have their infant's unique capacities seen and appreciated, to look at their own capacities and responses to the infant, and to be able to explore with a supportive caregiver their experience of being a new mother. Increasingly, women in industrialized countries find themselves without a close circle of supportive family and friends with which to form this matrix, and the nurse, nurse–midwife, or pediatric nurse practitioner frequently becomes an important or central figure in the affirming matrix. Within this important relationship, deep concerns about parenting, the child's development, and other vulnerabilities can be shared. Meeting this need in the postpartum period can have an impact on the health and well-being of this dyad well into the future.

## Clinical Vignette: A Six-Week Postpartum Visit with the Nurse–Midwife

At a postpartum visit, the certified nurse–midwife (CNM) talks with Yolanda about how her health, recovery from delivery, breast feeding, and adjustment to motherhood are going. They briefly reminisce about Yolanda's labor and the birth of Anna and how quickly Anna took to the breast. The CNM is warm and supportive, and Yolanda is quiet and a little guarded. It has taken the two of them several months to build their relationship. Yolanda says things are going well for both her and the infant. When asked about any signs of postpartum depression, Yolanda says that she has none and goes on to note that she has felt better than expected, is getting plenty of rest, and has a lot of family around to help. As they talk, 6-week-old Anna is in her mother's arms in a transitional state between sleep and awake. Before the physical examination, Yolanda puts Anna in a small crib next to the examination table.

After completing a physical examination, the CNM says that she thinks Yolanda is doing fine physically, and Yolanda agrees. As the visit concludes, the CNM says that she will see Yolanda for any problems or concerns in the coming months, but otherwise she does not need to return for a year. The CNM comments on the important events that they have shared together and says that she will miss seeing Yolanda so frequently.

✳

Clinical Comment: This is an important juncture in the relationship of the CNM and the client as the pattern of supportive and frequent contacts makes a transition to a new level of lesser intensity. The CNM is carefully making a space for the "out-the-door question," a phenomenon described by Dixon and Stein (1992) when pivotal moments in provider–client contact, such as the end of an office visit or major transitions in the care relationship, may create a sense of urgency to discuss important matters left unsaid until now. The CNM, aware that she has become an important part of Yolanda's affirming matrix, knows this moment is important for both of them and leaves time and space for an out-the-door question to emerge. The CNM also decides to make a strategic transition and shift focus to the infant as a way for nurse and client to acknowledge what they have shared together and to affirm Yolanda's success and competence in her role as Anna's mother.

✳

Anna now is wide-eyed and in a quiet alert state, staring at the examination light mounted on the wall. The CNM asks Yolanda's permission to do an NBO, and Yolanda quickly agrees. The CNM quietly shakes a rattle near Anna's ear, and the 6-week-old immediately turns toward the sound.

Yolanda smiles: "She can hear."

CNM: "Were you worried about that?"

Yolanda: "No, not really, but you know, you always wonder whether they're okay."

CNM: "Would you like to try it?"

The CNM hands the rattle to the mother, who gently shakes the rattle near Anna's other ear, and Anna turns to the sound.

Yolanda: "She's funny. She hears so well." Yolanda smiles and giggles in a delighted, almost child-like tone. "I can't believe she can do that. You know . . . hear so well."

The CNM observes that Yolanda is more talkative, engaged, and animated now than previously in their time together. The CNM takes a red ball and places it in Anna's line of vision. When Anna looks at the ball, the CNM slowly moves the ball in an arc away from her point of focus. Anna follows the ball nearly 180 degrees, from one side to the other.

Yolanda: "Oh, wow, she sees things so . . . so . . . well. I didn't know she could do that. She's great." Yolanda reaches down and strokes Anna's hair.

CNM: "Have you seen her do this before?"

Yolanda: "No. But she did watch the dog one day walking around the room, and I thought it was funny because everyone told me she can't see yet. But I thought she could see because sometimes she just looks at me for a long time when she's nursing. I kind of thought I was crazy to think that she could see because my mom said infants are like puppies or kittens . . . they don't see for a while. But, she can really see, can't she?"

Clinical Comment: As the NBO was being conducted, the CNM carefully watched Yolanda's response, including her comments, affect, and interactions with Anna. The CNM remained curious about Yolanda's experience of Anna and used the infant's behavior as a common language and their observations as a shared moment of delight in the infant. This sophisticated and well-paced use of the NBO, layered with curiosity, attention, and respect for Yolanda's observations and perceptions, brings client and nurse to a new therapeutic level, opening the moment for the safe discussion of grief and loss in the transition of the relationship, affirmation of the passage that they have shared, or other potent exchanges.

Yolanda now is looking at Anna with an expression of admiration and pleasure. After completing a few more elements of the NBO, the CNM notices that Yolanda's delight seemed to subside. When the CNM asks Yolanda what she is thinking, the new mother's eyes fill with tears.

Yolanda: "I've been a little worried. I've been really sad a lot lately. Like, not about Anna, you know, she's great. But, I've just felt sad and I wondered if it was hurting Anna that I haven't been myself since she was born. I tried to tell my sister about it, and she told me to snap out of it. My mom goes on and on about how happy I should be that Anna is so strong and healthy. I cry sometimes when Anna is sleeping and no one is around, and I'm worried that I'm not feeling okay. Mostly I've been worried that Anna will know how I feel . . . that somehow this will hurt her . . . you know, like change her development. But, I think she's okay. Don't you?"

Clinical Comment: With the use of the NBO, the nurse created a space in which the mother could voice intimate and feared topics. The CNM had expected that Yolanda would share thoughts about her sense of loss in the change in their relationship and did not expect that the issue of a postpartum mood disorder would arise, but the space was created for important issues to emerge in a moment in which Anna's developmental progress was acknowledged and Yolanda's competence as a mother affirmed through the infant's behavior and the clinician's respectful curiosity (Tronick, 1998). The triadic nature of the NBO also afforded both nurse and client the opportunity to encounter one another indirectly in approaching a period of sensitive transition.

## SUMMARY

The NBO is a simple, easily learned, quickly mastered, and rapidly administered tool that in the hands of skilled clinicians becomes a powerfully complex and rich interactive strategy for observing and showcasing the infant's behavioral repertoire and unique capacities. The NBO administration also provides for simultaneous exploration of the parents' awareness and response to the infant's behaviors and the meaning that a parent makes of these.

Self-correcting potential and the energy for adaptation probably are stronger in the newborn period than they ever will be again, and support and insight that are offered at this time can unleash potent positive forces for attachment and growth. The relationship and contact with an expert nurse or other professionals can be a powerful force for change as well as an effective measure to prevent future problems (Brazelton & Cramer, 1990).

In addition to the NBO's use for learning about the newborn and having a positive impact on parent–infant interaction, it is a catalyst for renewing and rejuvenating the clinician's sense of gratification and zest in working with newborns and their families. The NBO offers MCFNs a systemic and easily administered intervention that may have a lifelong impact on the lives of the infants and families whom they touch. The NBO also offers clinicians an invitation to enter into the family system in a more meaningful way and to be rewarded by giving parents what they need to do the best for their children.

# 8

# USING THE NEWBORN BEHAVIORAL OBSERVATIONS SYSTEM IN MULTICULTURAL ENVIRONMENTS

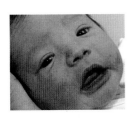

The question that this chapter addresses is how clinicians can use the Newborn Behavioral Observations (NBO) system to support families from very different backgrounds in a way that is authentic to the families and that helps them meet the needs of their young children, while validating and affirming them in their role as parents. How can the NBO be used to provide anticipatory child guidance in a way that respects the parents' cultural values and at the same time promotes their successful adaptation as a family? Questions about where infants sleep, how infants are fed, how crying is dealt with, what roles fathers and grandfathers play in child care, and whether infants can be spoiled all are culturally charged questions that emerge in the context of the NBO and demand both developmental and cultural competency from clinicians if they are to provide guidance to parents that is developmentally sound and culturally appropriate.

## CHANGING DEMOGRAPHIC PATTERNS

A recent review of a UNESCO report on international migration patterns reveals that for the first time, the majority of the world's families can be classified as migrants, headed by parents who are living in diasporic situations or cultural environments other than those in which they were raised (Timur, 2000). Moreover, there is no evidence that the worldwide movement of families from rural to urban centers, often crossing national boundaries, will be reversed in the future. Whether the family move is across national boundaries or within the country, every family shift constitutes a unique set of stresses and parenting challenges. The level of stress for these parents is compounded when this new environment is culturally and linguistically different from that of their community of origin. Inevitably, these parents have to face the challenge of reassessing their parenting goals and their child-rearing practices to help their children adapt successfully to the new cultural environment.

As a result of these demographic changes, it is likely that every society, in a very real sense, will be multicultural, and more and more parents will be facing the task of bringing up their children in a milieu that is alien to them (Garcia Coll & Meyer, 1993; Nugent, 2002). That these families have very different values, goals, expectations, practices, and beliefs about children and how they should be raised is indisputable. But, this new demographic reality also should challenge clinicians to reexamine the way in which they work with families from different cultural groups and, more important perhaps, to examine their own attitudes toward different cultures and their understanding of how culture shapes child and family development.

## Western Middle-Class Values

Just as child-rearing techniques are culturally bound, child guidance and parent support also are cultural constructions. Clinicians need to think about how they offer caregiving guidance to parents from different cultures and how responsive their guidance is to the particular cultural needs and challenges of the families with whom they are working. It is especially important for clinicians to appreciate fully the wide range of differences in the worlds that infants experience from birth in virtually every aspect of their daily lives. Equally important is the need to acknowledge that the principles that govern child and family development and medicine are based, in large part, on Western/middle-class/Euro-American values, which shape and fuel clinicians' caregiving advice to parents and do so in ways that are hidden from clinicians, masquerading as universal "common sense" principles. The assumptions on which the NBO system is based are that not only are there cultural differences in newborn behavior and in child-rearing practices but also that culture itself is the primary organizer of family experiences. This means that one of the major challenges for clinicians is to shift the focus of their interventions from the child or the family *in isolation* to the child and the family *in context*—in cultural context.

The NBO approach to working with families from different cultural communities is characterized by a nonjudgmental stance, emphasizing the separation of value judgments from explanations and avoiding the imposition of the practitioner's own cultural values on the parents' caregiving decision-making process.

To help the clinician do this effectively, this chapter summarizes the theoretical and empirical principles that describe the relationship between culture and child development. First, this chapter takes a closer look at the changing profile of families in contemporary society to provide a better appreciation of the challenges that families face and to understand how best clinicians can support them.

## PARENTING IN ISOLATION: THE CULTURE OF THE IN-BETWEEN

Although parents in all societies struggle with how to raise their children in a way that prepares them for the complexities of life, parenting in a culture with which they are unfamiliar or one in which they have minority status or where they may be subject to prejudice makes the task especially stressful (Garcia Coll & Meyer, 1993). Although many parents today feel isolated from their families and other cultural support systems, they also find themselves in environments in which their traditions, customs, and worldviews are different from and often at odds with those of the dominant "host" country. These parents are caught between cultures—born into one but living in a very different one—and thus face the daunting challenge of parenting in a culture other than the one on which they were brought up and one that they little understand. Homi Bhabha (1994) referred to this as the "culture of the in-between," the culture of liminality. Liminality is the transitional state between the two cultural communities in which these parents find themselves, so that while they no longer belong to their previous society, they are not yet incorporated into their new society. For these parents, "the culture of liminality" is a limbo, an ambiguous state characterized by feelings of isolation and anomie, as they learn that their own indigenous philosophy of child rearing is in conflict with that of the society in which they now are bringing up their children. These conflicts may involve attitudes and decisions about who will look after the infant, whether to breast-feed or bottle-feed, whom to ask for advice, or even which medication to use to cure a rash. These practical decisions touch on their own culturally rooted values and beliefs about children and how they should be treated.

## Cultural Discontinuity

There is evidence to suggest that many immigrant parents experience this sense of isolation and report feeling hopeless, ignored, and invisible to others (Reid, 2004). The parenting experience of many parents today therefore is characterized by both familial and cultural discontinuity. As a result, parents may forfeit their identity and sense of self and with that a sense of confidence in their ability to know what their children need to develop successfully. While child maltreatment has many causes, the relationship between social isolation and maltreatment has been well established in studies in a range of cultural environment (e.g., Gracia &

Musitu, 2003). Abusive parents show lower levels of community integration, participation in community social activities, and use of formal and informal organizations than parents who provide adequate care to their children. Similarly, the increase in postnatal depression has been attributed to parents' feelings of isolation and the absence of social and cultural support systems (e.g., Campbell, Cohn, Flanagan, Popper, & Meyers, 1992; Cutrona, 1983). If the immigrant experience is compounded by poverty, then the experience of social isolation, stigmatization, and powerlessness may become cyclical. It is not surprising that children of immigrant parents are more likely to experience developmental difficulties and various psychosocial problems than do children of indigenous populations.

Clinicians therefore need to be aware of the challenges that face parents who raise their children in a world that is substantially different from the world in which they and their forebears were raised. In this context, using the NBO preventively to support parents during the transition to parenthood may help to buffer the cumulative burden of multiple risk factors and sources of stress, which compromise the caregiver's capacity to promote sound health and development, because lower levels of parental stress and social support networks are connected to positive child outcomes (Fenichel & Mann, 2002; Hauser-Cram, Warfield, Shonkoff, & Krauss, 2001; Shonkoff & Phillips, 2000).

## CULTURE AND CHILD REARING

Many theoretical models have been applied to an examination of the role of culture on child development. There also is a long tradition of cross-cultural research that provides descriptions of the wide range of socialization practices in various cultures and that can inform clinical practice with families from different cultures. Other research has provided evidence that not only are there cultural differences in newborn behavior and development from the very beginning but also that the infant has a role in shaping and directing the socialization process itself (Nugent, Lester, & Brazelton, 1989, 1991; Rogoff, 2003). Cross-cultural studies have documented differences in the roles of fathers and mothers and differences and commonalities in how affection is expressed and how children learn and how they are taught (e.g., Price-Williams, 1975; Brazelton et al., 1976; Dixon, Tronick, Keefer, & Brazelton, 1982; Greenfield & Cocking, 1994; Ho, 1994; LeVine et al., 1994; Martini & Kirkpatrick, 1981; Super & Harkness, 1982, 1997; Whiting & Edwards, 1988). These studies also reveal that in many cultures, child rearing involves not only parents but also a wide array of community members, who feel a responsibility toward the growth and development of that child. In contemporary United States, whereas middle-class European American parents often live far away from their family and relatives, in African American, Native American, and Latino communities, grandparents and extended family play an important role in the everyday life of the children (Diamond, 2000). The role of fathers with infants also varies across cultural communities. Among Aka foragers in Central Africa, for example, almost half of the father's day is spent holding or being close to his infant (Hewlitt, 1991). In Cameroon, the care of infants is the responsibility of the community, whereas among the Efe in the Democratic Republic of the Congo, the care of infants is shared among the women of the community (Winn, Tronick, & Morelli, 1989).

## Socialization Goals and Practices

Ethnographic studies show, then, that although all societies use a range of child-rearing practices to instill desirable traits in their children, parents choose child-rearing practices (techniques) on the basis of beliefs about how children grow and develop and about what makes a good parent (LeVine et al., 1994; Whiting et al., 1975; Whiting & Edwards, 1988; Super & Harkness, 1997; Shweder, Goodnow, Hatano, LeVine, Markus, & Miller, 1998). Some of these differences depend on the likelihood of infant mortality or survival and the availability of siblings or grandparents or extended family, among other environmental variables. LeVine (1980) described a three-level hierarchy of parental child-rearing goals that varies across cultures to explain why child-rearing goals emerge and how they may vary across settings:

1.  In cultures where there is a high level of infant mortality, parents first must consider the child's physical survival and health.

2.  If this goal is met, then parents focus on preparing children to maintain themselves economically in maturity.

3.  When these goals have been met, parents then can consider the child's potential to maximize other cultural values, such as prestige, religious piety, intellectual achievement, personal satisfaction, and self-realization.

The working assumption, therefore, is that differences in child-rearing techniques are culturally based solutions to child care challenges that are specific to that culture, so what is successful in one culture may not apply to another, or what is successful at one time may not work when economic or social changes take place. These strategies, whether they involve where infants sleep or when solid foods are introduced or whether older siblings care for their younger siblings, are guided by cultural belief systems that have evolved over time in response to the goals of that particular social historical context.

Garcia Coll, for example, examined developmental skills such as tactile stimulation, verbal interaction, nonverbal interaction, and feeding routines in multicultural families, including African American, Chinese American, Hopi, Mexican American, and Navajo families. She concluded that parents' child-rearing practices differ, so that "minority infants are not only exposed to different patterns of affective and social interactions, but that their learning experiences might result in the acquisition of different modes of communication from those characterizing Anglo infants, different means of exploration of their environment, and the development of alternative cognitive skills" (1990, p. 274). In the United States and in many Western European societies, where most newborn infants sleep alone in a separate room apart from their parents, parents believe that this will promote the child's independence and self-sufficiency, which is seen as the key to successful adaptation in these societies. In many cultures, including the Gusii in Kenya studied by LeVine et al. (1994), the Mayans studied by Morelli, Rogoff, Oppenheim, and Goldsmith (1992), and Japanese infants studied by Kawasaki et al. (1994), mothers and infants sleep together. This practice generally lasts until the mother's next child is born or much later in the case of Japan. Sleeping together allows the mother to breast-feed the infant more easily, and breast feeding on demand both at night and during the day typically continues into the second year and even beyond. LeVine et al. (1994) argued that frequent breast feeding has played an essential role in cultures where infant mortality was very high, by helping to ensure early weight gain and the possible maintenance of hydration in the presence of diarrhea.

In summary, socialization goals—what parents want for their children—are shaped by economic, social, and cultural priorities and guide parents' beliefs about child-rearing practices. These goals are expressed in terms of who cares for the infant or what kind of care is appropriate and how behavior is managed and controlled. The studies of newborn behavior and parent–child relations in different cultural contexts confirm the dynamic bidirectional nature of development while they expand our understanding of the range of variability in newborn behavioral patterns and the diversity of child-rearing practices and belief systems. How, then, do clinicians provide to parents guidance that supports the child's adaptation to his or her new environment? How do clinicians provide child guidance that is culturally appropriate? What principles should guide clinicians' practice?

## CULTURAL CAPITAL: MOVING AWAY FROM THE "CULTURAL DEPRIVATION MODEL"

In the past, clinical work with families from other cultures tended to be based on a *cultural deprivation model*. Variations in other cultural communities were seen as deficits. Their practices and beliefs were seen as inferior, with little consideration of "their origins, meanings, functions from the perspective of the community" (Rogoff, 2003, p. 15). Because cultural differences were seen as deficits, early intervention programs were designed to compensate for the children's "cultural deprivation" (see Garcia Coll & Meyer, 1993; Garcia Coll & Magnuson, 1996; Ogbu, 1981; Rogoff, 2003). Although this approach characterized much of the clinical work with culturally different families in many Western societies in the past,

Rogoff (2003) warned that these deficit models still are present, while Super and Harkness (1997) pointed out that parents' beliefs and cultural worldview often are overlooked in clinicians' work with families.

One concept that can counterbalance the deprivation model approach and can help reframe clinicians' understanding of what parents from other cultures bring to the relationship is the notion of *cultural capital*. Cultural capital is a concept that was introduced by the French sociologist Pierre Bourdieu (1998) and is based on his analysis of the social and educational experiences of working-class immigrant families in France. This theory maintains that new parents and their families who come from different cultures possess cultural capital that can be defined as the knowledge, skills, education, customs, achievements, and expectations that are related to a family's social position in their own culture. This capital can be called on to promote their social and psychological growth in the new culture. LeVine et al. (1994) pointed out that parents typically do not face child rearing on their own but rely on cultural practices, their own socialization into parenting, their intuitive sense of right and wrong, and their overall cultural beliefs. This is their cultural capital. In their study of refugees from Bosnia-Herzegovina, Weine, Ware, and Klebic (2004) demonstrated that providing family-centered support to immigrant families was successful in assisting parents to convert cultural capital to help their children successfully meet the challenges of the new culture. Because parents are the repositories of cultural capital, it is they who provide children with the attitudes and knowledge that make the new culture a comfortable, familiar place in which they can succeed. When clinicians value the family's cultural strengths, families develop the confidence to convert cultural capital so as to enhance their own cultural vitality and social incorporation into the new society.

## Poverty and Cultural Capital

Parents who lack other valued forms of capital, such as economic capital, can use cultural capital to buffer the stress that is caused by poverty or lack of opportunity. Among both working-class Chinese American parents and African American parents in North America, social networks, including extended kin and co-ethnic friends, help to compensate for limited money and time for educational participation (Diamond, 2000). Diamond's research showed that among African American parents, extended family networks provided parents with scarce time, money, and educational resources for their children. In addition, communal child-rearing orientations among African Americans allowed multiple adults to influence children's education and to reinforce parental expectations for behavior and academic achievement. In both communities, access to these resources depended on immersion in the cultural traditions of the community, making this immersion a form of cultural capital. From this point of view, the very diversity of cultural practices within societies is seen as a resource for creativity and for enriching society, in general, and therefore, we as professionals should work toward helping families draw on their own unique cultural resources (Dunst et al., 1988).

As a relationship-building tool, which is intended to provide appropriate, culturally adapted caregiving guidance to parents, the NBO can be used to assist in converting cultural capital through building a partnership between the clinician and the parents. The aim of this partnership is to foster a positive parent–infant relationship by supporting and affirming the parents' own "intuitive" sense of parenting, thereby increasing parents' involvement in their children's development, social life, and cultural life. This respect for the parents' value system allows clinicians to collaborate actively with the parents in the articulation and development of caregiving strategies that are open and flexible and yet consistent with the parents' cultural values. The NBO can provide clinicians with a unique opportunity to support parents in this process by helping them make the kinds of child-rearing decisions that enable them to draw on the richness of their own cultural value system. The clinician can also help the parents retain their sense of continuity with their cultural values and beliefs and develop strategies to respond to the needs of their new community. In this way, their children's lives are enriched and the parents are affirmed in their ability to help their children grow and develop in the new cultural context.

## DEVELOPING CROSS-CULTURAL COMPETENCE

Nowhere is the model of supportive, culturally sensitive, family-centered services for infants and families more comprehensively exemplified than in services for infants with disabilities, which were mandated by the Individuals with Disabilities Education Act of 1990 (PL 101-476). Although programs differ in how services are delivered, in general, the early intervention approach recognizes that the family is the primary context of development and that every family has its own unique developmental and cultural context (Hauser-Cram, 2006). Clinicians are charged with the task of working with families in a nonjudgmental mode that at once respects families' varying functioning styles and also offers services that are consonant with the needs of the child and the parents' cultural beliefs.

The importance of respecting parents' values and beliefs and families' child-rearing practices is central to clinical practice with families from different cultures. This means that clinicians should know as much as they can about the cultures of the families with whom they are working. However, it is knowing how values and beliefs play out in the lives of families that is essential for relational care. Cultural competence training should be a sine qua non for clinicians who use the NBO in their work with families from different cultures.

### Respecting Cultural and Linguistic Diversity

Lynch and Hanson (2004) defined cross-cultural competence as "the ability to think, feel and act in ways that acknowledge, respect and build upon ethnic, [socio]cultural, and linguistic diversity." (p. 49) This includes being able to interact with ease with families and cultures that are different from one's own and being able to learn about the culture in the context of the relationship. In the context of the NBO, it means being able to acknowledge and appreciate the parents' cultural worldview and at the same time guide the parents in developing the kinds of caregiving techniques that they will use to promote their infant's development in accordance with their cultural values, without imposing one's own cultural values and beliefs. The approach on which the NBO is based is characterized by a nonjudgmental stance toward parents, emphasizing the separation of value judgments from explanations and avoiding the imposition of the clinician's own cultural values on the parents' caregiving decision making.

Bornstein and Cote (2004), in a survey of Japanese and South American mothers who lived in North America, pointed out that clinicians tend to know very little about immigrant parents' knowledge of child rearing. For that reason, clinicians should know as much as they can about the public information on any particular culture and find out as much as possible from the parents themselves in their encounters with them. To reach this level of understanding, clinicians need to see themselves as learners, because they are newcomers to the culture's meaning system (Kleinman, 1981). Only when clinicians approach parents with this kind of openness will parents feel free to share their own hopes and fears for themselves and their child, and only then can clinicians begin to understand and appreciate the parents' goals for their child. No a priori summary of a community's cultural beliefs can substitute for the quiet process of empathic listening that is inherent in the NBO approach. Clinicians need to make it possible for parents to share their hopes and goals with them so that clinicians can learn about the parents' culture.

## AWARENESS OF ONE'S OWN ASSUMPTIONS AND BIASES

Before clinicians can understand parents' assumptions about how children develop and their own role in that development, they need to understand their own cultural beliefs and worldview and have an integrated sense of their own cultural identity. However, a careful examination of the principles of child and family development, the very canon on which the principles and guidelines for working with children and families is based, reveals that much of one's information on child development is based on norms that almost exclusively are Western and middle class. Most of the studies that provide the foundation for theory and practice have been conducted in Western environments and scarcely can be said to be representative of the world's population. As such, this body of research has perpetuated "a middle-class, Western and male-centered view of the universe" (Greene, 2002, p.179; Lynch & Hanson, 2004; Shonkoff & Phillips, 2000; Rogoff, 2003). The classic dominant research tradition in child and family development reveals little about how children develop in many parts of the world and indeed has little to reveal about how children develop in the so-called minority cultures in Western societies (Garcia Coll & Meyer, 1993; LeVine, 1988; Rogoff, 2003; Valsiner, 1989; Whiting & Edwards, 1988). Clinicians not only must question the representativeness of their current knowledge base but also must acknowledge that much of the research on child and family development has been conducted within the classic empirical tradition and reveals little about the dynamic nature of child–culture relations or the social or political context of child and family development.

## Unconscious Ethnocentrism

Working with families from cultures that are different from one's own may serve to challenge the validity of one's current assumptions about human behavior and to free one from his or her own unconscious ethnocentrism. This form of ethnocentrism can be called unconscious or latent because it is not readily accessible to the conscious reasoning, and it plays a subtle and often unconscious role in one's interactions with families from cultures other than one's own (Nugent, 1994). Ethnocentrism involves "making judgments that another cultural community's ways are immoral, unwise, or inappropriate based on one's own cultural background" (Rogoff, 2003, p. 15). Clinicians, therefore, need to examine their own assumptions about the very nature of the child, about the contribution of genes and culture, and about the role of parents in shaping the child's growth and develop ment. This means that clinicians cannot prejudge or evaluate or guide parents without first having an understanding of the values and priorities of their own culture. For those reasons, using the NBO in such clinical environments can serve to challenge the validity of one's current assumptions about human behavior and to free one from his or her own ethnocentric world view.

## CROSS-CULTURAL COMMUNICATION

Following are principles and guidelines that can inform clinician–parent communication in a way that is compatible with cultural diversity. In Chapter 4, we stressed the importance of clinicians developing the kinds of listening and communication skills that enable parents to participate actively in the session and thereby promote a partnership between the clinician and the parents. Empathic listening enables the clinician to learn to see the world from the parents' perspective. Cultural competence addresses the added challenge of communicating with parents who may have a different language and a different communication style from the clinician and as well as very different values and priorities for their children.

## Low- and High-Context Cultures

In addressing the issue of intercultural communication, Hall (1973) referred to the divide between *low-context* and *high-context* cultures. Although the model is oversimplified, it is highly suggestive and may be helpful in sensitizing clinicians to contrasting communication styles between low-context cultures, which value an individualist, independent ethos, and high-context cultures, which value interdependence and collectivism (typically found in non-Western societies). Members of high-context cultures communicate allusively rather than directly. As important as the explicit content of the message is the context in which it occurs, the surrounding nonverbal cues, and the hinted-at nuances of meaning. Directness or bluntness is not valued. Indeed, language is seen as a social instrument, a device for preserving or promoting social relations as much as a means for giving information. Tone of voice, facial expressions, and gestures (body language) are as important as the actual context of the language. In low-context cultures, conversely, language is more direct and little meaning is implicit in the context. What is to be said must be stated clearly and explicitly. Language performs an informational rather than a social affiliative function. Indirection or subtlety is not valued, and straightforward talk—getting to the point with an economic use of well-selected words and phrases—is seen as the essence of good communication.

It will be difficult for parents from high-context cultures, for whom a collectivist ethos is central to their relations with others, to respond to a clinician who values direct communication and "getting to the point" as paramount. For that reason, clinicians may need to build in time to give parents the opportunity for "small talk," for preliminary greetings and exchange, both before and during the NBO. Working with families from other cultures requires a shift from thinking of the session as a form of parent education to seeing it more as the development of a working partnership in which trust must be established and the parents' voice and involvement are welcomed and embraced. This stance also may require a very different pace as the clinician attempts to become acquainted with the family's communication style and patterns and as he or she tries to understand the meaning of the family's gestures and nonverbal communication patterns. Observing, becoming aware of, and making sense of the parents' communication style and their looks, words, and gestures become critical for effective communication. The amount of eye contact; the nature of the body language and gestures, including what kind of physical touching is permissible; and how much talking and how much silence are appropriate vary by culture. The clinician's failure to understand the role of these elements of communication in a particular culture can lead to miscommunication and misunderstanding, however inadvertent.

## The Evil Eye

How the clinician is perceived also may influence the clinician–parent relationship. Members of an interdependent culture are more cautious in dealing with a stranger from outside their circle, so in clinical environments, more emphasis needs to be placed on cultivating a personal relationship with the parents and the family before any frank, open interchange can take place. In the context of the NBO, for example, small talk, involving a search for commonly shared interests and concerns, may precede the more formal administration of the NBO items. As was pointed out in Chapter 5, asking how the infant's name was chosen can serve such a purpose. Moreover, in many non-Western societies, newborns are considered to be reincarnated beings (ancestors or gods), and these societies stress the need to protect infants from dangerous evil spirits, which may include excluding all "outsiders" from direct contact with the infant. Berry Brazelton, in his work among the Zinacantecos, a Mayan group in Mexico, noted that even though he was a health care clinician in his own culture, as an outsider in that culture, he was automatically endowed with the "evil eye," which prohibited him from relating to the infant, as the infant got older (Brazelton, Robey, & Collier, 1969).

Using the NBO in a clinical environment with a family from a culture that is different from the clinician's should be seen as an ongoing negotiation and as an integral part of getting to know the infant and the family through their culture. The clinician's primary stance toward the family, therefore, is one of openness, demonstrating a readiness to listen and learn from the parents about how they see their infant and what their goals for their infant are. Although background information on the history, art, music, customs, and language of the culture of the family can provide the clinician with an invaluable starting point, it is the clinician's respect for the family in the session itself that can allow parents readily to provide him or her with the kind of information that is relevant to this infant and important for this family. Because the NBO session should allow the clinician to hear both the "infant's story" and the "family's story," clinicians need to give parents the opportunity to share their own thoughts and goals. By listening to the parents, clinicians can learn about their culture and its values and, more important, how the parents bring their child-rearing goals into conformity with their culture.

## Cultural Misunderstandings

It also must be acknowledged that no amount of openness and therapeutic skill can prevent misunderstandings or mistakes in clinicians' interactions with families from different cultures. No one can understand fully the complex and extensive body of shared knowledge of a culture other than his or her own, but because one of the goals of the NBO is to build a relationship of trust with the parents, mistakes and misunderstandings can be addressed and remedied. If the clinician, because of his or her lack of familiarity with the culture, uses the wrong word or gesture or makes the wrong attribution or judgment, then he or she readily can ask the parents to help him or her understand the phenomenon from the parents' perspective. Where relationship building is paramount, the clinician can ask parents to help him or her understand the meaning of the particular practice. In the context of a relationship, mistakes and misunderstanding can be forgiven, so despite the hurt and dissatisfaction of both the parents and the clinician, the clinician can use this opportunity to understand the family better and at the same time learn to be a more culturally competent clinician.

In summary, in the context of the NBO, the culturally competent clinician should be

- Respectful of cultural worldviews other than his or her own

- Ready to learn as much as he or she can about a specific culture

- Aware of his or her own cultural values

- Open to learning from parents

- Ready to give parents every opportunity to share their thoughts and feelings

- Nonjudgmental toward the child-rearing beliefs and practice of other cultures

- Ready to repair miscommunications, mistakes, or misunderstandings in communication with parents from different cultures

- Able to support parents in making their own decisions about caregiving strategies without imposing his or her own view

## CHILD GUIDANCE AND CULTURE

Are infants innately good, or are they "little devils" at heart? Should parents talk to their infants? Where should infants sleep? Is play a waste of valuable time? Do infants need a bath once a day or three times a day? Should a feverish infant be given aspirin or an amulet? Which is better? Every culture will provide several different—and sometimes contradictory—answers to each of these questions. The ethnographic research, reviewed previously in this chapter, highlights the vast diversity in how parents around the world go about caring for their infants and raising them to become members of their particular society. These studies show that cultural differences in caregiving practices often are related to differences in belief systems. To a great extent, parents' decisions about how to treat their offspring are based on deeply held beliefs and lay theories. This is true regardless of whether the decisions are singular, momentous ones, such as choosing a name and determining which religious rituals should be performed for a newborn, or important everyday matters, such as treating a sick infant or bathing, feeding, and painting designs on an infant. Clinicians therefore need to understand the meaning of these behaviors for the parents and how the behaviors fit into the local cultural framework. Clinicians cannot interpret infant behavior without regard for their meaning in terms of both their developmental and their cultural functions. This does not mean that judgments cannot be made about particular behaviors, because one cannot avoid making judgments. But these judgments must be informed by one's developmental perspective and by the cultural goals that the parents have for their infant, and clinicians need to be able to separate value judgments from observations of behavior.

It should be pointed out that because the caregiving guidelines that are offered through the NBO are based on the shared observation of the infant's behavior by the parents and the clinician, this guidance is both reliable and trustworthy, but it is how this objective information is interpreted by clinicians and applied by parents that is important for culturally sensitive practice. Because the underlying clinical principles of the NBO emphasize the importance of drawing on parents' knowledge and understanding of development, clinicians need to be aware that parents' perceptions and questions are mediated by their beliefs about children's development and their own child-rearing values. As pointed out in Chapters 1 and 4, the explanations that parents give for their child-rearing practices, their explanatory models, are cognitive, mental constructs that often are unconscious yet can have a strong effect on a family's behavior as parents (Harkness et al., 1992). In other words, when interpreting the information that parents provide, clinicians must take into consideration the sources and cultural contexts of this understanding.

## Avoiding Value Judgments

When it comes to interpreting the infant's behavior and offering guidelines for caregiving, the guidance that clinicians offer must be nonjudgmental. Clinicians need to separate value judgments from explanations and avoid the temptation to impose their own cultural values on the articulation of the caregiving strategies. Although in the context of the NBO, the clinician may single out a hand-to-mouth activity as an example of a refined motor skill and excellent self-regulation skills, parents from another culture may value this differently. Our own research in Japan, for example (Kawasaki et al., 1994), revealed that Japanese mothers seemed to place little value on the kinds of newborn self-regulating behaviors such as hand-to-mouth behaviors or self-consoling capacities that tend to be valued in Western societies. Although a Japanese mother sees her newborn as independent at birth, her goal is to bring the infant into her own relational orbit by fostering the infant's dependence on her, a cultural concept referred to as *Amae*. On the basis of the notion of *ai* in Japanese Buddhism, which is defined as passionate caring love, *Amae* means "indulgent dependence" and is described by Doi (1991) as the word that best describes the relationship between the child and the mother. The value of *Amae* may explain why Japanese mothers prefer to foster the infant's sense of dependence while not encouraging the kinds of "independence" skills that are seen to run counter to collectivist ideals of Japanese society. Indeed, it was found that parents valued this characteristic above all others as the primary goal of socialization (Takahashi et al., 1994).

In comparing the responsiveness of U.S. mothers and Gusii mothers (sub-Saharan East African agriculturalists) to their infants, Keefer, working with LeVine et al. (1994), pointed out that North American mothers are relatively tolerant of infant crying and believe that this is a way to foster independence or self-reliance. A Gusii mother, conversely, would not allow her infant to cry for more than a few seconds and would have little respect for a mother who would allow her newborn infant to cry any longer. Among Hausa mothers, for example, the custom is not to show affection for their infants in public (Price-Williams, 1975), and Gusii mothers do not see infants as capable of communicating or of understanding language and so do not engage in that type of stimulating face-to-face interaction with them. Making judgments about the quality of the parent–child relationship, without an understanding of the cultural context, can lead to mistaken diagnoses and inappropriate guidance (Donahue Finn, 2003).

Until one understands the values and interpretations of the child's behavior by the parents, clinicians do well to avoid applying their own values and interpretations. For example, one can say in observing an infant, "She is fussing or crying . . . now she is rooting . . . she gets her hand to her mouth . . . she has stopped fussing and now she opens her eyes"; that is a description of the behavior. To say, "How strong she is," or, "How capable she is," is to value the behavior. To say, "Look at how independently she consoles herself," is to give an interpretation to the behavior. To ask, "Isn't it wonderful that she can calm herself?" is to give value to the interpretation. Cultures vary in the value that they place on these behaviors. Whereas it may be seen as adaptive in one culture, it may be seen as maladaptive in another. The task for clinicians, who may subscribe to one or another of these beliefs themselves, is to allow the parents to express their own opinions and the underlying values that support this belief. Perhaps, if the parents express ambivalence over their practice or their exercise of the practice leads to struggle with the infant or other caregivers, then the clinician may help the parents explore other options. Great care should be taken, however, to avoid simply replacing the parents' belief and practice with that of the clinician.

## SUMMARY

Cross-cultural studies suggest that whereas the basic organizational processes in infancy may be universal, the range and form of these adaptations are shaped by the demands of each individual culture. However, the heuristic value of these studies for clinicians goes beyond the simple description or documentation of different patterns of behavior in unfamiliar cultures. These research findings should sensitize clinicians who use the NBO with infants and families from different cultures to the different trajectories of infant and family development, from birth onward. This body of research forces clinicians to revise and broaden their definitions of what is considered "normal" or "typical" behavior and what is considered "abnormal" or "atypical." Clinical work with infants and parents from different cultures therefore can serve to challenge clinicians' core assumptions about the nature of development and about what is thought of as good or bad, appropriate or inappropriate behavior. The concepts of normality and risk therefore are revealed as cultural constructs that may not have validity in cultures other than the one in which the concept was constructed.

Using the NBO with parents from different cultures challenges clinicians' assumptions about the very nature of child and family development. It urges introspection as it forces clinicians to examine their own belief systems and to unmask their own cultural biases by reviewing their attitudes toward children and families. It goes without saying that without an awareness and appreciation of one's own culture or without a firm sense of identity with one's own culture, it will be extremely difficult to be sensitive or open to the nuances of another culture. It will be equally difficult to have access to one's own biases and prejudices. Paradoxically, it is only in a person's engagement with other cultures that an understanding of his or her own culture is refined and an appreciation of other cultures simultaneously is enriched.

This chapter presented a set of principles and guidelines on how to use the NBO with families from cultures other than one's own in a way that is authentic to the parents and that helps them meet the developmental needs of their young children while validating them and affirming their role as parents. Also discussed was the need to be aware of the challenges that face parents who raise their children in a world that is substantially different from the world in which they and their forebears were raised and who are beset by a sense of cultural and familial discontinuity. Introduced was the notion of cultural capital as a potentially valuable construct for clinicians, because it enables them to value cultural strengths and thereby enables parents to convert cultural capital in a way that enhances their own cultural vitality and their own social incorporation into the new cultural community. Also described was the kind of developmental and cultural competencies that clinicians need to provide anticipatory child guidance in a way that respects the parents' cultural values and at the same time promotes their successful adaptation as a family.

The NBO approach to working with families from different cultural communities is characterized by a nonjudgmental stance that emphasizes the separation of value judgments from explanations and avoids the imposition of the clinician's own cultural values on the parents' caregiving decision making. Listening to and searching for the authentic voices of infants and their families through the NBO will allow parents to teach clinicians about themselves and their culture. As a relationship-building tool that is intended to provide appropriate, culturally adapted caregiving guidance to parents, the NBO can be used to assist in converting cultural capital through building a partnership between the clinician and the parents. Ultimately, the aim of this partnership is to foster a positive parent–infant relationship by supporting and affirming the parents' sense of themselves as parents, thereby increasing their involvement in their children's cognitive, motor, and socioemotional development and deepening their own social and cultural life.

# REFERENCES

Adams, R.J., Courage, M.L., & Mercer, M.E. (1994). Systematic measurement of human neonatal color vision. *Vision Research, 34,* 1691–1701.

Adamson, L.B. (1996). *Communication development during infancy.* Madison, WI: Brown and Benchmark.

Ainsworth, M.D.S., Blehar, M., Waters, E., & Wall, S. (1978). *Patterns of attachment: A psychological study of the strange situation.* Mahwah, NJ: Lawrence Erlbaum Associates.

Alberts, E., Kalverboer, A.F., & Hopkins, B. (1983). Mother–infant dialogue in the first days of life: An observational study during breastfeeding. *Journal of Child Psychology and Psychiatry, 24*(4) 145–161.

Aldridge, M.A., Stillman, R.D., & Bower, T.G.R. (2001). Newborn categorization of vowel-like sounds. *Developmental Science, 4,* 220–232.

Als, H. (1979). Social interaction: Dynamic matrix for developing behavioral organization. In I.C. Uzgiris (Ed.), Social interaction and communication in infancy, Vol 4 (pp. 21–41). San Francisco: Jossey Bass.

Als, H. (1982). Toward a synactive theory of development: Promise for the assessment and support of infant individuality. *Infant Mental Health Journal, 3*(4), 229–243.

Als, H. (1986). A synactive model of neonatal behavioral organization: Framework for the assessment of neurobehavioral development in the premature infant and for support of infants and parents in the neonatal intensive care unit. In J.K. Sweeney (Ed.), *The high-risk neonate: Developmental therapy perspectives* (pp. 3–53). New York: Haworth Press.

Als, H., Duffy, F., McAnulty, G., Rivkin, M., Vajapeyam, S., Mulkern, R., et al. (2004). Early experience alters brain function and structure. *Pediatrics, 113*(4), 846–857.

Als, H., Gilkerson, L., Duffy, F.H., McNulty, G.B., Buehler, D.M., Vandenberg, K., et al. (2003). A three-center, randomized, controlled trial of individualized developmental care for very low birth weight preterm infants: Medical, neurodevelopmental, parenting, and caregiving effects. *Developmental and Behavioral Pediatrics, 24*(6), 399–408.

Als, H., Lawhon, G., Duffy, F.H., McAnulty, G.B., Gibes-Grossman, R., & Blickman, J.G. (1994). Individualized developmental care for the very low-birth-weight preterm infants. *Journal of the American Medical Association, 272*(111), 853–105.

Als, H., Lester, B.M., Tronick, E., & Brazelton, T.B. (1982). Manual for the Assessment of Preterm Infants' Behavior (APIB). In H.E. Fitzgerald, B.M. Lester, & M.W. Yogman (Eds.), *Theory and research in behavioral pediatrics* (Vol. 1, pp. 65–132). New York: Plenum.

American Academy of Pediatrics Committee on Hospital Care. (2003). Family-centered care and the pediatricians role. *Pediatrics, 112,* 691–696.

American Academy of Pediatrics Committee on Practice and Ambulatory Medicine. (2000). Recommendations for preventive pediatric healthcare. *Pediatrics, 105,* 645.

American Academy of Pediatrics Task Force on Sudden Infant Death Syndrome. (2005). The changing concept of sudden infant death syndrome: Diagnostic coding shifts, controversies regarding the sleeping environment, and new variables to consider in reducing risk. *Pediatrics, 116*(5), 1245–1255.

American Committee on Hospital Care. (2003). Family-centered care and the pediatricians' role. *Pediatrics, 112*(3), 691–696.

American Psychiatric Association. (1994). *Diagnostic and statistical manual of mental disorders* (4th ed.). Washington, DC: Author.

Amiel-Tison, C., & Grenier, A. (1986). *Neurological assessment during the first year of life.* New York: Oxford University Press.

Amy, E. (2001). Reflections on the interactive newborn bath demonstration. *The American Journal of Maternal Child Nursing, 26*(6), 320–322.

Anders, T., Halpern, L., & Hua, J. (1992). Sleeping through the night: A developmental perspective. *Pediatrics, 90,* 554–590.

Anderson C.J., & Sawin, D. (1983). Enhancing responsiveness in mother–infant interaction. *Infant Behavior and Development, 6*(3), 361–368.

Anderson, G.C. (1991). Current knowledge about skin-to-skin (kangaroo) care for preterm infants. *Journal of Perinatology, 11*(3), 216–226.

Anderson, J.L., Morgan, J.L., & White, K.S. (2003). A statistical basis for speech–sound discrimination. *Language and Speech, 46,* 155–182.

Andre-Thomas, C.I., & Dargassies, S.S. (1960). *The neurological examination of the infant.* London: The Spastic Society Medical Education and Information Unit.

Anisfield, E., & Pincus, M. (1978). The post-partum support project: Serving young mothers and older women through home visiting. *Zero to Three, 8,* 13–15.

Ayres, A.J. (1979). *Sensory integration of the child.* Los Angeles: Western Psychological Services.

Banks, M.S. (1980). The development of visual accommodation during early infancy. *Child Development, 51,* 646–666.

Barclay, L., & Lupton, D. (1999). The experiences of new fatherhood: A socio-cultural analysis. *Journal of Advanced Nursing, 29*(4), 1013–1020.

Barnard, K.E., Morisset, C.E., & Speiker, S. (1993). Preventive interventions: Enhancing parent–infant relationships. In C.H. Zeanah (Ed.), *Handbook of infant mental health* (pp. 386–410). New York: Guilford Press.

Barr, R.G. (1990). The normal crying curve: What do we really know? *Developmental Medicine and Child Neurology, 32,* 356–362.

Barr, R.G. (1998). Reflections on N-shaped curves in early infancy: Regulated or re-organized development? [Special issue] *Infant Behavior and Development, 21,* 184.

Barr, R.G., Chen, S., Hopkins, B., & Westra, T. (1996). Crying patterns in preterm infants. *Developmental Medicine and Child Neurology, 38,* 345–355.

Barr, R.G., Konner, M., Bakeman, R., & Adamson, L. (1991). Crying in Kung San infants: A test of the cultural specificity hypothesis. *Developmental Medicine and Child Neurology, 33,* 601–610.

Barr, R.G., Rotman, A., Yaremko, J., Leduc, D., & Francoeur, T.E. (1992). The crying of infants with colic: A controlled empirical description. *Pediatrics, 90*(1), 21.

Barr, R.G., St. James-Roberts, I., & Keefe, M.R. (Eds.). (2001). *New evidence on unexplained early infant crying: Its origins, nature and management.* Skillman, NJ: Johnson and Johnson Pediatric Institute.

Barrera, M.E., & Maurer, D. (1981). The perception of facial expressions by the three-month-old. *Child Development, 52*(1), 203–206.

Barrows, P. (1999). Fathers in parent–infant psychotherapy. *Infant Mental Health Journal, 20*(3), 333–345.

Barrows, P. (2004). Fathers and families: Locating the ghosts in the nursery. *Infant Mental Health Journal, 25*(5), 408–423.

Bates, J.E. (1986). On the relation between temperament and behavior problems. In G.A. Kohnstamm (Ed.), *Temperament discussed: Temperament and development in infancy and childhood* (pp. 181–189). Lisse, Netherlands: Swets & Zeitlinger.

Beal, J.A. (1986). The Brazelton Neonatal Behavioral Assessment: A tool to enhance parental attachment. *Journal of Pediatric Nursing, 1,* 170–177.

Becker, M., Palfrey, J.S., & Wise, P.H. (1998). Evaluation of a program to improve the transition from birth hospital to primary care. *Ambulatory Child Health, 4,* 189.

Beckwith, L. (2000). Prevention science and prevention programs. In, C.H. Zeanah (Ed.), *Handbook of infant mental health* (2nd ed., pp. 439–456). New York: Guilford Press.

Beckwith, L., Cohen, S.E., & Hamilton, C.E. (1999). Maternal sensitivity during infancy and subsequent life events relate to attachment representation at early adulthood. *Developmental Psychology, 35,*(3), 693–700.

Beebe, B., & Lachman, F.M. (2002). *Infant research and adult treatment: Co-constructing interactions.* Hillsdale, NJ: The Analytic Press.

Beeghly, M., Brazelton, T.B., Flannery, K., Nugent, J.K., Barrett, D., & Tronick, E.Z. (1995). Specificity of preventative pediatric intervention effects in early infancy. *Journal of Developmental and Behavioral Pediatrics, 16*(3), 158–166.

Bell, S.M., & Ainsworth, M.D. (1972). Infant crying and maternal responsiveness. *Child Development, 43*(4), 1171–1190.

Belsky, J. (1985). Experimenting with the family in the newborn period. *Child Development, 56,* 407–414.

Belsky, J. (1993) Etiology of child maltreatment: A developmental-ecological analysis. *Psychological Bulletin, 114,* 413–434.

Benoit, D., & Parker, K. (1994). Stability and transmission of attachment across three generations. *Child Development, 65,* 1444–1456.

Bernal, J. (1972). Crying during the first ten days of life and maternal responses. *Developmental Medicine and Child Neurology, 14*, 362–372.

Bethell, C., Peck, C., Abrams, M., Halfon, N., Sareen, H., & Collins, K.S. (2002). *Partnering with parents to promote the healthy development of young children enrolled in Medicaid: Results from a survey assessing the quality of preventive and developmental services for young children enrolled in Medicaid in three states.* New York: The Commonwealth Fund.

Bethell, C., Peck, C., & Schor, E. (2001). Assessing health system provision of well-child care: The Promoting Healthy Development Survey. *Pediatrics, 107*(5), 1084–1094.

Bhabha, H. (1994). *The location of culture.* London: Routledge.

Bigelow, A.E. (2003). The development of joint attention in blind infants. *Development and Psychopathology, 15*, 259–275.

Blanchard, Y., & Mouradian, L. (2000). Integrating neurobehavioral concepts into early intervention eligibility evaluation. *Infants and Young Children, 13*(2), 41–50.

Blass, E.M., & Camp, C.A. (2003). Biological bases of face preference in 6-week-old infants. *Developmental Science, 6*(5), 524–536.

Blumberg, M.S., & Lucas, D.E. (1996). A developmental and component analysis of active sleep. *Developmental Psychobiology, 29*, 1–22.

Blumberg, S.J., Olson, L., Frankel, M., Osborn, L., Becker, C.J., Srinath, K.P., et al. (2003). Design and operation of the National Survey of Children with Special Health Care Needs. *Vital Health Statistics 1, 41*,1–136.

Boger, K., & Kurnetz, R. (1985). Perinatal positive parenting: Hospital-based support for first-time parents. *Pediatric Basics, 41*, 4–15.

Bokhorst, C.L., Bakermans-Kranenburg, M.J., Fearon, R.M., van IJzendoorn, M.H., Fonagy, P., & Scheungel, C. (2003). The importance of shared environment in mother–infant attachment security: A behavioral genetic study. *Child Development, 74*(6), 1769–1782.

Bornstein, M.H., & Cote, L.R. (2001). Mother–infant interaction and acculturation: I. Behavioural comparisons in Japanese American and South American families. *International Journal of Behavioral Development, 25*(6), 549–563.

Bornstein, M.H., & Cote, L.R. (2004). "Who is sitting across from me?" Immigrant mothers' knowledge of parenting and children's development. *Pediatrics, 114*(5), 557–564.

Bornstein, M.H., & Suess, P.H. (2000). Physiological self-regulation and information processing in infancy: Cardiac vagal tone and habituation. *Child Development, 71*, 273–287.

Boukydis, C.F.Z. (Ed.). (1986). *Supports for parents and infants.* New York: Routledge & Kegan Paul.

Boukydis, C.F.Z. (1999). The NICU network neurobehavioral scale: Clinical use with drug-exposed infants and their mothers. In B.M. Lester (Ed.), *Clinics in perinatology* (pp. 213–220). Philadelphia: W.B. Saunders.

Boukydis, C.F.Z., & Lester, B.M.L. (1998). Infant crying, risk status and social support in families of preterm and term infants. *Early Development and Parenting, 7*, 31–39.

Bourdieu, P. (1986). The forms of capital. In John Richardson (Ed.), *Handbook of theory and research for the sociology of education* (pp. 241–258). New York: Greenwood Press.

Bourdieu, P. (1998). *Practical reason: On the theory of action.* Stanford, CA: Stanford University Press.

Bower, T.G.R. (1974). *Development in infancy.* San Francisco: Freeman.

Bowlby, J. (1982). *Attachment and loss: Vol. 1. Attachment.* New York: Basic Books. (Original work published 1969)

Brazelton, T.B. (1962). Crying in infancy. *Pediatrics, 29*, 579–588.

Brazelton, T.B. (1973). Neonatal Behavioral Assessment Scale. Clinics in Developmental Medicine, No. 50. Spastics International Medical Publications. London: Wm. Heinemann Medical Books Ltd., Philadelphia: J.P. Lippincott.

Brazelton, T.B. (1981). Precursors for the development of emotion in early infancy. In R. Plutchik & H. Kellerman (Eds.), *Emotion: Theory, research, and experience* (Vol. II, pp. 35–55). New York: Academic Press.

Brazelton, T.B. (1982). Early intervention: What does it mean? In H.E. Fitzgerald, B.M. Lester, & M.W. Yogman (Eds.), *Theory and research in behavioral pediatrics* (Vol. 1, pp. 1–34). New York: Plenum.

Brazelton, T.B. (1984). *Neonatal Behavioral Assessment Scale* (2nd ed.). Clinics in Developmental Medicine, No. 88. London: Spastics International Medical Publications.

Brazelton, T.B. (1990). Parent–infant co-sleeping revisited. *Ab Initio, 2*(1), 1–2.

Brazelton, T.B. (1992). *Touchpoints.* Reading, MA: Addison Wesley Longman.

Brazelton, T.B. (1995). Working with families: Opportunities for early intervention. *Family-Focused Pediatrics, 42*(1), 1–9.

Brazelton, T.B., & Als, H. (1979). Four early stages in the development of mother–infant interaction. *Psychoanalytic Study of the Child, 34,* 349–369.

Brazelton, T.B., & Cramer, B.G. (1990). *The earliest relationship.* Reading, MA: Addison Wesley Longman.

Brazelton, T.B., Koslowski, B., & Main, M. (1974). The origins of reciprocity: The early mother–infant interaction. In M. Lewis & L. Rosenblum (Eds.), *The effect of the infant on its caregivers* (pp. 49–77). New York: Wiley Interscience.

Brazelton, T.B., Koslowski, B., & Tronick, E. (1976). Neonatal behavior among urban Zambians and Americans. *Journal of the American Academy of Child Psychiatry, 15,* 97–107.

Brazelton, T.B., & Nugent, J.K. (1987). Neonatal assessment as intervention. In H. Rauh & H.C. Steinhausen (Eds.), *Psychobiology and early development* (pp. 215–229). Amsterdam: North Holland.

Brazelton, T.B., & Nugent, J.K. (1995). *The Neonatal Behavioral Assessment Scale.* London: McKeith Press.

Brazelton, T.B., Nugent, J.K., & Lester, B.M. (1987). The Neonatal Behavioral Assessment Scale. In J. Osofsky (Ed.), *The handbook of infant development* (2nd ed., pp. 780–817). New York: John Wiley & Sons.

Brazelton, T.B., Robey, J.S., & Collier, G.A. (1969). Infant behavior in the Zinacanteco Indians in southern Mexico. *Pediatrics, 44,* 274–281.

Britton J.R. (2005). Pre-discharge anxiety among mothers of well newborns: Prevalence and correlates. *Acta Pediatrica, 94*(12), 1704–1705.

Bronfenbrenner, U. (2002). Preparing a world for the infant in the twenty-first century: The research challenge. In J. Gomes-Pedro, J.K. Nugent, J.G. Young, & T.B. Brazelton (Eds.), *The infant and family in the twenty-first century* (pp. 45–53). New York: Brunner-Routledge.

Bronson, G. (1974). The postnatal growth of visual capacity. *Child Development, 45,* 873–890.

Bronson, G. (1994). Infants' transitions to adult-like scanning. *Child Development, 65,* 1243–1261.

Brousseau, D.C., Meurer, J.R., Isenberg, M.L., Kuhn, E.M., & Gorelick, M.H. (2004). Association between infant continuity of care and pediatric emergency department utilization. *Pediatrics, 113,* 738–741.

Brown, A.M. (1990). Development of visual sensitivity to light and color vision in human infants: A critical review. *Vision Research, 30*(8), 1159–1188.

Brown, A.M. (1994). Intrinsic contrast noise and infant visual contrast discrimination. *Vision Research, 34*(15), 1947–1964.

Browne, J.V. (2000). Considerations for touch and massage in the neonatal intensive care unit. *Neonatal Network, 19,* 61–64.

Browne, J.V., & Talmi, A. (2005). Family-based intervention to enhance infant–parent relationship in the neonatal intensive care unit. *Journal of Pediatric Psychology, 30*(8), 667–677.

Bruner, J. (1990). *Acts of meaning.* Cambridge, MA: Harvard University Press.

Bruschweiler-Stern, N. (1997). Mère à terme et mère premature [The full-term and preterm mother]. In M. Dugnat (Ed.), *Le monde relationnel du bébé* [The relational world of the newborn] (pp. 19–24). Ramonville Saint-Agne, France: ERES.

Bruschweiler-Stern, N. (2004). A multifocal neonatal intervention. In A.J. Sameroff, S.C. McDonough, & K.L. Rosenblum (Eds.), *Treating parent–infant relationship problems* (pp. 188–212). New York: Guilford Press.

Buss, A.H., & Plomin, R. (1984). *Temperament: Early developing personality traits.* Mahwah, NJ: Lawrence Erlbaum Associates.

Campbell, S.B., Cohn, J.F., Flanagan, C., Popper, S., & Meyers, T. (1992). Course and correlates of postpartum depression during the transition to parenthood. *Development and Psychopathology, 4,* 29–47.

Candilis-Huisman, D. (1997). La NBAS, un paradigme pour l'etude des premieres relations du nouveau-ne [The NBAS, a new paradigm for the study of early parent–child relations]. In M. Dugnat (Ed.), *Le monde relationnel du bebe* [The relational world of the newborn] (pp. 93–100). Ramonville Saint-Agne, France: ERES.

Carbajal, R., Veerapen, S., Couderc, S., Jugie, M., & Ville, Y. (2003). Analgesic effect of breast feeding in term neonates: Randomised controlled trial. *British Medical Journal,* (326), 13–17.

Cardone, I.A., & Gilkerson, L. (1990). Family administered neonatal activities: A first step in the integration of parental perceptions and newborn behavior. *Infant Mental Health Journal*, 11, 127–131.

Cardone, I.A., & Gilkerson, L. (1990). Family administered neonatal activities (FANA). In T.B. Brazelton & J.K. Nugent, *The Neonatal Behavioral Assessment Scale* (3rd ed., pp. 111–116). London: McKeith Press.

Carey, W.B. (1999). "Colic" prolonged or excessive crying in young infants. In W.B. Carey (Ed.), *Developmental-behavioral pediatrics* (3rd ed., pp. 365–369). Philadelphia: W.B. Saunders.

Carey, W.B., & McDevitt, S.C. (1995). *Coping with children's temperament. A guide for professionals.* New York: Basic Books.

Carlson, E.A., & Sroufe, L.A. (1995). Contribution of attachment theory to developmental psychopathology. In D. Cicchetti & D. Cohen (Eds.), *Developmental psychopathology: Vol. 1. Theory and methods* (pp. 581– 617). Oxford, England: John Wiley & Sons.

Carter, P. (2003). "Black" cultural capital, status positioning, and schooling conflicts for low-income African American youth. *Social Problems, 50*(1), 136–155.

Cernoch, J.M., & Porter, R.H. (1985). Recognition of maternal auxiliary odors by infants. *Child Development, 56,* 1593–1598.

Chisholm, J. (1989). Biology, culture, and the development of temperament: A Navajo example. In J.K. Nugent, B.M. Lester, & T.B. Brazelton (Eds.), *The cultural context of infancy* (Vol. 1, pp. 341–345). New York: Ablex.

Clark, R., Tluczek, A., & Gallagher, K.C. (2004). Assessment of parent–child early relational disturbances. In R. Delcarmen-Wiggins & A. Carter (Eds.), *Handbook of infant, toddler, and preschool mental health assessment* (pp. 25–60). New York: Oxford University Press.

Clarkson, M.G., & Clifton, R.K. (1995). Infants' pitch perception: Inharmonic tonal complexes. *Journal of the Acoustical Society of America, 98,* 1372–1379.

Cohen, L.J., & Slade, A. (2000). The psychology and psychopathology of pregnancy: Reorganization and transformation. In C.H. Zeanah, Jr. (Ed.), *Handbook of infant mental health* (pp. 20–36). New York: Guilford Press.

Cole, J.G., & Frappier, P. (1985). Infant stimulation reassessed. *Journal of Obstetric, Gynecologic, & Neonatal Nursing, 14*(6), 471–477.

Costa, G. (2006). Mental health principles, practices, strategies, and dynamics pertinent to early intervention practitioners. In G.M. Foley & J.D. Hochman (Eds.), *Mental health in early intervention: Achieving unity in principles and practice.* Baltimore: Paul H. Brookes Publishing Co.

Costello, A., & Chapman, J. (1998). Mothers' perceptions of the care-by-parent program prior to hospital discharge of their preterm infants. *Neonatal Network, 17*(7), 37–42.

Cowan, C.P., & Cowan, P.A. (1995). Interventions to ease the transition to parenthood: Why they are needed and what they can do. *Family Relations, 44,* 412–423.

Cowan, C.P., & Cowan, P.A. (2000). *When partners become parents.* Mahwah, NJ: Lawrence Erlbaum Associates.

Craig, C.M., & Lee, D.N. (1999). Neonatal control of sucking pressure: Evidence from an intrinsic tau-guide. *Experimental Brain Research, 124,* 371–382.

Cramer, B. (1987). Objective and subjective aspects of parent–infant relations. In J. Osofsky (Ed.), *The handbook of infant development* (2nd ed., pp. 1037–1059). New York: John Wiley & Sons.

Crockenberg, S. (1981). Infant irritability, mother responsiveness, and social support influences on the security of infant–mother attachment. *Child Development, 52,* 857–865.

Crockenberg, S. (1986). Professional support for adolescent mothers: Who gives it, how adolescent mothers evaluate it, what they would prefer. *Infant Mental Health Journal, 7*(1), 49–58.

Cutrona, C.E. (1983). Causal attributions and perinatal depression. *Journal of Abnormal Psychology, 92,* 161–172.

Dannemiller, J.L., & Freedland, R.L. (1991). Detection of relative motion by human infants. *Developmental Psychology, 27,* 67–78.

D'Apolito, K. (1991). What is an organized infant? *Neonatal Network, 10*(1), 23–29.

Dargassies, S.S. (1977). Long-term neurological follow-up of 286 truly premature infants. I. Neurological sequelae. *Developmental Medicine and Child Neurology, 19,* 462–478.

Das Eiden, R., & Reifman, A. (1996). Effects of Brazelton demonstrations on later parenting. *Journal of Pediatric Psychology, 21,*(6), 857–868.

Davis, K.F., Parker, K.P., & Montgomery, G.L. (2004). Sleep in infants and young children. Part 1: Normal sleep. *Journal of Pediatric Healthcare, 18,* 65–71.

DeCasper, A.J., & Fifer, W.P. (1980). Of human bonding. *Science, 208,* 1174–1176.

DeCasper, A.J., & Spence, M.J. (1991). Auditorily mediated behavior during the perinatal period: A cognitive view. In M.J.S. Weiss & P.R. Zelazo (Eds.), *Newborn attention: Biological constraints and the influence of experience* (pp. 142–176). Stamford, CT: Ablex.

DeGangi, G.A. (2002). An integrated intervention approach to treating infants and young children with regulatory, sensory processing, and interactional problems. In Interdisciplinary council on developmental and learning disorders (Ed.), *Clinical Practice Guidelines* (pp. 215–242). Bethesda, MD: The American Occupational Therapy Association.

DeGangi, G.A., Craft, P., & Castellan, J. (1991). Treatment of sensory, emotional, and attentional problems in regulatory disordered infants. Part 2. *Infants and Young Children, 3,* 9–19.

Denhoff, E. (1981). Current status of infant stimulation or enrichment programs for children with developmental disabilities. *Pediatrics, 67*(1), 32–37.

Desantis, A., Coster, W., Bigsby, R., & Lester, B. (2004). Colic and fussing in infancy, and sensory processing at 3 to 8 years of age. *Infant Mental Health Journal, 25*(6), 522–539.

De Wolff, M.S., & van IJzendoorn, M.H. (1997). Sensitivity and attachment: A meta-analysis on parental antecedents of infant attachment. *Child Development, 68,* 571–591.

Diamond, J.B. (2000). Beyond social class: Cultural resources and educational participation among low-income black parents. *Berkeley Journal of Sociology, 44*(15), 54.

Diego, M.A., Field, T., & Hernandez-Reif, M. (2005, July). Vagal activity, gastric motility, and weight gain in massaged preterm neonates. *Journal of Pediatrics, 147*(1), 50–55.

Dieter, J.N.I., Field, T., Hernandez-Reif, M., Emory, E.K., & Redzepi, M. (2003). Stable preterm infants gain more weight and sleep less after five days of massage therapy. *Journal of Pediatric Psychology, 28*(6), 403–411.

DiPietro, J.A., Hodgson, D.M., Costigan, K.A., & Hilton, S.C. (1996). Fetal neurobehavioral development. *Child Development, 67,* 2553–2567.

Dixon, S., & Stein, M. (1992). *Encounters with children: Pediatric behavior and development.* St. Louis: Mosby.

Dixon, S., Tronick, E.Z., Keefer, C., & Brazelton, T.B. (1982). Perinatal circumstances and newborn outcome among the Gusii of Kenya: Assessment of risk. *Infant Behavior and Development, 5,* 11–37.

Dobbing, J. (1990). Vulnerable periods in the developing brain. In J. Dobbing (Ed.), *Brain, behavior, and iron in the infant diet* (pp. 1–17). London: Springer-Verlag.

Dodrill, P., McMahon, S., Ward, E., Weir, K., Donovan, T., & Riddle, B. (2004). Long-term oral sensitivity and feeding skills of low-risk pre-term infants. *Early Human Development, 76*(1), 23–37.

Doi, T. (1991). *The anatomy of dependence.* Tokyo: Kodansha International.

Donahue Finn, C. (2003). Cultural models for early caregiving. *Zero to Three, 5,* 40–45.

Donovan, E.G., Perlstein, P.H., Atherton, H.D., & Kotagal, U.R. (2000). Prenatal care and infant emergency department use. *Pediatric Emergency Care, 16*(3), 156–159.

Drillien, C.M. (1972). Abnormal neurologic signs in the first year of life in low-birthweight infants: Possible prognostic significance. *Developmental Medicine and Child Neurology, 14,* 575–584.

Dube, S.R., Felitti, V.J., Dong, M., Giles, W.H., & Anda, R.F. (2003). The impact of adverse childhood experiences on health problems: Evidence from four birth cohorts dating back to 1900. *Preventive Medicine, 37*(3), 268–277.

Dubowitz, L.M.S., Dubowitz, V., & Mercuri, E. (1999). *The neurological assessment of the preterm & full-term newborn infant.* London: MacKeith Press.

Dunn, J. (1977). *Distress and comfort.* Cambridge, MA: Harvard University Press.

Dunst, C.J., Trivette, C.M., & Deal, A.G. (1988). *Enabling and empowering families: Principles and guidelines for practice.* Cambridge, MA: Brookline.

Dworkin, P.H. (1992). Developmental screening: (Still) expecting the impossible? *Pediatrics, 89,* 1253–1255.

Ecklund-Flores, L., & Turkewitz, G. (1996). Asymmetric head-turning to speech and nonspeech in human newborns. *Developmental Psychobiology, 29*(3), 205–217.

Eisenberg, R.B. (1976). *Auditory competencies in early life: The roots of communicative behavior.* Baltimore: University Park Press.

Eisengart, S.P., Singer, L.T., Fulton, S., & Baley, J.E. (2003). Coping and psychological distress in mothers of very low birthweight young children. *Parenting: Science and Practice, 3,* 49–72.

Eliot, L. (1999). *What's going on in there? How the brain and mind develop in the first five years of life.* New York: Bantam Books.

Emde, R.N. (1983). The prerepresentational self and its affective core. *Psychoanalytic Study of the Child, 38,* 165–192.

Emde, R.N. (1987). Infant mental health: Clinical dilemmas, the expansion of meaning and opportunities. In J. Osofsky (Ed.), *The handbook of infant development* (2nd ed., pp. 1297–1320). New York: John Wiley & Sons.

Emde, R.N., Korfmacher, J., & Kubricek, L.F. (2000). Towards a theory of early relationship-based intervention. In J.D. Osofsky & H. Fitzgerald (Eds.), *WAIMH handbook of infant mental health* (pp. 3–32). New York: John Wiley & Sons.

Emde, R.N., & Robinson, J. (1979). The first two months: Recent research in developmental psychobiology and the changing view of the newborn. In J. Noshpitz (Ed.), *Basic handbook of child psychiatry.* New York: Basic Books.

Epperson, N. (2002). Postpartum mood changes: Are hormones to blame? *Zero to Three, 22*(6), 17–23.

Erikson, E.H. (1963). *Childhood and society.* New York: W.W. Norton & Company. (Original work published 1950)

Erickson, M.F., Korfmacher, J., & Egeland, B. (1992). Attachments past and present: Implications for therapeutic intervention with mother–infant dyads. *Development and Psychopathology, 4* 495–507.

Fabre-Grenet, M. (1997). L'echelle de Brazelton au quotidien dans un service de neonatologie. Le point de vue du pediatre [The use of the Brazelton Scale in neonatal practice: The pediatrician's perspective]. In M. Dugnat (Ed.), *Le Monde relationnel du bebe [The relational world of the newborn].* Ramonville, Saint-Agne, France: ERES.

Fantz, R.L. (1961). The origin of form perception. *Scientific American, 204,* 66–72.

Fantz, R.L., & Miranda, S. (1975). Newborn infant attention to form and contour. *Child Development, 46,* 224–228.

Farroni, T., Massaccesi, S., Pividori, D., & Johnson, M.H. (2004). Gaze following in newborns. *Infancy, 5,* 39–60.

Feldman, H.M., Ploof, D., & Cohen, W. (1999). Physician–family partnerships: The adaptive practice model. *Developmental and Behavioral Pediatrics, 20*(2), 111–116.

Feldman, R., Keren, M., Gross-Rozval, M.A., & Tyano, S. (2004). Mother–child touch patterns in infant feeding disorders: Relation to maternal, child and environmental factors. *Journal of the American Academy of Child and Adolescent Psychiatry, 35,* 733–748.

Fenichel, E. (Ed.). (1992). *Learning through supervision and mentorship to support the development of infants toddlers and their families. A source book.* Arlington, VA: ZERO TO THREE: National Center for Infants, Toddlers, and Families.

Fenichel, E., & Mann, T.L. (2002). Early head start for low-income families with infants and toddlers. *The Future of Children, 11*(1), 135–141.

Ferber, S.G., Kuint, J., Weller, A., Feldman, R., Dollberg, S., Arbel, E., & Kohelet, D. (2002). Massage therapy by mothers and trained professionals enhances weight gain in preterm infants. *Early Human Development, 67*(1/2), 37–45.

Ferber, S.G., Laudon, M., Kuint, J., Weller, A., & Zisapel, N. (2002). Massage therapy by mothers enhances the adjustment of circadian rhythms to the nocturnal period in full-term infants. *Journal of Developmental and Behavioral Pediatrtics, 23*(6), 410–415.

Ferri, R., Chiaramonti, R., Elia, M., Musumeci, S.A., Ragazzoni, A., & Stam, C.J. (2003). Nonlinear EEG analysis during sleep in premature and full-term newborns. *Journal of Clinical Neurophysiology, 114*(7), 1176–1180.

Ferry, P.C. (1986). Infant stimulation programs: A neurologic shell game? *Archives of Neurology, 43*(3), 281–282.

Field, T.M. (1987). Affective and interactive disturbances in infants. In J. Osofsky (Ed.), *The handbook of infant development* (2nd ed., pp. 972–1005). New York: John Wiley & Sons.

Field, T.M. (1998). Early interventions for infants of depressed mothers. *Pediatrics, 102*(5, Suppl. E), 1305–1310.

Field, T.M., Dempsey, J., Hallock, N., & Shuman, H.H. (1978). Mothers' assessments of the behaviors of their infants. *Infant Behavior and Development, 1,* 156–167.

Field, T.M., Grizzle, N., Scafidi, F., Abrams, S., & Richardson, S. (1996). Massage therapy for infants of depressed mothers. *Infant Behavior and Development, 19,* 107–112.

Field, T.M., Schanberg, S.M., Scafidi, F., Bauer, C.R., Vega-Lahr, N., Garcia, R., et al. (1986). Tactile/kinesthetic stimulation effects on preterm neonates. *Pediatrics, 77,* 654–658.

Field, T.M., Woodson, R., Greenberg, R., & Cohen, C. (1982). Discrimination and imitation of facial expressions in newborns. *Science, 218,* 179–181.

Fifer, W.P. (1993) The fetus, the newborn, and the mother's voice. In J. Gomes-Pedro, J.K. Nugent, J.G. Young, & T.B. Brazelton (Eds.), *The infant and family in the twenty-first century* (pp. 79–86). New York: Brunner-Routledge.

Fifer, W.P., & Moon, C.M. (1994). The role of mother's voice in the organization of brain function in the newborn. *Acta Paediatrica, 97*(Suppl.), 86–93.

Fish, M., & Stifter, C.A. (1995). Patterns of mother–infant interaction and attachment: A cluster-analytic approach. *Infant Behavior and Development, 18*(4), 435–446.

Floccia, C., Christophe, A., & Bertoncini, J. (1997). High-amplitude sucking in newborns: The quest for underlying mechanisms. *Journal of Experimental Child Psychology, 64,* 175–198.

Foege, W.H. (1998). Adverse childhood experiences: A public health perspective (editorial). *American Journal of Preventive Medicine, 14,* 354–355.

Fonagy, P. (2002). Understanding of mental states, mother–infant interaction and the development of the self. In J.M. Maldonado-Duran (Ed.), *Infant and toddler mental health, models of clinical intervention with infants and their families* (pp. 57–74). Washington, DC: American Psychiatric Publishing.

Fox, N.A., & Polak, C.P. (2001). The possible contribution of temperament to understanding the origins and consequences of persistent excessive crying. In R.G. Barr, I. St. James-Roberts, & M.R. Keefe (Eds.), *New evidence on unexplained early crying: Its origins, nature and management.* Stillman, NJ: Johnson and Johnson Pediatric Institute.

Fraiberg, S. (1980). *Clinical studies in infant mental health: The first year of life.* New York: Basic Books.

Fraiberg, S., Adelson, E., & Shapiro, V. (1980). Ghosts in the nursery: A psychoanalytic approach to the problems of impaired infant–mother relationships. In S. Fraiberg (Ed.), *Clinical studies in infant mental health: The first year of life* (pp. 164–196). New York: Basic Books.

Freedman, D. (1980). Maturational and developmental issues in *the first* year. In S.I. Greenspan & G.H. Pollock (Eds.), *The course of life, Vol. 1: Infancy and early childhood* (pp. 787–796). Washington, DC: Government Printing Office.

Furman, E. (1992). On feeling and being felt with. *Psychoanalytic Study of the Child, 47,* 67–84.

Garbarino, J. (1982). Sociocultural risk: Dangers to competence. In C.B. Kopp & J.B. Crakow (Eds.), *The child: Development in a social context* (pp. 630–687). Reading, MA: Addison Wesley Longman.

Garbarino, J. (1992). *Children and families in the social environment.* Chicago: Aldine.

Garcia Coll, C.T. (1990). Developmental outcome of minority infants: A process-oriented look into our beginnings. *Child Development, 61*(2), 270–289.

Garcia Coll, C.T., Kagan, J., & Reznick, S. (1984). Behavioral inhibition in young children. *Child Development, 55,* 1005–1019.

Garcia Coll, C.T., & Magnuson, K. (1996). Cultural differences in beliefs and practices about pregnancy and childbearing. *Medicine and Health, Rhode Island, 79*(7), 257–260.

Garcia Coll, C.T., & Meyer, E. (1993). The sociocultural context of infant development. In C.H. Zeanah (Ed.), *Handbook of infant mental health.* New York: Guilford Press.

Gavin, N.I., Gaynes, B.N., Lohr, K.N., Meltzer-Brody, S., Gartlehner, G., & Swinson, T. (2005). *Perinatal depression: A systematic review of prevalence and incidence.* Obstetrics & Gynecology, 106, 1071–1083.

George, C., Kaplan, N., & Main, M. (1985). *Adult attachment interview.* Unpublished protocols, University of California, Berkeley.

George, C., & Solomon, J. (1999). Attachment and caregiving: The caregiving behavioral system. In J. Cassidy & P.R. Shaver (Eds.), *Handbook of attachment: Theory, research, and clinical applications* (pp. 649–670). New York: Guilford Press.

George, L. (2005). Lack of preparedness: Experience of first-time mothers. *The American Journal of Maternal Child Nursing, 30*(4), 251–255.

Georgieff, M.K., & Bernbaum, J.C. (1986). Abnormal shoulder girdle muscle tone in premature infants during their first 18 months of life. *Pediatrics, 77*(5), 664–669.

Georgieff, M.K., Bernbaum, J.C., Hoffman-Williamson, M., & Daft, A. (1986). Abnormal truncal muscle tone as a useful early marker for developmental delay in low birth weight infants. *Pediatrics, 77*(5), 659–663.

Gilkerson, L., & Shamoon-Shanook, R. (2000). Relationship for growth: Cultivating reflective practice in infant, toddler and preschool programs. In J. Osofsky & H.E. Fitzgerald (Eds.), *WAIMH handbook of infant mental health (Vol. II, pp. 33–79).* New York: John Wiley & Sons.

Gill, N.E., White, M.A., & Anderson, G.C. (1984). Transitional newborn infants in a hospital nursery: From first oral cue to first sustained cry. *Nursing Research, 33*(4), 213–217.

Goeb, J-L., LeBlanc-Deshayes, M., Coin, L., Malka, J., Bouderlique, C., Duverger, P. (2004). Neonatal death of a newborn twin. *Archives of Pediatric, 11,* 1135–1138.

Gomes-Pedro, J., Nugent, J.K, Young, G., & Brazelton, T.B. (Eds.). (2002). *The infant and family in the 21st century.* New York: Brunner/Mazel.

Gomes-Pedro, J., Patricio, M., Carvalho, A., Goldschmidt, T., Torgal-Garcia, F., & Monteiro, M.B. (1995). Early intervention with Portuguese mothers: A two year follow-up. *Developmental and Behavioral Pediatrics, 16,* 21–28.

Goodlin-Jones, B.L., Burnham, M.M., & Anders, T.F. (2000). Sleep and sleep disturbances: Regulatory processes in infancy. In A.J. Sameroff, M. Lewis, & S.M. Miller (Eds.), *Handbook of developmental psychology* (2nd ed., pp. 309–325). New York: Kluwer.

Goren, G.C., Sarty, M., & Wu, P.Y.K. (1975). Visual following and pattern discrimination of facelike stimuli by newborn infants. *Pediatrics, 56,* 544–549.

Gormally, S., Barr, R.G., Wertheim, L., Alkawaf, R., Calinoui, N., & Young, S.N. (2001). Contact and nutrient caregiving effects on newborn infant pain responses. *Developmental Medicine and Child Neurology, 43,* 28–38.

Gracia, E., & Musitu, G. (2003). Social isolation from communities and child maltreatment: A cross-cultural comparison. *Child Abuse and Neglect, 27*(2), 137–140.

Gray, J.E., Safran, C., Davis, R.B., Pompilio-Weitzner, G., Stewart, J.E., Zaccagnini, L., et al. (2000). Baby CareLink: Using the internet and telemedicine to improve care for high-risk infants. *Pediatrics, 106,* 1318–1324.

Gray, L., Miller, L.W., Philipp, B.L., & Blass, E.M. (2002). Breastfeeding is analgesic in healthy newborns. *Pediatrics, 109*(4), 590–593.

Green, M., & Palfrey, J. (Eds.). (2000). *Bright futures: Guidelines for health supervision of infants, children and adolescents* (2nd ed.). Arlington, VA: National Center for Education in Maternal and Child Health.

Greene, S. (2002). Child development: Old themes and new directions. In J. Gomes-Pedro, J.K. Nugent, J.G. Young, & T.B. Brazelton (Eds.), *The infant and family in the 21st century.* New York: Brunner/Mazel.

Greenfield, P.M., & Cocking, R.R. (Eds.) (1994). *Cross-cultural roots of minority child development.* Hillsdale, NJ: Lawrence Erlbaum Associates.

Greenspan, S.I. (1981). *The clinical interview of the child.* New York: McGraw-Hill.

Greenspan, S.I. (1992). *Infancy and early childhood: The practice of clinical assessment and intervention with emotional and developmental challenges.* Madison, CT: International Universities Press.

Greenspan, S.I., & Wieder, S. (1993). Regulatory disorders. In C.H. Zeanah (Ed.), *Handbook in infant mental health.* New York: Guilford Press.

Greenspan, S.I., & Wieder, S. (2001). The DIR (developmental, individual-difference, relationship-based) approach to assessment and intervention planning, *Zero to Three, 21*(4), 11–19.

Grossman, K., Grossman, K.E., & Kindler, H. (2005). Early care and the roots of attachment and partnership representations: The Bielefeld and Regensburg Longitudinal Studies. In K.E. Grossman, K. Grossman, & E. Waters (Eds.), *Attachment from infancy to adulthood: The major longitudinal studies* (pp. 98–136). New York: Guilford Press.

Gurwitt, A.R. (1976). Aspects of prospective fatherhood. In S.H. Cath, A.R. Gurwitt, & J.M. Ross (Eds.), *Father and child: Developmental and clinical perspectives* (pp. 275–299). Boston: Little, Brown.

Gurwitt, A.R. (1988). On becoming a family man. *Psychoanalytic Inquiry, 8,* 261–279.

Gustafson, G.E., Wood, R.M., & Green, J.A. (2000). Can we hear the causes of infants' crying? In R. Barr, B. Hopkins, & J. Green (Eds.), *Crying as a sign, symptom, and a signal. Clinics in Developmental Medicine, 152,* 8–22.

Hafler, J. (2005). *Facilitator's guide for pediatrics in practice.* Iowa City, Iowa: Henry Bernstein, DO for the Health Promotion Work Group. Retrieved May 20, 2006, from http://www.pediatricsin-practice.org/pdfs/FacilitatorsGuide.pdf

Haith, M. (2004). Progress and standardization in eye movement work with human infants. *Infancy, 6*(2), 257–265.

Hall, E.T. (1973). *The silent language.* New York: Anchor Books.

Hamilton, C.E. (2000). Continuity and discontinuity of attachment from infancy through adolescence. *Child Development, 71*(3), 690–694.

Hannon, P., Willis, S., & Scrimshaw, S. (2001). Persistence of maternal concerns surrounding neonatal jaundice. An exploratory study. *Archives of Pediatric and Adolescent Medicine, 155,* 1357–1363.

Harkness, S., Super, C.M., & Keefer, C.H. (1992). Learning to be an American parent: How cultural models gain directive force. In R.G. D'Andrade & C. Strauss (Eds.), *Human, motives and cultural models.* Cambridge, MA: Cambridge University Press.

Harkness, S., Super, C.M., Keefer, C.H., Rahgavan, C., & Kipp, E.H. (1995). Ask the doctor: The negotiation of cultural models in American parent–pediatrician discourse. In S. Harkness & C.M. Super (Eds.), *Parents' cultural belief systems: Their origins, expressions, and consequences.* New York: Guilford Press.

Harrison, H. (1993). The principles of family-centered neonatal care. *Pediatrics, 92*(5), 643–650.

Hauck, F.R., Herman, S.M., Donovan, M., Iyasu, S., Merrick Moore, C., Donoghue, E., et al. (2003). Sleep environment and the risk of sudden death syndrome in an urban population: The Chicago Infant Mortality Study. *Pediatrics, 111,* 1207–1214.

Hauser-Cram, P. (2006). Young children with developmental disabilities and their families: Needs, policies and services. In K.M. Theis & J.F. Travers (Eds.), *Handbook of human development for health care professionals* (pp. 287–305). Sudbury, MA: Jones and Bartlett.

Hauser-Cram, P., Warfield, M.E., Shonkoff, J., & Krauss, M.W. (2001). Children with disabilities: A longitudinal study of child development and parent well-being. *Monographs of the Society for Research in Child Development, 66*(3), i–viii, 1–114, discussion 115–126.

Hawthorne-Amick, J.A. (1989). The effects of different routines in a special care baby unit on the mother–infant relationship. In J.K. Nugent, B.M. Lester, & T.B. Brazelton (Eds.), *The cultural context of infancy: Vol. 1. Biology, culture, and infant development* (pp. 237–267). Stamford, CT: Ablex.

Hecox, K.E., & Deegan, D.M. (1985). Methodological issues in the study of auditory development. In G. Gottlieb & N.A. Krasnegor (Eds.), *Measurement of audition and vision in the first year of postnatal life: A methodological overview.* Westport, CT: Ablex Publishing.

Heinicke, C.M., Feinman, N.R., Ponce, V.A., Guthrie, D., & Rodning, C. (1999). Relationship-based intervention with at-risk mothers: Outcome in the first year of life. *Infant Mental Health Journal, 20,* 349–374.

Hepper, P.G. (1991). An examination of fetal learning before and after birth. *Irish Journal of Psychology, 12,* 95–107.

Herzog, J.M. (1984). Fathers and young children: Fathering daughters and fathering sons. In J.D. Call, E. Galenson, & R.L. Tyson (Eds.), *Frontiers of infant psychiatry* (Vol. II, pp. 335–342). New York: Basic Books.

Hesse, E. (1999). The adult attachment interview. In J. Cassidy & P.R. Shaver (Eds.), *Handbook of attachment: Theory, research, and clinical applications* (pp. 395–433). New York: Guilford Press.

Hewlitt, B.S. (1991). *Intimate fathers.* Ann Arbor: University of Michigan Press.

Higley, E., Cole, J.G., Howland, E., Ranuga, T., & Nugent, J.K. (1999). *Neonatal Behavioral Assessment Scale (NBAS) Handbook.* Boston: Brazelton Institute, Children's Hospital.

Hinde, R. (1976). On describing relationships. *Journal of Child Psychology and Psychiatry, 17,* 1–19.

Hinshaw, S.P., & Lee, S.S. (2003). Conduct and oppositional defiant disorders. In E.J. Mash & R.A. Barkley (Eds.), *Child Psychopathology* (2nd ed., pp. 144–198). New York: Guilford Press.

Hirschberg, L.M. (1993). Clinical interviews with infants and their families. In C.H. Zeanah (Ed.), *Handbook of infant mental health* (pp. 173–190). London: Guilford Press.

Ho, F. (1994). Cognitive socialization in Confucian heritage cultures. In P. Greenfield & R. Cocking (Eds.), *Cross cultural roots of minority child development* (pp. 285–314). Hillsdale, NJ: Lawrence Erlbaum Associates.

Hopkins, B. (1998). Moving into the two-month revolution: An action-based account [Special issue]. *Infant Behavior and Development, 21,* 183.

Hopkins, B. (2000). Development of crying in normal infants: Method, theory and some speculations. In R.G. Barr, B. Hopkins, & J.A. Green (Eds.), *Crying as a sign, a symptom and a signal* (pp. 71–85). London: MacKeith Press.

Hrdy, S.B. (1999). *Mother nature: A history of mothers, infants, and natural selection.* New York: Pantheon Books.

Hughes, R.B., Townsend, P.A., & Branvin, Q.K. (1988). Relationship between neonatal behavioral responses and lactation outcomes. *Issues in Comprehensive Pediatric Nursing, 11*(5–6), 271–281.

Hunnius, S., & Geuze, R. (2004). Developmental change in visual scanning of dynamic faces and abstract stimuli in infants: A longitudinal study. *Infancy, 6*(2), 231–255.

Huppi, P.S., Warfield, S., Kikinis, R., Barnes, P.D., Zientara, G.P., Jolesz, F.A., et al. (1998). Quantitative magnetic resonance imaging of brain development in premature and mature newborns. *Annals of Neurology, 43*(2), 224–235.

Huttenlocher, P.R. (2002). *Neural plasticity: The effects of environment on the development of the cerebral cortex.* Cambridge, MA: Harvard University Press.

Ikonomov, O.C., Stoynev, A.G., & Shisheva, A.C. (1998). Integrative coordination of circadian mammalian diversity: Neuronal networks and peripheral clocks. *Progress in Neurobiology, 54*(1), 87–97.

Illingworth, R.S. (1983). *The development of the infant and the young child.* Edinburgh: Churchill Livingstone.

Individuals with Disabilities Education Act (IDEA) of 1990, PL 101-476, 20 U.S.C. §§ 1400 *et seq.*

Inui, T.S. (1996). What are the sciences of relationship-centered primary care? *The Journal of Family Practice, 42*(2), 171–177.

Johnson, S.P., Slemmer, J.A., & Amso, D. (2004). Where infants look determines how they see: Eye movements and object perception performance in 3-month-olds. *Infancy, 6,* 185–201.

Jordan, J.V. (1986). *The meaning of mutuality.* Wellesley, MA: Wellesley Centers for Women.

Jordan, J.V. (1989). *Relational development: Therapeutic implications of empathy and shame.* Wellesley, MA: Wellesley Centers for Women.

Jordan, J.V., & Dooley, C. (2000). *Relational practice in action: A group manual.* Wellesley, MA: Wellesley Centers for Women.

Kagan, J., & Snidman, N. (1998). Childhood derivatives of high and low reactivity in infancy. *Child Development, 69*(6), 1183–1193.

Kagan, J., & Snidman, N. (2004). *The long shadows of temperament.* Cambridge, MA: Harvard University Press.

Karl, D.J. (1999). The interactive newborn bath: Using infant neurobehavior to connect parents and newborns. *MCN: The American Journal of Maternal Child Nursing, 24*(6), 280–298.

Karl, D.J. (2004). Using principles of newborn behavioral state organization to facilitate breast-feeding. *MCN: The American Journal of Maternal Child Nursing, 29*(5), 292–298.

Karl, D.J., Beal, J.A., & Rissmiller, P.N. (1995). A model for integrating the NBAS into nursing practice. In T.B. Brazelton & J.K. Nugent (Eds.), *Neonatal behavioral assessment scale* (3rd ed., pp. 92–101). London: MacKeith Press.

Karl, D.J., Limbo, D., & Ricker, V.J. (1998). Healthy connections: A relational model to extend primary care into the perinatal period. *Journal of Pediatric Health Care, 12*(4), 176–182.

Kavanaugh, K., & Moro, T. (2006). Supporting parents after stillborn or newborn death: There is much that nurses can do. *American Journal of Nursing, 106,* 74–79.

Kawasaki, K., Nugent, J.K., Miyashita, H., Miyahara, H., & Brazelton, T.B. (1994). The cultural organization of infant's sleep. *Children's Environments, 11,* 134–141.

Kaye, K. (1982). *The mental and social life of babies: How parents create persons.* Chicago: University of Chicago Press.

Kaye, K., & Brazelton, T.B. (1971, April). *The ethological significance of the burst-pause pattern in infant sucking.* Paper presented at Society for Research in Child Development, Minneapolis, MN.

Kaye, K., & Wells, A.J. (1980). Mothers' jiggling and burst-pause pattern in neonatal feeding. *Infant Behavior and Development, 3,* 29–46.

Keefer, C.H. (1995). The combined physical and behavioral neonatal examination: A parent-centered approach to pediatric care. In T.B. Brazelton & J.K. Nugent (Eds.), *The neonatal behavioral assessment scale* (pp. 92–101). London: McKeith Press.

Keefer, C.H., Tronick, E., Dixon, S., & Brazelton, T.B. (1982). Specific differences in motor performance between Gusii and American newborns and a modification of the Neonatal Behavioral Assessment Scale. *Child Development, 53,* 554–559.

Kemper, K., Forsyth, B., & McCarthy, P. (1989). Jaundice, terminating breast-feeding, and the vulnerable child. *Pediatrics, 84*(55), 773–778.

Kennell, J., & McGrath, S.K. (2003). Beneficial effects of postnatal skin-to-skin contact. *Acta Paediatrica, 92,* 272–273.

Kennell, J., & Rolnick, A. (1960). Discussing problems in newborn babies with their parents. *Pediatrics, 26,* 832–838.

Klaus, M., & Kennell, J. (2002). Commentary: Routines in maternity units: Are they still appropriate for 2002? *Birth, 28*(4), 270–273.

Klaus, M.H., Kennell, J.H., & Klaus, P.H. (1995). *Bonding.* Reading, MA: Addison Wesley Longman.

Klaus, M., & Klaus, P.H. (1998). *Your amazing newborn.* Cambridge, MA: Perseus Books.

Kleberg, A., Westrup, B., & Stjernqvist, K. (2000). Developmental outcome, child behaviour and mother–child interaction at 3 years of age following Newborn Individualized Developmental Care and Intervention Program (NIDCAP) intervention. *Early Human Development, 60,* 123–135.

Kleinman, A. (1981). *Patients and healers in the context of culture.* Berkeley: University of California Press.

Kobak, R. (1999). The emotional dynamics of disruptions in attachment relationships: Implications for theory, research, and clinical intervention. In J. Cassidy & P.R. Shaver (Eds.), *Handbook of attachment: Theory, research, and clinical applications* (pp. 21–43). New York: Guilford Press.

Konner, M. (1998). Behavioral changes around two months of age in a population of African hunter-gatherers [Special issue]. *Infant Behavior and Development, 21,* 185.

Korner, A.F., & Thoman, E.B. (1972). The relative efficacy of contact and vestibular-proprioceptive stimulation in soothing neonates. *Child Development, 43,* 443–453.

Kron, R.E., Stein, M., & Goddard, K.E. (1966). Newborn sucking behavior affected by obstetric medication. *Pediatrics, 37,* 1012–1016.

Langer, A., Campero, L., Garcia, C., & Reynoso, S. (1998). Effects of psychosocial support during labour and childbirth on breastfeeding, medical interventions, and mother's wellbeing in a Mexican public hospital: A randomized clinical trial. *British Journal of Obstetrics and Gynaecology, 105*(10), 1056–1063.

Laplante, D., Orr, R., Neville, K., Vorkapich, L., & Sasso, D. (1996). Discrimination of stimulus rotations by newborns. *Infant Behavior and Development, 19*(3), 271–279.

Lavelli, M., & Fogel, A. (2005). Developmental changes in the relationship between the infant's attention and emotion during early face-to-face communication: The two month transition. *Developmental Psychology, 41*(1), 265–280.

Lawhon, G. (2002). Facilitation of parenting the premature infant within the newborn intensive care unit. *Journal of Perinatal & Neonatal Nursing, 16*(1), 71–83.

Leckman, J.F., & Mayes, L.C. (1999). Preoccupations and behaviors associated with romantic and parental love: The origin of obsessive-compulsive disorder? *Child and Adolescent Psychiatry Clinics of North America, 8,* 635–665.

Lerner, R.M., Rothbaum, F., Boulos, S., & Castellino, D.R. (2000). Developmental systems perspective on parenting. In M.H. Bornstein (Ed.), *Handbook of parenting: Vol 2. Biology and ecology of parenting.* Mahweh, NJ: Lawrence Erlbaum Associates.

Lester, B.M. (1984a). A biosocial model of crying. In L. Lipsitt & C. Rovee-Collier (Eds.), *Advances in infancy research* (Vol. 3, pp. 167–212). Stamford, CT: Ablex.

Lester, B.M. (1984b). Data analysis and prediction. In T.B. Brazelton (Ed.), *Neonatal behavioral assessment scale* (2nd ed., pp. 85–96). London: MacKeith Press.

Lester, B.M., Boukydis, C.F., Garcia Coll, C., & Hole, W. (1990). Colic for developmentalists. *Infant Mental Health Journal, 11,* 321–333.

Lester, B.M., Hoffman, J., & Brazelton, T.B. (1985). The rhythmic structure of mother–infant interaction in term and preterm infants. *Child Development, 51,* 15–27.

Lester, B.M., & Tronick, E.Z. (2005). *NICU network neurobehavioral scale (NNNS) manual.* Baltimore: Paul H. Brookes Publishing Co.

Lester, B.M., & Zeskind, P.S. (1978). Brazelton scale and physical size correlates of neonatal cry features. *Infant Behavior and Development, 1,* 393–402.

Levine, M. (summer, 2006). The NBO promotes family-centered care in early intervention. *Ab Initio*; www.brazelton-institute.com/abinitio2006summer/art3/html

LeVine, R.A. (1980). Cross-cultural perspectives on parenting. In M. Fantini & R. Cardinas (Eds.), *Parenting in a multicultural society* (pp. 17–26). New York: Longman.

LeVine, R.A. (1988). Human parental care: Universal goals, cultural strategies and individual behavior. In R.A. LeVine, P. Miller, & M. Maxwell (Eds.), *New directions for child development, 40,* 3–12.

LeVine, R.A., LeVine, S., Dixon, S., Richman, A., Leiderman, P.H., Keefer, C.H., et al. (1994). *Child care and culture: Lessons from Africa.* Cambridge, UK: Cambridge University Press.

Lieberman, A.F. (1991). Attachment theory and infant–parent psychotherapy: Some conceptual, clinical and research considerations. In D. Cicchetti & S. Toth (Eds.), *Models and integrations Rochester Symposium on developmental psychopathology* (Vol. 3, pp. 261–288). Hillsdale, NJ: Lawrence Erlbaum Associates.

Lieberman, A.F., Padron, E., Van Horn, P., & Harris, W.W. (2005). Angels in the nursery: The intergenerational transmission of benevolent parental influences. *Infant Mental Health Journal, 26,* 504–520.

Linn, P.L., & Horowitz, F.D. (1984). The relationship between infant individual differences and mother–infant interaction in the neonatal period. *Infant Behavior and Development, 6,* 415–427.

Loo, K.K., Espinosa, M., Tyler, R., & Howard, J. (2003). Using knowledge to cope with stress in the NICU: How parents integrate learning to read the physiologic and behavioral cues of the infant. *Neonatal Network, 22*(1), 31–37.

Lothian, J.A. (1995). It takes two to breastfeed: The baby's role in successful breastfeeding. *Journal of Nurse Midwifery, 49*(4), 328–334.

Lozoff, B., Wolf, A.W., & Davis, A.W. (1984). Co-sleeping in urban families with young children. *Pediatrics, 74*(2), 172–182.

Lundqvist, C., & Sabel, K. (2000). The Brazelton Neonatal Behavioral Assessment Scale detects differences among newborn infants of optimal health. *Journal of Pediatric Psychology, 25,* 577–582.

Lynch, E.W., & Hanson, M.J. (2004). *Developing cross-cultural competence: A guide for working with young children and their families* (2nd ed.). Baltimore: Paul H. Brookes Publishing Co.

Lyons-Ruth, K., Zeanah, C.H., & Benoit, D. (2003). Disorder and risk for disorder during infancy and toddlerhood. In E.J. Mash & R.J. Barkley (Eds.), *Childhood Psychopathology* (pp. 589–631). New York: Guilford Press.

Macfarlane, A. (1975). Olfaction in the development of social preferences in the human neonate. In Ciba Foundation Symposium (Ed.), *Parent–infant interaction* (pp. 103–117). New York: Elsevier.

Mahoney, G., & Perales, F. (2005). Relationship-focused early intervention with children with pervasive developmental disorders and other disabilities: A comparative study. *Developmental and Behavioral Pediatrics, 26*(2), 77–85.

Main, M. (2000). The adult attachment interview: Fear, attention, safety and discourse processes. *Journal of the American Psychoanalytic Association, 48*(4), 1055–1096.

Main, M., Kaplan, N., & Cassidy, J. (1985). Security in infancy, childhood, and adulthood: A move to the level of representation. *Monographs of the Society for Research in Child Development, 50,* 66–104.

Main, M., & Solomon, J. (1990). Procedures for identifying infants as disorganized/disoriented during the Ainsworth Strange Situation. In M.T. Greenberg, D. Cichetti, & E.M. Cummings (Eds.), *Attachment in the preschool years* (pp. 121–160). Chicago: University of Chicago Press.

Mainous, A., Goodwin, M., & Slange, K. (2004). Patient–physician shared experiences and value patients place on continuity of care. *Annals of Family Medicine, 2*(5), 452–454.

Makoul, G. (2001). Essential elements of communication in medical encounters: The Kalamazoo consensus statement. *Academic Medicine, 76*(4), 390–393.

Maldonado-Duran, M., & Sauceda-Garcia, J.M. (1996). Excessive crying in infants with regulatory disorders. *Bulletin of the Menninger Clinic, 60,* 62–78.

Martini, M., & Kirkpatrick, J. (1981). Early interactions in the Marquesas Islands. In T.M. Field, A.M. Sostek, P. Vietze, & P.H. Liederman (Eds.), *Culture and early interactions* (pp. 189–213). Hillsdale, NJ: Lawrence Erlbaum Associates.

Mattingly, C., & Garro, L. (Eds.). (2000). *Narrative and the cultural construction of illness and healing.* Berkeley: University of California Press.

Maurer, D., & Barrera, M. (1981). Infants' perception of natural and distorted arrangements of a schematic face. *Child Development, 52*(1), 196–202.

Mayes, L.C. (2002). Parental preoccupation and perinatal mental health. *Zero to Three, 22*(6), 4–9.

McDonough, S.C. (1993). Interaction guidance: Understanding and treating early infant–caregiver disturbances. In C.H. Zeanah (Ed.), *Handbook of infant mental health* (pp. 414–426). New York: Guilford Press.

McDonough, S.C. (2000a). Interaction guidance: An approach for difficult-to-engage families. In C.H. Zeanah (Ed.), *Handbook of infant mental health* (2nd ed., pp. 485–493). New York: Guilford Press.

McDonough, S.C. (2000). Preparing infant mental health personnel for twentieth century practice. In J. Osofsky & H.E. Fitzgerald (Eds.), *WAIMH handbook of infant mental health* (Vol. II, pp. 535–546). New York: John Wiley & Sons.

McHaffie, H.E. (1990). Mothers of very low birthweight babies: How do they adjust? *Journal of Advanced Nursing, 15,* 6–11.

McKenna, J.J. (2000). Cultural influences on infant and childhood sleep biology and the science that studies it: Toward a more inclusive paradigm. In J. Loughlin, J.L. Carroll, & C.L. Marcus (Eds.), *Sleep in development and pediatrics* (pp. 99–124). New York: Marcel Dekker.

McKenna, J.J., & Moskol, S. (2001). Mother infant cosleeping: Toward a new beginning. In R. Byard & H. Krous (Eds.), *Sudden infant death syndrome: Problems, puzzles, possibilities* (pp. 258–272). New York: Arnold Publishing.

McQuiston, S., Kloczko, N., Johnson, L., O'Brien, S., & Nugent, J.K. (2006, Summer). Training pediatric residents in the Newborn Behavioral Observations (NBO) system: A follow-up study. *Ab Initio*; www.brazelton-institute.com/abinitio2006summer/art10.html

Medoff-Cooper, B., McGrath, J., & Shults, J. (2002). Feeding patterns of full-term and preterm infants at forty weeks postconceptual age. *Developmental and Behavioral Pediatrics, 23*(4), 231–236.

Meier-Kohl, A., Hall, V., Hellwig, U., Kott, G., & Meier-Koll, V. (1978). Biological oscillator system and the development of sleep-waking behavior during early infancy. *Chronobiologia, 5,* 425–440.

Meisels, S., Dichtelmiller, M., & Fong-Ruey, L. (1993). A multidimensional analysis of early childhood intervention programs. In C.H. Zeanah (Ed.), *Handbook of infant mental health* (pp. 361–385). New York: Guilford Press.

Melnyk, B.M., Feinstein, N.F., & Fairbanks, E. (2002). Effectiveness of informational/behavioral interventions with parents of low birth weight (LBW) premature infants: An evidence base to guide clinical practice. *Pediatric Nursing, 28,* 511–516.

Meltzoff, A.N., & Moore, M.K. (1994). Imitation, memory and the representation of persons. *Infant Behavior and Development, 17,* 83–99.

Meltzoff, A.N., & Moore, K. (1999). Persons and representation: Why infant imitation is important for theories of human development. In J. Nadel & G. Butterworth (Eds.), *Imitation in infancy.* Cambridge, UK: Cambridge University Press.

Miller, J.B. (1986). *What do we mean by relationships?* Wellesley, MA: Wellesley Centers for Women.

Miller, J.B., Jordan, J., Stiver, I.P., Walker, M., Surrey, J.L., & Eldridge, N.S. (1999). *Therapists' authenticity.* Wellesley, MA: Wellesley Centers for Women.

Miller, L.J., Reisman, J.E., Mcintosh, D.N., & Simon, J. (2001). An ecological model of sensory modulation: Performance of children with fragile-X syndrome, autistic disorder, attention-deficit/hyperactivity disorder and sensory modulation dysfunction. In R. Schaaf (Ed.), *Understanding the nature of sensory integration with diverse populations* (pp. 57–82). San Antonio, TX: Therapy Skill Builders.

Minde, K. (2000). The assessment of infants and toddlers with medical conditions and their families. In J. Osofsky & H. Fitzgerald (Eds.), *Handbook of infant mental health* (Vol. 2). New York: John Wiley & Sons.

Minuchin, B. (1985). Families and individual development: Provocations from the field of family therapy. *Child Development, 59,* 289–302.

Mirmiran, M., & Lunshof, S. (1996). Perinatal development of human circadian rhythms. *Progress in Brain Research, 111,* 217–226.

Mishler, E. (1985). Attending to the voice of the lifeworld: Alternative practices and their functions. In *Discourse of Medicine* (pp. 137–185). Stamford, CT: Ablex.

Moon, C.M., Bever, T.G., & Fifer, W.P. (2002). Canonical and non-canonical syllable discrimination by 2-day-old infants. *Journal of Child Language, 19*(1), 1–17.

Moon, C.M., Cooper, R.P., & Fifer, W. (1993). Two-day-olds prefer their native language. *Infant Behavior and Development, 16,* 495–500.

Moon, C.M., & Fifer, W.P. (2000). Evidence of transnatal auditory learning. *Journal of Perinatology, 20*(8 Part 2), S37–S44.

Morelli, G.A., Rogoff, B., Oppenheim, D., & Goldsmith, D. (1992). Cultural variation in infants' sleeping arrangements: Questions of independence. *Developmental Psychology, 28,* 604–613.

Morrongiello, B., Fenwick, K.D., Hillier, L., & Chance, G. (2004). Sound localization in newborn human infants. *Developmental Psychobiology, 27*(8), 519–538.

Morton, J., & Johnson, M. (1991). CONSPEC and CONLERN: A two-process theory of infant face recognition. *Psychological Review, 98,* 164–181.

Mouradian, L.E., & Als, H. (1994). The influence of neonatal intensive care unit caregiving practices on motor functioning of preterm infants. *American Journal of Occupational Therapy, 48,* 527–533.

Mouradian, L.E., Als, H., & Coster, W.J. (2000). Neurobehavioral functioning of healthy preterm infants of varying gestational ages. *Journal of Developmental and Behavioral Pediatrics, 21*(6), 408–414.

Muir, D., & Field, J. (1979). Newborn infants orient to sounds. *Child Development, 50,* 431–436.

Munck, H. (1985, January). *Reflections on qualitative aspects in a study of preterm infants and their parents.* Paper presented at the International Symposium on Psychobiology and Early Development, West Berlin.

Munck, H., Mirdal, G., & Marner, G. (1991). Mother–infant interaction in Denmark. In J.K. Nugent, B.M. Lester, & T.B. Brazelton (Eds.), *The cultural context of infancy: Vol. 2. Multicultural and interdisciplinary approaches to parent–infant relations* (pp. 169–199). Stamford, CT: Ablex.

Murray, L. (1994, June). *The infant's contribution to the mother–infant relationship in the context of postnatal depression.* Paper presented at the 9th International Conference on Infant Studies, Paris, France.

Murray, L., & Cooper, P.J. (1997). The role of infant and maternal factors in postpartum depression, mother–infant interactions, and infant outcomes. In L. Murray & P.J. Cooper (Eds.), *Postpartum depression and child development* (pp. 111–135). New York: Guilford Press.

Myers, B.J. (1982). Early intervention using Brazelton training with middle class mothers and fathers of newborns. *Child Development, 53,* 462–471.

Napell, S. (1976). Six common non-facilitating teaching behaviors. *Contemporary Education, 47*(2), 199–202.

National Mental Health Association (2006); retrieved January 2007 from www.nmha.org/infoctr/factsheets/postpartum.cfm

National Scientific Council on the Developing Child. (2004). *Young children develop in an environment of relationships* (Working Paper No. 1). Waltham, MA: Brandeis University; www.developingchild.com

Nazzi, T., Floccia, C., & Bertoncini, J. (1998). Discrimination of pitch contours by neonates. *Infant Behavior and Development, 21*(4), 779–784.

Nobile, C., & Drotar, D. (2003). Research on the quality of parent–provider communication in pediatric care: Implications and recommendations. *Journal of Developmental and Behavioral Pediatrics, 24,* 279–290.

Notman, M.T., & Lester, E.P. (1988). Pregnancy: Theoretical considerations. *Psychoanalytic Inquiry, 8*(2), 139–159.

Nugent, J.K. (1985). *Using the NBAS with infants and their families: Guidelines for intervention.* White Plains, NY: March of Dimes Birth Defects Foundation.

Nugent, J.K. (1991). Cultural and psychological influences on the father's role in infant development. *Journal of Marriage and the Family, 53*(2), 475–485.

Nugent, J.K. (1994). Cross-cultural studies of child development: Implications for clinicians. *Zero to Three, 15*(2), 1–8.

Nugent, J.K. (2002). The cultural context of child development: Implications for research and practice in the twenty-first century. In J. Gomes-Pedro, J.K. Nugent, J.G. Young, & T.B. Brazelton (Eds.), *The infant and family in the twenty-first century* (pp. 87–98). New York: Brunner-Routledge.

Nugent, J. D., & Alhaffer, D. (2006, Summer). The NBO and the March of Dimes NICU Family Support program: The effects of the NBO as an educational and emotional support system for parents of premature infants. *Ab Initio*; www.brazelton-institute.com/abinitio2006summer/art5.html

Nugent, J.K., & Blanchard, Y. (2006). Newborn behavior and development: Implications for health care professionals. In J.F. Travers & K. Theis (Eds.), *The handbook of human development for health care professionals* (pp. 79–94). Boston: Jones and Bartlett.

Nugent, J.K., Blanchard, Y., & Stewart, J.S. (2007). Supporting parents of premature infants: An infant-focused family-centered approach. In D. Brodsky & M.A. Ouellette (Eds.), *Primary care of the premature infant.* New York: Elsevier.

Nugent, J.K., & Brazelton, T.B. (1989). Preventive intervention with infants and families: The NBAS model. *Infant Mental Health Journal, 10,* 84–99.

Nugent, J.K., & Brazelton, T.B. (2000). Preventive infant mental health: Uses of the Brazelton scale. In J. Osofsky & H.E. Fitzgerald (Eds.), *WAIMH handbook of infant mental health* (Vol. II, pp. 159–202). New York: John Wiley & Sons.

Nugent, J.K., Hoffman, J., Barrett, D., Censullo, M., & Brazelton, T.B. (1987, April). *The effects of early intervention on IUGR infants.* Paper presented at the Biennial Meeting of the Society for Research in Child Development, Baltimore, Maryland.

Nugent, J.K., Keefer, C.H., O'Brien, S., Johnson, L., & Blanchard, Y. (2005). *The newborn behavioral observations (NBO) system.* Boston: The Brazelton Institute, Children's Hospital.

Nugent, J.K., Killough, J., Gonzalez, J., & Wides, J. (2005, November). *The effect of the Newborn Behavioral Observations (NBO) system on postpartum mother–infant interaction.* Paper presented at the ZERO TO THREE 21st National Training Institute, Washington, DC.

Nugent, J.K., Lester, B.M., & Brazelton, T.B. (Eds.). (1989). *The cultural context of infancy: Vol. 1. Biology, culture, and infant development.* Stamford, CT: Ablex.

Nugent, J.K., Lester, B.M., & Brazelton, T.B. (Eds.). (1991). *The cultural context of infancy: Vol. 2. Multicultural and interdisciplinary approaches to parent–infant relations.* Stamford, CT: Ablex.

Nugent, J.K., Snidman, S., Kagan, J., Shih, M.S., Ming, S., Matson, C., et al. (2006). Brief report: Using the revised NBAS (NBAS-R) to examine the relationship between newborn behavior and temperament categories at four months of age. *Ab Initio;* www.brazelton-institute.com/abinitio2006summer/art4.html

Nugent, J.K., Valim, C., Killough, J., Gonzalez, J., Wides, J., & Shih, M.C. (2006, July). *Effect of the Newborn Behavioral Observations (NBO) system on postpartum maternal depression.* Paper presented at the 10th World Congress of the World Association for Infant Mental Health, Paris, France.

Nugent, J.K., Yogman, M., Lester, B.M., & Hoffman, J. (1988). The father's impact on infant development in the first critical year of life. In E. James Anthony & Colette Chiland (Eds.), *The child in his family* (Vol. 8). New York: John Wiley & Sons.

Ogbu, J. (1981). Origins of human competence: A cultural-ecological perspective. *Child Development, 52,* 413–429.

Ohgi, S., Fukada, M., Moriuchi, H., Kusumoto, T., Akiyama, T., Nugent, J.K., et al. (2002). Comparison of kangaroo care: Behavioral organization, development, and temperament in healthy low-birth weight infants through 1 year. *Journal of Perinatology, 22,* 374–379.

Okami, P., Weisner, T., & Olmstead, R. (2002). Outcome correlated of parent–child bedsharing: An eighteen year longitudinal study. *Developmental and Behavioral Pediatrics, 23,* 244–253.

Olds, D.L. (2002). Prenatal and Infancy home visiting by nurses: From randomized trials to community replication. *Prevention Science, 3*(3), 153–172.

Olds, D.L., & Kitzman, H. (1993). Review of research on home visiting for pregnant women and parents of young children. *The Future of Children, 3*(3), 53–92.

Onozawa, K., Glover, V., Adams, D., Modi, N., & Kumar, R.C. (2001). Infant massage improves mother–infant interaction for mothers with postnatal depression. *Journal of Affective Disorders, 63,* 201–207.

Owen, M.T., Ware, A.M., & Barfoot, B. (2000). Caregiver–mother partnership behavior and the quality of caregiver–child and mother–child interactions. *Early Childhood Research Quarterly, 15*(3), 413–428.

Papousek, M. (1998). Persistent crying in early infancy: A non-trivial condition of risk for the developing mother–infant relationship. *Child: Care, Health and Development, 24*(5), 395–424.

Papousek, H., & Papousek, M. (1987). Intuitive parenting: A dialectic counterpart to the infant's integrative competence. In J. Osofsky (Ed.), *The handbook of infant development* (2nd ed., pp. 669–720). New York: John Wiley & Sons.

Papousek, M., & Papousek, H. (1990). Excessive Infant crying and intuitive parental care: Buffering support and its failures in parent–infant interaction. *Early Child Development and Care, 65,* 117–126.

Papousek, M., & Papousek, H. (2002). Parent–infant speech patterns. In J. Gomes-Pedro, J.K. Nugent, J.G. Young, & T.B. Brazelton (Eds.), *The infant and family in the twenty-first century* (pp. 101–108). New York: Brunner-Routledge.

Parke, R.D., & Buriel, R. (1998). Socialization in the family: Ethnic and ecological perspectives. In N. Eisenberg (Ed.), *Handbook of child Psychology: Vol. 3. Social, emotional and personality development* (4th ed., pp. 463–552). New York: Wiley.

Parker, S., Zahr, L.K, Cole, J.C.D., & Brecht, M.L. (1992). Outcome after developmental intervention in the neonatal intensive care unit for mothers of preterm infants with low socioeconomic status. *Journal of Pediatrics, 120,* 780–785.

Pascalis, O., de Schonen, S., Morton, J., Deruelle, C., & Fabre-Grenet, M. (1995). Mother's face recognition by neonates: A replication and an extension. *Infant Behavior and Development, 18,* 79–85.

Pawl, J., St. John, M., & Pekarsky, J.H. (2000). Training mental health and other professionals in infant mental health: Conversations with trainees. In H.E. Fitzgerald & J.D. Osofsky (Eds.), *Handbook of infant mental health* (pp. 380–401). New York: John Wiley & Sons.

Peiper, A. (1963). *Cerebral function in infancy and childhood* (3rd ed.). New York: Consultants Bureau.

Percy, M.S., Stadtler, A.C., & Sands, D. (2002). Touchpoints: Changing the face of pediatric nurse practitioner education. *American Journal of Child Nursing, 27*(4), 222–228.

Philliber Research Associates. (2001, March). *The clinical neonatal behavioral assessment scale: Training outcomes.* New York: Accord.

Piper, M.C., & Darrah, J. (1994). *Motor assessment of the developing infant.* Philadelphia: W.B. Saunders.

Porges, W., Doussard-Roosevelt, J.A., Stifter, C.A., McClenny, B.D., & Riniolo, T.C. (1999). Sleep state and vagal regulation of heart period patterns in the human newborn: An extension of polyvagal theory. *Psychophysiology, 36,* 14–21.

Postpartum Disorders Factsheet (2006). National Mental Health Association Website, wwww.nmha.org/infoctr/factsheets/postpartum.cfm

Prechtl, H.F.R. (1977). *The neurological examination of the full-term newborn infant* (2nd ed.). Spastics International Medical Publications. London: William Heinemann; Philadelphia: J.B. Lippincott.

Prechtl, H.F.R., & Beintema, D.J. (1964). The neurological examination of the full term newborn infant. *Clinics in Developmental Medicine, 12,* 1–49.

Price-Williams, D. (1975). *Explorations in cross-cultural psychology.* San Francisco: Chandler and Sharp.

Pruett, K.D. (1983). Infants of primary nurturing fathers. *The Psychoanalytic Study of the Child, 38,* 257–277.

Querleu, D., Lefebre, C., Titran, M., Renard, X., Morillon, M., & Crepin, G. (1984). Reaction of the newborn infant less than two hours after birth to the maternal voice (in French). *Journal de Gynécologie, Obstétrique et Biologie de la Reproduction (Paris), 13*(2), 125–134.

Querleu, D., Renard, X., Boutteville, C., & Crepin, G. (1989). Hearing by the human fetus? *Seminars in Perinatology, 13,* 409–420.

Rakic, P. (1977). Prenatal development of the visual system in rhesus monkeys. *Philosophical Transactions of the Royal Society of London. Series B, Biological Sciences, 278,* 245–260.

Rakic, P. (1995). Corticogenesis in human and nonhuman primates. In M.S. Gazzaniga (Ed.), *The cognitive neurosciences* (pp. 127–145). Cambridge, MA: MIT Press.

Raphael-Leff, J. (2001). *Pregnancy: The inside story.* London: Karnac Books.

Rauh, V., Achenbach, T., Nurcombe, B., Howell, C., & Teti, D. (1988). Minimizing adverse effects of low birthweight: Four-year results of an early intervention program. *Child Development, 59,* 544–553.

Redshaw, M.E. (1997). Mothers of babies requiring special care: Attitudes and experiences. *Journal of Reproductive & Infant Psychology, 15*(2), 109–121.

Reid, C. (2004). *The wounds of exclusion: Poverty, women's health & social justices.* Edmonton, Alberta, Canada: Qualitative Institute Press.

Robb, M.P., & Goberman, A.M. (1997). Application of an acoustic cry template to evaluate at-risk newborns: Preliminary findings. *Biology of the Neonate, 71,* 131–136.

Rochat, P. (1998). The newly objectified world of 2-month olds [Special issue]. *Infant Behavior and Development, 21,* 182.

Rochat, P., & Goubet, N. (1995). Development of sitting and reaching in 5- to 6-month-old infants. *Infant Behavior and Development, 18,* 53–686.

Rochat, P., & Hespos, S. (1997). Differential rooting response by neonates: Evidence for an early sense of self. *Early Development and Parenting, 6,* 105–112.

Rogoff, B. (2003). *The cultural nature of child development.* Oxford, England: Oxford University Press.

Rommel, N., De Meyer, A.M., Feenstra, L., & Veereman-Wauters, G. (2003). Complexity of feeding problems in 700 infants and young children presenting to a tertiary care institution. *Journal of Pediatric Gastroenterology and Nutrition, 37*(1), 75–84.

Rooks, J.P. (1999). The midwifery model of care. *Journal of Nurse Midwifery, 44*(4), 370–374.

Rothbart, M.K., Posner, M.I., & Boylan, A. (1994). Orienting in normal and pathological development. *Development and Psychopathology, 6,* 635–652.

Rubin, R. (1967). Attainment of the maternal role. *Nursing Research, 16,* 237–245.

Rubin, R. (1984). *Maternal identity and the maternal experience.* New York: Springer Publishing Co.

Rutter, M. (1990). Psychosocial resilience and protective mechanisms. In J. Rolf (Ed.), *Risk and protective factors in the development of psychopathology* (pp. 42–73). New York: Cambridge University Press.

Saint-Anne Dargassies, S. (1977). Long-term neurological follow-up of 286 truly premature infants. I. Neurological sequelae. *Developmental Medicine and Child Neurology, 19,* 462–478.

Sameroff, A.J. (1997). Models of development and developmental risk. In C.H. Zeanah (Ed.), *Handbook of infant mental health* (pp. 3–13). New York: Guilford Press.

Sameroff, A.J., & Emde, R.N. (Eds.). (1989). *Relationship disturbances in early childhood.* New York: Basic Books.

Sameroff, A.J., & Fiese, B.H. (2000). Transactional regulation and early intervention. In J.S. Meisels & J.P. Shonkoff (Eds.), *Handbook of early childhood intervention* (pp. 119–149). New York: Cambridge University Press.

Sander, L.W. (1961). Issues in early mother–child interaction. *Journal of the American Academy of Child Psychiatry, 1,* 141–165.

Sander, L.W, Stechler, G., Burns, P., & Lee, A. (1979). Change in infant caregiver variables over the first two months of life: Integration of action in early development. In E.B. Thoman (Ed.), *Origins of the infant's social responsiveness* (pp. 349–407). Hillsdale, NJ: Lawrence Erlbaum Associates.

Sanders, L.W., & Buckner, E.B. (2006). The newborn behavioral observations system as a nursing intervention to enhance engagement in first-time mothers: Feasibility and desirability. *Pediatric Nursing, 32*(5), 455–459.

Sansavini, A., Bertoncini, J., & Giovanelli, G. (1997). Newborns discriminate the rhythm of multisyllabic stressed words. *Developmental Psychology, 33,* 3–11.

Scafidi, F.A., Field, T., & Schanberg, S.M. (1993). Factors that predict which preterm infants benefit most from massage therapy. *Developmental and Behavioral Pediatrics, 14,* 176–180.

Schon, D.A. (1983). *The reflective practitioner.* New York: Basic Books.

Schore, A.N. (1994). *Affect regulation and the origin of the self.* Hillsdale, NJ: Lawrence Erlbaum Associates.

Seifer, R., & Dickstein, S. (2000). Parental mental illness and infant development. In C.H. Zeanah (Ed.), *Handbook of infant mental health* (2nd ed., pp. 145–160). New York: Guilford Press.

Seligman, S. (2000). Clinical interviews with families of infants. *Journal of Infant, Child, and Adolescent Psychotherapy, 1*(1), 77–96.

Shelton, T. (1999). Family centered care in pediatric practice: When and how. *Journal of Developmental and Behavioral Pediatrics, 20*(2), 117–119.

Shimizu, H., & LeVine, R.A. (Eds.). (2001). *Japanese frames of mind: Cultural perspectives on human development.* Cambridge, UK: Cambridge University Press.

Shonkoff, J.P., & Meisels, S.J. (2000). *Handbook of early intervention.* Cambridge, UK: Cambridge University Press.

Shonkoff, J.P., & Phillips, D.A. (Eds.). (2000). *From neurons to neighborhoods: The science of early childhood development* (p. 28). Washington, DC: National Academies Press.

Shweder, R.A., Goodnow, J.J., Hatano, G., LeVine, R.A., Markus, H.R., & Miller, P. (1998). The cultural psychology of development: One mind, many mentalities. In R.L. Lerner (Ed.), *Handbook of child psychology: Vol. 1. Theoretical models of human development* (pp. 865–938). New York: John Wiley & Sons.

Siegel, D.J. (1999). *The developing mind.* New York: Guilford Press.

Simkin, P. (1991). Just another day in a woman's life? Women's long-term perceptions of their first birth experience. Part I. *Birth, 18,* 203–210.

Simkin P. (1992). Just another day in a woman's life? Nature and consistency of women's long-term memories of their first birth experience. Part II. *Birth, 19,* 64–81.

Simkin, P. (1996). The experience of maternity in a woman's life. *Journal of Obstetric, Gynecologic, & Neonatal Nursing, 25*(3), 247–252.

Slade, A. (2002). Keeping the baby in mind: A critical factor in perinatal mental health. *Zero to Three, 22*(6), 10–16.

Slater, A. (2001). Visual perception. In G. Bremner & A. Fogel (Eds.), *Blackwell handbook of infant development* (pp. 5–34). Oxford, England: Blackwell.

Slater, A., Morison, V., Town, C., & Rose, D. (1985). Movement perception and identity constancy in the new-born baby. *British Journal of Developmental Psychology, 3,* 211–220.

Small, M.F. (1998). *Our babies, ourselves.* New York: Anchor Books.

Sobotkova, D., Dittrichova, J., & Mandys, F. (1996). Comparison of maternal perceptions of preterm and fullterm infants. *Early Development and Parenting, 5*(2), 73–79.

Spence, M.J., & Freeman, M.S. (1996). Newborn infants prefer the maternal low-pass filtered voice, but not the maternal whispered voice. *Infant Behavior and Development, 19,* 199–212.

Spielman, E. (2002). Early connections: Mother–infant psychotherapy in support of perinatal mental health. *Zero to Three, 22*(6), 26–30.

Spiker, D., Ferguson, J., & Brooks-Gunn, J. (1993). Enhancing maternal interactive behavior and child social competence in low birthweight, premature infants. *Child Development, 64,* 754–768.

Spock, B., & Needleman, R. (2004). *Dr. Spock's baby and child care, 8th Edition.* New York and London: Simon and Schuster.

Sroufe, L.A., & Waters, E. (1977). Attachment as an organizational construct. *Child Development, 48,* 1184–1199.

Stadtler, A., O'Brien, M.A., & Hornstein, J. (1995). The Touchpoints model: Building supportive alliances between parents and professionals. *Zero to Three, 15*(1), 24–28.

Standley, K., Soule, A.B., Copans, S.A., & Klein, R.P. (1978). Multidimensional sources of infant temperament. *Genetic Psychology Monographs, 98,* 203–231.

Stein, M.T., Kennell, J.H., & Fulcher, A. (2004). Benefits of a doula present at the birth of a child. *Pediatrics, 114*(5), 1488–1491.

Stern, D.N. (1977). *The first relationship: Infant and mother.* Cambridge, MA: Harvard University Press.

Stern, D.N. (1985). *The interpersonal world of the infant: A view from psychoanalysis and developmental psychology.* New York: Basic Books.

Stern, D.N. (1995). *The motherhood constellation: A unified view of parent–infant psychotherapy.* New York: Basic Books.

Stern, D.N., & Bruschweiler-Stern, N. (1998). *The birth of a mother: How the motherhood experience changes you forever.* New York: Basic Books.

Stern-Bruschweiler, N., & Stern, D.N. (1989). A model for conceptualizing the role of the mother's representational world in various mother–infant therapies. *Infant Mental Health Journal, 10*(3), 16–25.

Stewart, M.A. (1995). Effective physician–patient communication and health outcomes: A review. *Canadian Medical Association Journal, 152,* 1423–1433.

Stewart, M.A., Brown, J.B., Weston, W.W., McWhinney, I.R., McWilliam, C.L., & Freeman, T.R. (1995). *Patient-centered medicine: Transforming the clinical method.* Thousand Oaks, CA: Sage Publications.

Stifter, C. (2002). Individual differences in emotion regulation in infancy: A thematic collection. *Infancy, 3,* 129–132.

St. James-Roberts, I. (2001). Infant crying and its impact on parents. In R.G. Barr, I. St. James-Roberts, I., & M.R. Keefe (Eds.), *New evidence on unexplained early infant crying: Its origins, nature and management.* NJ: Skillman, NJ: Johnson and Johnson Pediatric Institute.

St. James-Roberts, I., & Plewis, I. (1996). Individual differences, daily fluctuations and developmental changes in the amount of waking, fussing, crying, feeding and sleeping. *Child Development, 67,* 2527–2540.

Suchman, A.L. (2006). A new theoretical foundation for relationship-based care. *Journal of General Internal Medicine, 21,* 40–44.

Super, C.M., & Harkness, S. (1982). The infant's niche in rural Kenya and metropolitan America. In L. Adler (Ed.), *Cross-cultural research at issue* (pp. 47–55). New York: Academic Press.

Super, C.M., & Harkness, S. (1997). The cultural structuring of child development. In J.W. Berry, Y.P. Poortinga, J. Pandey, P.R. Dason, & T.S. Saraswathi (Eds.), *Handbook of cross-cultural psychology* (Vol. 2, pp. 1–39). Needham Heights, MA: Allyn & Bacon.

Swain, I., Zelazo, P., & Clifton, R. (1993). Newborn infants' memory for speech sounds retained over 24 hours. *Developmental Psychology, 29,* 312–323.

Sweet, M.A., & Applebaum, M.I. (2004). Is home visiting an effective strategy? A meta-analytic review of home visiting programs for families with young children. *Child Development, 75*(5), 1435–1456.

Takahashi, S., Nugent, J.K., Kawasaki, C., Greene, S., Wieczorek-Deering, D., & Brazelton, T.B. (1994, September). Parents socialisation goals and father involvement in caregiving in Japan and some comparisons with Ireland. Paper presented at the 14th Annual Conference of the Society for Reproductive and Infant Psychology, Dublin, Ireland.

Teller, D.Y. (1998). Spatial and temporal aspects of infant color vision. *Vision Research, 38,* 3275–3282.

Thoman, E.G. (1975). Sleep and wake behaviors in neonates: Consistencies and consequences. *Merrill-Palmer Quarterly, 21,* 293–313.

Thomas, A., & Chess, S. (1977). *Temperament and development.* New York: Brunner/Mazel.

Thomas, J. (1998). Summary of the practice parameters for the psychiatric assessment of infants and toddlers. *Journal of the American Academy of Child and Adolescent Psychiatry, 37*(1), 127–132.

Thoyre, S.M. (2003). Developmental transition from gavage to oral feeding in the preterm infant. *Annual Review of Nursing Research, 21,* 61–92.

Timur, S. (2000). Changing trends and major issues in international migration: An overview of UNESCO programmes. *International Social Science Journal, 52,* 165, 255–268.

Trehub, S.E. (2001). Musical predispositions in infancy. *Annals of the New York Academy of Sciences, 930,* 1–16.

Tresolini C.P., & Pew-Fetzer Task Force (1994). *Health professions education and relationship-centered care.* San Francisco: Pew-Health Professions Commission.

Tresolini, C.P. (1996). Health care relationships: Instruments for effective patient-focused care in the academic health center. *Journal of Dental Education, 60*(12), 945–950.

Trevarthen, C. (1979). Communication and cooperation in early infancy: A description of early subjectivity. In M. Bullowa (Ed.), *Before speech: The beginning of interpersonal communication* (pp. 321–349). Cambridge, England: Cambridge University Press.

Trevarthen, C. (1993). The functions of emotions in early infant communication and development. In J. Nadel & L. Camaioni (Eds.), *New perspectives in early communicative development* (pp. 48–81). London: Routledge.

Trevarthen, C., Kokkinaki, T., & Faimonghi, G. (1999). What infants' communications communicate: With mothers, with fathers and with peers. In J. Nadel & G. Butterworth (Eds.), *Imitation in infancy.* Cambridge, UK: Cambridge University Press.

Tronick, E.Z. (1989). Emotions and emotional communication in infants. *American Psychologist, 44*(2), 112–119.

Tronick, E.Z. (1998). Dyadically expanded states of consciousness and the process of therapeutic change. *Infant Mental Health Journal, 19,* 290–299.

Tronick, E.Z. (2003). Emotions and emotional communication in infants. In J. Raphael-Leff (Ed.), *Parent–infant psychodynamics, wild things, mirrors and ghosts* (pp. 35–53). London: Whurr Publishers.

Tronick, E.Z., Als, H., & Brazelton, T.B. (1980). Monadic phases: A structural descriptive analysis of infant–mother face-to-face interaction. *Merrill-Palmer Quarterly, 26,* 3–13.

Tronick, E.Z., & Cohn, J.F. (1989). Infant–mother face-to-face interaction: Age and gender differences in coordination and occurrence of miscoordination. *Child Development, 60,* 85–92.

Turati, C. (2004). Why faces are not special to newborns: An account of the face preference. *Current Directions in Psychological Science, 13,* 5–8.

Turati, C., Simion, F., & Zanon, L. (2003). Newborns' perceptual categorization for closed and open geometric forms. *Infancy, 4*(3), 309–325.

U.S. Public Health Service. (2000). *Report of the Surgeon General's conference on children's mental health: A national action agenda.* Washington, DC: Author.

Valsiner, J. (1989). *Development and culture.* Lexington, MA: Lexington Books.

Vandenberg, K. (1997). Basic principles of developmental caregiving. *Neonatal Network, 16*(7), 69–71.

Van den Boom, D.C. (1991). The influence of infant irritability on the development of the mother–infant relationship in the first 6 months of life. In J.K. Nugent, B.M. Lester, & T.B. Brazelton (Eds.), *The cultural context of infancy: Vol. 2. Multicultural and interdisciplinary approaches to parent–infant relations* (pp. 63–89). Stamford, CT: Ablex.

Van den Boom, D.C. (1994). The influence of temperament and mothering on attachment and exploration: An experimental manipulation of sensitive responsiveness among lower class mothers with irritable infants. *Child Development, 65,* 1457–1477.

Van den Boom, D.C. (1995). Do first-year intervention effects endure? Follow-up during toddlerhood of a sample of Dutch irritable infants. *Child Development, 66,* 1798–1816.

Van den Boom, D.C., & Hoeksma, J.B. (1994). The effect of infant irritability on mother–infant interaction: A growth curve analysis. *Developmental Psychology, 30,* 581–590.

van IJzendoorn, M., & De Wolff, M.S. (1997). In search of the absent father—Meta-analyses of infant–father attachment: A rejoinder to our discussants. *Child Development, 68,* 604–609.

Varendi, H., & Porter, R.H. (2001). Breast odour as the only maternal stimulus elicits crawling towards the odour source. *Acta Paediatrica, 90,* 372–375.

Vareny, H., Kriebs, J.M., & Gegor, C.L. (2003). *Vareny's midwifery* (4th ed.). Boston: Jones & Bartlett.

Vergara, E.R., & Bigsby, R. (2004). *Developmental & therapeutic interventions in the NICU.* Baltimore: Paul H. Brookes Publishing Co.

Vickers, A., Ohlsson, A., Lacy, J.B., & Horsley, A. (2002). Massage for promoting growth and development of preterm and/or low birth-weight infants (Cochrane review). In *The Cochrane Library* (Issue 3). Oxford, England: Update Software.

Von Klitzing, K., Simoni, H., Amsler, F., & Burgin, D. (1999). The role of the father in early family interactions. *Infant Mental Health Journal, 20*(3), 222–237.

Vuorenkoski , V., Wasz-Hockert, O., Koivisto, E., & Lind, J. (1969). The effect of cry stimulus on the temperature of the lactating breast of primipara: A thermographic study. *Experientia, 25,* 1286–1287.

Vygotsky, L.S. (1987). *The collected works of L.S. Vygotsky: Vol. 1. Problems of general psychology.* New York: Plenum.

Warren, S.L., Huston, L., Egeland, B., & Sroufe, L.A. (1997). Child and adolescent anxiety disorders and early attachment. *Journal of the American Academy of Child and Adolescent Psychiatry, 36,* 637–644.

Waters, E., Merrick, S., Treboux, D., Crowell, J., & Albersheim, L. (2000). Attachment security in infancy and early adulthood: A twenty-year longitudinal study. *Child Development, 71*(3), 684–702.

Waters, E., Vaughn, B.E., & Egeland, B. (1980). Individual differences in infant–mother attachment relationships at age one: Antecedents in neonatal behavior in an urban, economically disadvantaged sample. *Child Development, 51,* 208–216.

Weatherston, D.J. (2000). Infant mental health assessment through careful observation and listening: Unique training approaches. In J. Osofsky & H.E. Fitzgerald (Eds.), *WAIMH handbook of infant mental health* (Vol. II, pp. 119–155). New York: John Wiley & Sons.

Weber, C., Hahne, A., Friedrich, M., & Friederici, A. (2004). Discrimination of word stress in early infant perception: Electrophysiological evidence. *Cognitive Brain Research, 18,* 149–161.

Weinberg, M.K., Olson, K.L., Beeghly, M., & Tronick, E.Z. (2006). Making up is hard to do, especially for mothers with high levels of depressive symptoms and their infant sons. *Journal of Child Psychology and Psychiatry, 47,* 670–683.

Weinberg, M.K., & Tronick, E.Z. (1996). Infant affective reactions to the resumption of maternal interaction after the still-face. *Child Development, 67,* 905–914.

Weinfield, N.S., Sroufe, L.A., & Egeland, B. (2000). Attachment from infancy to early adulthood in a high-risk sample: Continuity, discontinuity, and their correlates. *Child Development, 71*(3), 695–702.

Weine, S.M., Ware, N., & Klebic, A. (2004). Converting cultural capital among teen refugees and their families from Bosnia-Herzegovina. *Psychiatric Services, 55,* 923–927.

Weiss, J.S., & Wagner, S.H. (1998). What explains the negative consequences of adverse childhood experiences on adult health? Insights from cognitive and neuroscience research (editorial). *American Journal of Preventive Medicine, 14,* 356–360.

Weissbourd, B., & Kagan, S. (1989). Family support programs: Catalysts for change. *American Journal of Orthopsychiatry, 59,* 20–31.

Wessel, M.A., Cobb, J.C., Jackson, E.B., Harris, G.S., & Detwiler, A.C. (1954). Paroxysmal fussing in infancy, sometimes called "colic." *Pediatrics, 14,* 421–433.

Wheeden, A., Scafdi, F.A., Field, T., Ironson, G., Valdeon, C., & Bandstra, E. (1993). Massage effects on cocaine-exposed preterm neonates. *Journal of Developmental and Behavioral Pediatrics, 14*(5), 318–322.

White, C., Simon, M., & Bryan, A. (2002). Using evidence to educate birthing center nursing staff about infant states, cues, and behaviors. *MCN: The American Journal of Maternal Child Nursing, 27*(5), 294–298.

White, K. (2004). *Touch: Attachment and the body. The John Bowlby Memorial Conference Monograph.* London: Karnac Books for the Centre for Attachment-based Psychoanalytic Psychotherapy.

Whiting, B.B., & Edwards, C.P. (1988). *Children of different worlds: The formation of social behavior.* Cambridge, MA: Harvard University Press.

Whiting, B.B., Fischer, J.L., Longabaugh, R., & Whiting, J.W.M. (1975). *Children of six cultures.* Cambridge, MA: Harvard University Press.

Widmayer, S., & Field, T. (1981). Effects of Brazelton demonstrations for mothers on the development of preterm infants. *Pediatrics, 67,* 711–714.

Williamson, G.G., Anzalone, M.E., & Hanft, B.H. (2000). Assessment of sensory processing, praxis, and motor performance. In Interdisciplinary Council on Developmental and Learning Disorders (Ed.), *Clinical Practice Guidelines* (pp. 155–184). Bethesda, MD: American Occupational Therapy Association.

Winn, S., Tronick, E., & Morelli, G. (1989). The infant and the group: A look at Efe caretaking practices in Zaire. In J.K. Nugent, B.M. Lester, & T.B. Brazelton (Eds.), *The cultural context of infancy: Vol. I. Biology, culture, and infant development* (pp. 87–110). Stamford, CT: Ablex.

Winnicott, D.W. (Ed.). (1975). *Primary maternal preoccupation.* In D.W. Winnicott, *Through paediatrics to psycho-analysis* (pp. 300–305). New York: Basic Books.

Wolf, L.S., & Glass, R.P. (1992). *Feeding and swallowing disorders in infancy.* San Antonio, TX: Therapy Skill Builders.

Wolff, P.H. (1959). Observations on human infants. *Psychosomatic Medicine, 221,* 110–118.

Wolff, P.H. (1966). *The causes, controls, and organization of behavior in the neonate.* New York: International Universities Press.

Wolke, D., Dave, S., Hayes, J., Townsend, J., & Tomlin, M. (2002). Routine examination of the newborn and maternal satisfaction: A randomized controlled trial. *Archives of Diseases in Childhood: Fetal and Neonatal Edition, 86*(3), F155–F160.

Wolke, D., Gray, P., & Meyer, R. (1994). Excessive infant crying: A controlled study of mothers helping mothers. *Pediatrics, 94,* 322.

Wolke, D., Rizzo, P., & Woods, S. (2002). Persistent infant crying and hyperactivity problems in middle childhood. *Pediatrics, 109*(6), 1054–1060.

Worchel, F.F., & Allen, M. (1997). Mothers' ability to discriminate cry types in low-birthweight premature and full-term infants. *Children's Health Care, 26*(3), 183–195.

Worobey, J. (1997). Convergence between temperament ratings in early infancy. *Journal of Developmental and Behavioral Pediatrics, 18*(4), 260–263.

Worobey, J., & Belsky, J. (1982). Employing the Brazelton Scale to influence mothering: An experimental comparison of three strategies. *Developmental Psychology, 18,* 736–743.

Yogman, M.W. (1982). Development of the father–infant relationship. In H. Fitzgerald, B.M. Lester, & M.W. Yogman (Eds.), *Theory and research in behavioral pediatrics* (Vol. 1, pp. 221–279). New York: Plenum.

Young-Taffe, K., Davis, K., Schoen, C., & Parker, S. (1998). Listening to parents: A national survey of parents with young children. *Archives of Pediatrics and Adolescent Medicine, 152,* 254–262.

Zeanah, C.H. (Ed.). (1993). *Handbook of infant mental health.* New York: Guilford Press.

Zeanah, C.H., & Anders, T.F. (1987). Subjectivity in parent–infant relationships: A discussion of internal working models. *Infant Mental Health Journal, 8*(3), 237–250.

Zeanah, C.H., & Boris, N.W. (2000). Chapter 22: Disturbances and disorders of attachment in early childhood. In C.H. Zeanah (Ed.), *Handbook of infant mental health* (2nd ed., pp. 353–368). New York: Guilford Press.

Zeanah, C.H., Boris, N.W., & Larrieu, J.A. (1997). Infant development and developmental risk: A review of the past ten years. *Journal of the American Academy of Child and Adolescent Psychiatry, 36*(2), 165–178.

Zeanah, C.H., & McDonough, S.C. (1989). Clinical approaches to families in early intervention. *Seminars in Perinatology, 13,* 513–522.

Zuckerman, B., & Zuckerman, P. (2005). The pediatrician as ghostbuster: Angels voices and kisses. *Infant Mental Health Journal, 26*(6), 529–532.

# INDEX

Page numbers followed by "*f*" indicate figures; numbers followed by "*t*" indicate tables.